I Remember Me – The Mom Chronicles

An Alzheimer's Journey Sharing Lessons Learned and Challenges Conquered as a Caregiver

Lori Aden

ISBN: 978-1-7373463-1-9

DEDICATION

I dedicate this book to my family who made numerous sacrifices to help take care of my mother. First, my sister, Sheila Parsley, drove 3 hours to Dallas every other weekend to spend time with Mom and give my husband and me some "away" time as caregivers. We grew so much as sisters during this journey, and I love her more now than I ever thought possible. Second, my son, Joshua Aden, who struggled with slowly watching his grandmother lose the essence of what he remembered as a grandmother, was always there to step in and take care of her if we needed help. Third, his fiancé, Leigha Gaines, was there with us to help him get through his struggles in this journey towards the end of his grandmother's life. Finally, my husband, Bruce Aden, made considerable sacrifices to let me do what I believed were the best care options for Mom. He stuck by me when we decided to sell our beautiful home and downsize to an RV to afford memory care. He never made me feel bad for this decision ever. He was my rock every step of the way. Sheila, Josh, Leigha, and Bruce - I love you all so much. Thank you for doing everything possible for Mom and our family during this difficult time in our lives.

We interacted with tons of people over the years who sent well-received suggestions and advice to us and then also sent greeting cards, gift cards, jewelry, and nail polish strips to Mom. I wish I could name each one of you. You know who you all are, and you are in my heart forever. I tagged many of you in the Mom Chronicle posts in this book to try and honor you in some small way.

Last but not least, I want to list one special person who helped guide me through the memory care days, and that person is Jenni Knutson. She was the director at Mom's first memory care center, and I honestly could not have gone through this journey without her advice, love, and commitment to her patients and their families. I have included a lot of advice I learned from her over the years in this book. Jenni - thank you for being a true friend and an advocate for people who can no longer speak for themselves. You are a bright light in this universe, and I love you dearly.

CONTENTS

FOREWORD

"Your mom got lost on her way back from the nail salon today. She ended up 30 minutes south of town and couldn't remember how to get back home." This was the text I received from my stepsister Robin in 2014. At this point, we knew Mom's memory problems were too serious to leave her safely in California. Our combined families decided it was time to move Mom and Ted back home to Texas from California so that we could take care of them. We had no idea what we were about to go through for the next 5 ½ years.

Let's back up about 15 years for a moment. My grandmother Daphne (Mom's mom) started showing signs of dementia in the early 2000s. I took care of her for a while by making a 2-hour drive every month from Huntsville, Tx to Ennis, Tx to refill her meds, take her to doctor appointments and hospitalizations, and handle any errands that she needed to be completed. But as the disease progressed, we realized she had Alzheimer's like at least one of her siblings had experienced. So when assisted living in Ennis no longer worked for her, we moved her in with us down in Huntsville. Mom lived in California, and my uncle lived in Boston. Grandma was here in Texas with us, so my husband, son, and I were the only caregiving options.

I loved my grandmother dearly and would do anything for her, so we didn't think twice about moving her in with us. But as a caregiver, we were not expecting all that goes along with caring for a patient with Alzheimer's. Who knows this stuff? It's not taught anywhere. Legal things like powers of attorney, physical caregiving - diapers for adults? Yikes! There were hours and hours of doctor appointments. The list goes on and on.

At the time, I was a college instructor for the local prison system. As the doctor appointments kept piling on, I missed more and more work, which required substitute teachers. I was called into the office one day and was told that I would need to find another job if I had to keep missing work. My heart sank. My boss did not like telling me this, but it is the nature of the beast. I had a job to do, and I wasn't fulfilling my part. It was not fair to my students who were not getting direct instruction from me. I understood completely.

I had to make a horrible choice of earning an income for my family versus taking care of my wonderful grandmother. I called my mom, who was retired in California, and told her that I would need to move Grandma out there for her to take care of now. I hated that. I absolutely hated that because I was already missing time with my mom, but now I was going to be missing precious time with my grandmother, whom I considered a second mother to me. Traveling to California was difficult on our budget, so I knew my time with her was going to be next to nothing now.

Mom and Ted cared for Grandma for four years before the disease took her. I remember watching the progression through the yearly visits we made out there and how Alzheimer's was taking my grandmother away from me. My last visit with her was one month before she passed. Grandma was just a shell of the former lady I knew: vacant eyes, frail, skin and bones, and so on. She died July 18, 2006.

Now, fast forward to 2014. My beautiful mother, who had been showing signs of dementia for about a year (she was constantly repeating stories over and over during phone calls), had progressed to the next stage. She forgot how to navigate to familiar places she visited all the time. We knew it was time.

Our dilemma? Robin, Ted's daughter, lived down in Magnolia. I lived in Dallas. Mom and Ted loved each other dearly, but they both missed their families from years and years of living in California. Ted wanted to be near his daughter and grandchildren, and Mom wanted to live with me and be near her grandson, Josh.

We compromised. Ted moved to Magnolia, and Mom moved in with me. (My husband Bruce supported this decision 100%. Family is family.) We promised that we would arrange for them to see each other as often as possible. Sometimes Ted would come up for a weekend. Most of the time, though, it was a halfway visit in Fairfield, or I would drive Mom down to Magnolia for lunch and a few hours of visit time. They did have phones and would call each other every day, several times a day. I know Ted would get frustrated with Mom's repeated conversations over and over, but he loved her and patiently talked to her every day.

At some point, I started "chronicling" our experiences with Mom so that we could remember the journey. As caregivers, we learned, we laughed, we cried, we got angry, we got frustrated, we got desperate at times, we worked hard, we shared, we lost, we gained, and we loved. At first, I only posted every now and then on Facebook when something happened with Mom. Then, as she progressed further in the disease, I started posting more regularly and titling the posts "Mom Chronicles." My sister Sheila would come up every other weekend from Huntsville to visit Mom and give Bruce and me a little break. She also started chronicling some of her experiences with Mom.

Along the way, we made terrific friends like Jenni Knutson and Shauna Sweetser in the Alzheimer's industry, who helped guide us when we had questions or let us cry on their shoulders. As a career educator, I also dug into a lot of research by reading books on Alzheimer's, following bloggers, digging into websites such as Alz.org and, reading posts on Alzheimer caregiver groups on Facebook. I wanted to learn as much as I could every step of the way to know how to take care of Mom. Believe me, we made a ton of mistakes, but in the end, I think we did the absolute best we could do for her and allowed her to live her life in the fullest way possible.

We also ended up becoming friends with many folks we would have never met outside of this world. Friends would message me and ask if I would allow their friend(s) to "friend" me on Facebook so that they could follow the Mom Chronicles. I was glad that some of my experiences with Mom helped others. I had the mindset that we could all learn from each other on this journey.

I have included most but not all the posts I wrote during the 5 ½ year journey as her caregiver. I tried to divide the chapters up into the various stages of Alzheimer's. There are different ways of categorizing the stages. Some use Early (mild), Middle (moderate), and Late (severe). Others use a 7-stage process. That is the one I preferred because it seemed to help me understand more clearly where Mom was in the "timeline."

I have also added tips and tricks I learned along the way to help fill in gaps that may be missing from the Chronicles. It was wonderful to hear from so many folks about how they fell in love with my mom through the Mom Chronicles. They felt like they knew her even though they never met her face to face. You will have a chance to get to know a special lady through the eyes of my family and me. You will laugh and maybe, just maybe, even cry a little. But most importantly, I hope you learn how to help someone dealing with this horrible disease, either as a patient or a caregiver. Because trust me, you WILL know someone like this in your lifetime - one way or another.

I have included QR codes to view short video clips I filmed of Mom to show her progression in the disease. Use your phone's camera or a QR code reader app to open the photos/videos to experience the entire journey. I will admit I was not an excellent videographer. But it is what it is. I still have many beautiful memories that I can now share to help you learn from our Alzheimer's journey.

I do have a few final notes:

- the thoughts and ideas shared in this book are not intended to substitute for medical or legal advice. Please consult with appropriate professionals in those areas.
- My family and I are Christians, so you will see me mention God quite a bit in this book. If you are not, feel free to gloss over those references and concentrate on the story. I just couldn't leave Him out because I personally believe He guided our hands throughout this whole journey.
- I occasionally use the phrase "Alzheimer's sucks" in my posts. It's not nice, but many times, that was the only phrase I could emotionally use to get through the experience. I apologize if that word offends anyone reading this book.

My mom moved in with us in December 2014. Let the chronicles begin.

CHAPTER 1: STAGES 1-4 ♥ THE BEGINNING

So what exactly is Alzheimer's? According to the Alzheimer's Association, "Alzheimer's is the most common cause of dementia, a general term for memory loss and other cognitive abilities serious enough to interfere with daily life. Alzheimer's disease accounts for 60-80% of dementia cases." (What is Alzheimer's Disease, n.d.)

Notice, they say 60-80% of dementia cases. This fact was something I learned along the way. I had no idea that there are different types of dementias AND different types of physical conditions that can mimic dementia. Here is just a sampling of various types of dementia:

- Lewy Body Dementia
- Frontotemporal Dementia
- Huntington's Disease
- Parkinson's Disease Dementia
- Vascular Dementia.

Without getting too far into the weeds, Alzheimer's is a brain disease. In a nutshell, the nerve cells in the brain start to break down. It slowly spreads in a specific order, which is why we see certain parts of the body systems affected during each stage since different parts of the brain control different systems in our bodies. Many books and websites dig deeper into the "plaques and tangles" if you want to learn more about this. I'm a doctor, but NOT in medicine, so I don't pretend to understand what this all means. All I know is that the damage is irreversible. Some medications can slow it down, but for now, there is no cure.

Alzheimer's is primarily experienced in advanced age, but it is not a normal process of growing old. There are many people younger than 65 who have "Early Onset Alzheimer's." Another interesting fact is that not everyone will experience the same symptoms in each stage. One example is wandering. My mom never wandered or escaped from our home or the memory care center, but many patients WILL do this. Upon diagnosis, the average lifespan is four to eight years. Some can live longer than eight years. After being officially diagnosed, my mom lived about five more years.

As mentioned in the Foreword, I like using the 7-Stage Identification model of the Alzheimer's stages developed by Dr. Barry Reisberg. Because I lived in Texas and Mom lived in California, I didn't see the day-to-day decline that she was experiencing. I could only tell that her memory was declining through the phone calls we had. She would repeat herself over and over and over and over during each phone call. Then I would hear the same stories over and over and over and over in each subsequent call.

The repeated stories got old fast, and I almost dreaded talking to her on the phone. Looking back now, I soooo wish I had recorded some of these conversations. I wish I had asked her more about her childhood to document things that were slowly being eaten away by this disease. I should have realized that Alzheimer's was now affecting her because of what we experienced with my grandmother.

There are several sources likeWebMD.com and Alzheimers.net that offer ways to explain the 7 stages. I pulled Dr. Reisberg's study to try and explain the first four Alzheimer's stages. The patient can experience the following indicators or signs:

Stage 1: No Impairment. The brain is starting to die, but it's not noticeable at all by loved ones. They are not experiencing any memory decline, and the physical symptoms from parts of the brain dying are not apparent yet.

Stage 2: Very Mild Decline. In this stage, we will start to notice minor memory issues or losing things around the house. They may have a hard time finding the right word while speaking. It's hard to distinguish between this decline and normal aging. Face it, we all lose our keys or our glasses, or forget a word in a conversation as we get older. So, this type of memory loss is still hard to determine if it's Alzheimer's. The person can still do well on memory tests, and the family physician will not be able to diagnose Alzheimer's yet.

Stage 3: Mild Decline. We are now in the stage where family members or close friends may notice changes in cognition and memory. Doctors may be able to start noticing cognition issues using memory tests. Here are some areas that we can see changes at this stage:

- If they are still working, their job performance may start declining.
- They may have trouble concentrating.
- They may repeat questions or stories over and over.
- They may have a hard time remembering names.
- They may forget where they placed things.
- They may start experiencing anxiety.

Dr. Reisberg believes that Stage 3 is the "border" stage. Patients experiencing these memory issues may not progress to Stage 4. They may just be experiencing normal aging signs. I believe Stage 3 is where we first realized Mom was experiencing dementia when we noticed she was repeating stories. Because I wasn't living near her, I couldn't tell if she was experiencing any other signs mentioned.

Stage 4: Moderate Decline. Dr. Reisberg believes that Alzheimer's can be diagnosed at this stage. In this stage, we see significant problems. For example, when Mom got lost while driving home, we had the clear-cut signal that she was in trouble. As you will see in some of the chronicle posts, we now knew that she had short-term memory issues and life history recall issues. Here are some common signs of Stage 4:

- Difficulty with grocery shopping or preparing meals.
- Choosing from a menu at a restaurant becomes hard. I can clearly remember when Mom would hand me a menu and ask me to pick something for her.
- Poor short-term memory. Dementia patients may forget the day, month, or season. They may also forget what they ate for breakfast.
- Difficulty with managing finances and paying bills. If your loved one is still living independently, are utilities being turned off? Are there debt-collection bills coming in the mail? Are bills being overpaid, causing the checking account to dwindle?
- Putting objects in unusual places (example: an article of clothing in the refrigerator)
- Forgetting life history details. I will add to this by saying not only are details being forgotten, but experiences that never happened become very real in their minds. You will read a couple of these types of stories in the chronicles. I especially loved Mom's story of being friends with Michelle Obama as a child and the story of when she visited Hawaii. (She never met Mrs. Obama nor visited Hawaii.)
  (VISN 21 MIRECC, n.d.)

I love the Alzheimer's Association website (www.alz.org). They have a list of 10 early signs and symptoms of Alzheimer's compared to normal aging changes. Here is a synopsis: (10 Early Signs and Symptoms of Alzheimer's, n.d.)

- Memory loss that disrupts daily life.
  - Common Alz Signs: Forgetting learned information or important dates/events; asking questions over and over; relying on memory aids or relying on family members to handle things they usually used to do themselves.
  - Normal Aging: Forgetting names or appointments but remembering them later.
- Challenges in planning or solving problems.
  - Common Alz Signs: difficulty following a favorite recipe or keeping track of monthly bills; difficulty concentrating and taking longer to do things than they did before.
  - Normal Aging: making occasional errors with finances or bills.

- Difficulty completing familiar tasks.
  - Common Alz Signs: completing daily tasks becomes difficult; forgetting how to drive to a familiar place; creating a grocery list; forgetting rules to a favorite game.
  - Normal Aging: forgetting how to use microwave settings or recording a TV show on occasion.
- Confusion with time or place.
  - Common Alz Signs: losing track of dates, seasons, and passage of time; forgetting where they are or how they got there; trouble understanding something if it is not happening at the current moment.
  - Normal Aging: forgetting the day of the week but remembering it later.
- Trouble understanding visual images and spatial relationships.
  - Common Alz Signs: difficulty with balancing or reading; difficulty judging distance and determining color or contrast. These signs could lead to driving issues.
  - Normal Aging: cataracts can mimic many of the early visual symptoms of Alzheimer's.
- New problems with words in speaking or writing.
  - Common Alz Signs: trouble following or participating in a conversation; struggling with vocabulary and remembering the name of an everyday object. For example, the website mentions a patient calling a "watch" a "hand-clock."
  - Normal Aging: trouble finding the right word on occasion.
- Misplacing things and losing the ability to retrace steps.
  - Common Alz Signs: putting things in unusual places; losing items and forgetting how to retrace steps to find them; accusing friends and family of stealing.
  - Normal Aging: misplacing things occasionally but can retrace steps to find them.
- Decreased or poor judgment.
  - Common Alz Signs: exhibiting poor judgment with money; not grooming or cleaning themselves as regularly as before.
  - Normal Aging: making bad decisions on occasion like forgetting to change the oil in the car.
- Withdrawing from work or social activities.
  - Common Alz Signs: because holding a conversation is more difficult, they may withdraw from favorite hobbies or social activities.
  - Normal Aging: feeling uninterested in the family or social activities sometimes.
- Changes in mood or personality.
  - Common Alz Signs: becoming confused, suspicious, depressed, fearful, or anxious.
  - Normal Aging: becoming irritable when a routine is disrupted.

Here is my first post about my mom from the beginning of our journey:

November 20, 2014
I need help from my older friends on Medicare. I am about to move my mother in with us. She is currently on California's MediCal insurance, so I need to switch her to Medicare to be covered here. I looked at the site, and it is crazy to try and figure out what is the best plan. If any of you are on Medicare, can you please guide me in the right direction on what I need to do for her????

♥

This post should clue you into the massive undertaking it will take to get insurance and finances set up for your loved one. I highly, highly, highly recommend that you and your loved one (if possible) visit with an Elder Law Attorney. Things like wills, power of attorneys, medical power of attorneys, advanced directives, bank accounts, real estate, savings, IRAs, etc., are all HUGE areas that need to be planned as soon as possible. **Everything** you do, from whose names are on the bank accounts and how you pay for her bills and expenses to handling her home, car, life insurances, etc., may affect the level of care needed in the later stages.

Please keep in mind that if Medicaid is an option you are considering for nursing home care in the later stages, there are many rules in place for how your loved one's money is spent. Medicaid also has an estate recovery program (MERP) designed to recoup money that Medicaid spent on a senior's care. Therefore, it's imperative to learn how MERP works and consult with an Elder Law Financial Planner/Attorney to minimize the program's financial impact after your loved one passes.

Another thing I learned after it was too late was to consider getting a Personal Care Agreement drawn up. As mentioned a moment ago, please consider visiting with an Elder Law Attorney asap to ask if this is a good option for you and your family. The AgingCare.com site has information that can explain Personal Care Agreements further._(Heiser, n.d.)

To recap, here are some documents you need to get set up as soon as possible before your loved one's cognitive abilities are too diminished, in my humble opinion:

- Will
- Power of Attorney
- Medical Power of Attorney
- Advanced Directive
- Personal Care Agreement

After that fateful day of learning that Mom had gotten lost while driving, it was now time to start the process of moving Mom to Texas. As God's timing would have it, Bruce had just lost his job due to his employer's leadership restructuring in November, and I had vacation time around Thanksgiving. His job loss allowed Bruce the time needed to go with me to California to pack Mom's belongings and drive back to Texas. So we told Mom it was time to move her to Texas to live with us and asked her to start packing her things.

November 21, 2014

Leaving on a jet plane! Bruce and I are heading to California to pack my mom's belongings up and move her in with us. We are ready for the next adventure in our lives and are glad she won't be so far away now.

♥

We flew to California on November 21 and arrived at Mom and Ted's home. When we got there, we were in shock. One word: HOARDING!

I later learned through research that hoarding is a big sign of Alzheimer's. Here is what Alzheimer's Association says:

"Hoarding for a person with dementia may be more likely to happen in the early and middle stages of dementia and often stems from trying to have some control in their lives. People with dementia may be driven to search or rummage for something that they believe is missing."

https://www.alz.org/media/greatermissouri/Rummaging_Hiding_and_Hoarding_Behaviors.pdf

Of course, we were still rookies and didn't know a thing about hoarding. We knew she was a packrat before her Alzheimer's diagnosis, but this level of hoarding was extreme. We didn't know how to deal with it.

I included the following post just to point out that interacting with an Alzheimer's patient, who happens to be your mother-in-law (DOUBLE WHAMMY!), can be stressful for your spouse. We were extremely frustrated when we got there to learn that Mom had not done any packing at all - which we had asked her to do. We later understood that this task was just too monumental for her to understand and handle. Mom insisted on so much stuff to be packed to go back to Texas with us. Since we had limited space in the moving truck (and at home), we wanted to leave things there that we knew were junk, but it made her so upset. Because she couldn't process this mentally, we decided to go ahead and pack things into the moving truck and then either trash it or donate it when we got back to Dallas. But this sure did put poor Bruce over the edge with a migraine. And boy did he get a doozy of one, which caused us to pause packing and go to the ER to get it under control.

November 22, 2014
We are down for the count. Too much stress, heavy lifting, and not enough water lead to an ER trip for Bruce out here in California with a bad migraine. Unfortunately, they are busy, so it will be a while before they can see him.

♥

After filling up the moving truck with Mom's belongings, Bruce and I made the trip back to Dallas over the Thanksgiving holidays. Mom stayed behind with Ted since Robin and one of her daughters would be going out in a few weeks to pack Ted's belongings and get the house ready to sell.

When she arrived in California, she went through the same frustration since Ted hoarded too. She also had to deal with many things we couldn't pack in the moving truck that Mom insisted be included in the move. If I remember correctly, Robin ended up with two large dumpsters of junk to be trashed and had to "fight" with Mom and Ted about what was getting thrown away. Mom didn't make it easy because, in her mind, every single slip of paper or knick-knack was priceless and couldn't be left behind. It was not an easy time for any of us.

On their way back to Texas, Robin and her daughter were in a moving truck while Mom and Ted followed in their car. Robin was a nervous wreck making sure Mom was driving safely behind them. I believe there were a few close calls if I remember the stories correctly!

December 16, 2014
Well, today is the day. Mom and Ted have made it in from California to my stepsister's home. Bruce and Josh are driving to Magnolia today to get the rest of her belongings and bring her back to her new home with us. Thanks to Robin for taking good care of my mom this past week. I know it was a stressful time for all of you. Bruce, Josh, Sheila, and I are excited to have Mom "home" now. She has been away from us for way too long. There will be lots of family adjustments to be made, but it will all be okay.

December 18, 2014
Success! She likes word search puzzles!! Now that we are around her more, we see just how much dementia is taking over. The stress of all the changes is hitting her hard. We are praying she feels settled in soon and her mind eases up some. We will take this one day at a time!

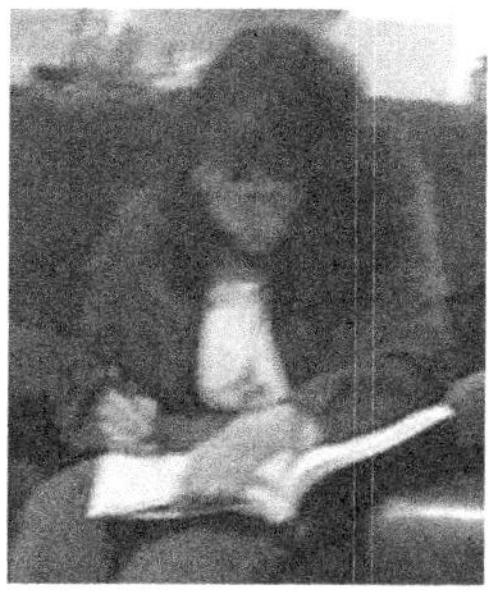

♥

Now that we had her home and could see the level of dementia she was experiencing, we believed she needed companionship and a little caregiving while we were at work. We didn't think she should be by herself. Finding companionship was a challenge. I started with a caregiver who didn't work out, as you will see in a post. I had to use a few friends and neighbors to help until we found someone who could work weird schedules. Bruce had found a new job and was working 24-hour shifts on alternating days as a paramedic. That made finding companionship and caregiving more difficult because most people want a set schedule.

I also wanted to mention here to please be sure and check out your state and county's senior citizen care resources. Some counties have fabulous resources that can assist with caregiving and possibly supplies for your loved one. For example, my friend Cathy lived in Dallas County and could get assistance for her mother, who has dementia, but I lived in Collin County and didn't have the same aid that she had. So it never hurts to check!

December 30, 2014
Here is another lesson learned on how to live with someone with dementia - lock up medications! We learned Mom got up in the middle of the night to take something to help her sleep. Luckily, she only took a chewable

vitamin, but it taught us quickly that we had to do something different. In the two short weeks she has been with us, we have learned a lot about dementia, and we know that there is more to come.

♥

Because of this scare, we purchased a hidden magnetic lock system since we had the type of cabinets that didn't have handles. We locked away all medicines and vitamins behind this locked cabinet door to keep Mom safe. We realized we had a 70+-year-old toddler in the home now and had to "toddler" proof it.

January 6, 2015
I am looking for someone (preferably female) part-time to stay with my mom in my home. She is in the beginning/middle stages of dementia and needs companionship during the day while we work (to keep her safe, take her to doctor appointments and the Senior Citizen Center for activities, etc.) Days aren't set in stone yet, but so far, it looks like Tues/Thurs and Wed/Fri (alternating weeks) - possibly some Mondays now and then.

♥

Notice that I asked for someone to help with doctor appointments. I later learned that I needed to be at every doctor appointment simply because I was the primary caregiver and could answer the doctor's questions that my mother couldn't answer. I say this to prepare you that you or someone in your family who knows all the details of your loved one's daily routine will probably need to be the one who takes her to the appointments.

January 15, 2015
We bought a nanny-cam last night to check in on a new caregiver today. (She was 25 minutes late on Tuesday, so we were uneasy about her.) After checking in on the nanny cam often during the 4 hours this morning, I left work to relieve her of her duties. Not only did she just sit the entire time, but she also watched Mom empty the dishwasher and didn't get up to lend a hand. She never interacted with her other than a few small chit-chat conversations, and then she had Mom fix the sandwiches for them both at lunchtime instead of getting up and helping. When I got home, she was taking a nap on the couch. I was livid. I am thankful for Jocelynn Clark and Dani Gray, who both are taking care of Mom on the other days they are available. They do a fantastic job with her. Now it is back to the drawing board to find someone reliable to fill in the days that Jocelynn and Dani can't be here. I'm going to try a caregiving agency this time that has extra vetting measures.

♥

Now that Mom was living with us, it was time to start getting her healthcare up to speed. There was no telling what all was wrong with her, in addition to her dementia. I needed to get a physician set up locally and her medications correct. I also needed a game plan for how to deal with her dementia. After the first appointment, I learned that the doctor wanted to run all kinds of tests to rule out physical issues that could be causing or mimicking dementia symptoms. For example, she wanted to check for vitamin deficiencies, thyroid issues, a UTI (urinary tract infection), strokes, etc. Mom had a whole battery of tests prescribed over the next several weeks/months to narrow down what all was wrong.

I found an article on the AgingCare.com site that shares tips on how to get a loved one to go to the doctor if she is refusing to go. Luckily, my mom never refused to go. It's essential to get a Power of Attorney and Medical Power of Attorney as soon as possible. This site mentions that the loved one may not want to visit the doctor because she denies that anything is even wrong. Because of the damage happening to the brain, they are not aware. The medical term for this is anosognosia.

Some suggested ideas are:

- Enlist the help of a trusted primary care physician that your loved one visits and have the doctor sing praises galore about the specialist your loved one needs to visit.

- Use a little white lie and take your loved one out on a fun activity. While heading home, stop by the doctor's office and tell your loved one that since we are driving by, let's just stop by and run in to put his name on the waiting list for a checkup. While inside, explain you just learned they had a cancellation and can get seen now. Be excited that you both are having good luck getting seen so quickly. They suggested giving the front desk staff a heads-up about what you are trying to accomplish to overcome your loved one's reluctance.
- Check out other options like house calls and telemedicine.

The article, What Do I Do If My Elderly Parent Refuses to Go to the Doctor? by Jacqueline Marcell was contributed by AgingCare.com. (Marcel, n.d.)

January 16, 2015
I learned that Mom is severely claustrophobic now. She didn't use to be. She had a brain MRI this afternoon, and about halfway through, she had a bad panic attack. She couldn't breathe and was crying. The technician let me stand by her since I wouldn't be in the way of the imaging and hold her hand to try to help her through it. I felt so bad for her! We got her through it, though! I'm hoping to get some answers soon for her memory issues.

♥

I also needed ideas for keeping Mom busy and entertained during the day. Dementia patients need to feel useful and needed in the household. They need a purpose. Along with jigsaw puzzles, word search puzzles, and black velvet poster art with markers, I had her helping me with folding clothes and loading/unloading the dishwasher. She could still cognitively play Solitaire on the computer, so that was one of her favorite pastimes to keep her busy.

Because she could still read, I labeled the cabinets and drawers in the kitchen so that she would know where glasses, plates, silverware, etc., get stored. There are tons of ideas out there for keeping a dementia patient busy. Do some simple searches for activities. There are ideas for both men and women with varied backgrounds to keep them active and feeling productive. Things like sorting colored plastic ware, sorting nuts, bolts, and screws, sorting coins in a change counter, and so on can keep them busy and productive. Just be careful that you aren't treating them like a child. A children's coloring book at this early stage may only upset them. They still need to be treated like an adult-they just need easier activities to do. Heck, in one of the Alzheimer's support groups on Facebook, I even read how one daughter had her mother tear apart paper towels at the seams and fold them to keep her busy. Reach out to friends, scour garage sales, become resourceful. Some activities can get expensive!

A word of warning, though. Some of the activities listed above may be good for these early stages but as your loved one progresses in the disease, be careful about the items you give them to sort or handle. For example, as their cognitive level decreases, they may not be safe handling knives when sorting silverware. You will read in a future post that my mom tried to use a screwdriver to get a hearing aid out of her ear. So some tools or objects may not be safe for them to handle.

January 19, 2015
Mom loves 100–piece to 300-piece jigsaw puzzles (500-piece is too hard for her), but unfortunately, these suckers are expensive in stores. If anyone has used puzzles you would like to sell me, let me know. If you are in the Huntsville area, I can arrange for my sister to get them from you. In the meantime, I will scour garage sales!! Thanks in advance!

♥

Along with activities, be sure to accept help from friends and family when you need a break. I had a conference out of town one week, and I knew I couldn't leave her at home because Bruce worked 24-hour shifts. My stepsister, Robin, agreed to care for my mom during that week. It allowed Mom and Ted to visit and enjoy each other's company. Your mental health as a caregiver is essential. You need to take care of yourself to be able to help your loved one physically. I was blessed with family and friends who helped us throughout the entire journey. Unfortunately, though, I have learned that MANY people do not have that luxury. I've heard of so many families where the siblings left all the caregiving for the parent to one person. It truly is heart-breaking.

If you do not need to care for someone, might I suggest that you volunteer time for a friend you know who IS taking care of someone? Trust me; they need some time just to go to the store by themselves, a dinner and movie night out, a mani/pedi afternoon, and so on. Couples who are caregivers need date nights. The stress level in marriages goes up when caregiving for a parent is brought into the relationship. A few hours here and there will mean the world to them. Consider creating caregiver night out events with your church or circle of friends.

If you are a sibling to one who is handling the lion's share of the caregiving, volunteer time and offer to help financially (if you can) to pay for some expenses and "babysitters" from time to time. Caregiving is EXPENSIVE and can be physically and emotionally draining! I may ruffle some feathers with the following sentence, but it is how I feel. Please do not use the excuse that you can't handle seeing your parent(s) in that shape. Your loved one can't help the condition he's in, and it's not fair to him. If he doesn't remember you, that's okay. It will "sting" at first, but you will get used to it. You can still bring some sunshine to his day just by allowing him to talk to you and interact with you. Dementia can be a lonely disease for both the loved one AND the caregiver.

"Oh, but my dad is mean! I don't like him!" Or maybe you never had a loving relationship with your parent. Unfortunately, I don't have experience with this. I wish I had words of advice because I can only imagine the heartache, frustration, and anger this causes. I see many folks in the support groups who harbor huge resentment for caring for a loved one who never was a loving, responsible parent. I do have experience with not liking my mom sometimes, but I never stopped loving her. She also was not a mean person to us other than some outbursts as the disease progressed. On the flip side, I have also seen caregivers experience forgiveness by caring for a parent they did not have a good relationship with during their past. Each family will have a set of unique experiences to work through on this journey.

February 3, 2015
Mom is safely tucked away this week with my stepsister. Bruce is enjoying an estrogen-free home for the week, and I am enjoying a few days in Austin at the TCEA conference. I scored a nice hotel this time under the state rate.

♥

If you remember some of the physical signs mentioned earlier, cataracts can cause visual distortions. It turns out Mom did have cataracts in both eyes, so we arranged to have this condition fixed to at least help with this part of her physical health. By having her cataracts fixed, she no longer needed to wear glasses. Her glasses were one less thing she needed to keep up with and not worry about losing around the house.

February 12, 2015
Mom is scheduled for cataract surgery on her left eye this morning, the right eye next Thursday, and then all four wisdom teeth removed in a couple of weeks. These three surgeries, plus a multitude of follow-up appointments, are making me tired of doctor's offices!! But, at least she should be all fixed up in a few weeks!

February 14, 2015
I'm so happy to have a date night with my honey. We are going to see a movie. A very special thank you to one of our sweetest friends Ken Krippner for hanging out with Mom tonight to let Bruce and me have a date night. We love you and appreciate you!

February 18, 2015
I took Mom for froyo at [a local frozen yogurt shop] after her doctor's appt. She loves frozen yogurt!

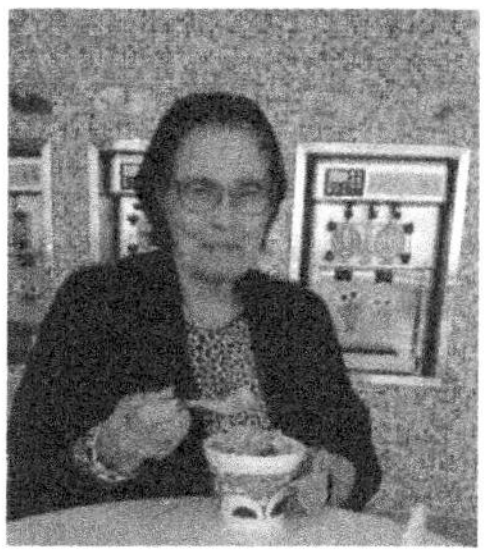

February 19, 2015
We had to sit in a 45-minute traffic jam because of a bad wreck this morning to get Mom to the clinic for her cataract surgery appointment. I was getting frustrated but then stopped myself because I realized those folks in the bad wreck (hoping they survived) were in a much more difficult situation than me. If we had to reschedule, that is okay. At least we are alive and healthy. I'm working on that bad, selfish attitude that I get sometimes! Mom is about ready to go back for her surgery. All is well in our lives!

February 21, 2015
Mom just had her hair fixed at the salon. Also, she no longer needs to wear glasses because of the cataract surgeries. Mom is in total amazement at how well she can see without glasses. She has worn glasses since she was a little girl. What a beautiful lady!

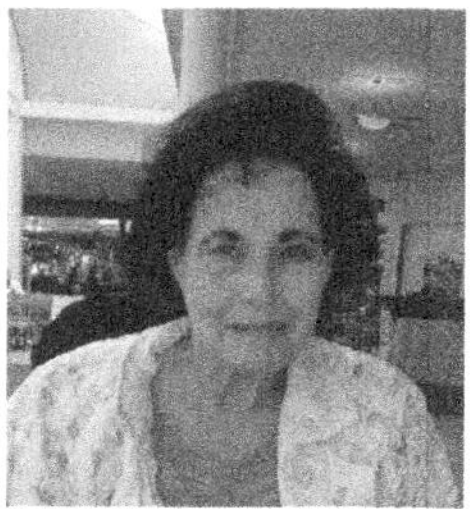

March 3, 2015
Joshua came over for dinner and a game - we played his new "Big Bang Theory Monopoly." We had lots of fun tonight! Mom did well with playing the game. It was a good exercise for her brain.

March 14, 2015
My sister is taking care of my mom tonight while Bruce and I have a date night! Woo hoo!!

March 17, 2015
Without explaining too much, I could use some prayers for patience with my mom tonight, please.

♥

I don't remember what the problem was that night that was testing my patience. I do know we had LOTS of those events when she lived with us! Patience will be stretched quite a bit as caregivers. Trust me!

After the doctor ran various tests to rule out strokes, vitamin deficiencies, thyroid issues, etc., we were finally referred to a neurologist to help determine what kind of dementia she was experiencing.

March 27, 2015
I took Mom to a neurologist today. The neurologist did several tests and said that he thinks she has Alzheimer's instead of vascular dementia. He will know for sure in a few months after several follow-ups. Since my grandmother had dementia, he said that Alzheimer's tends to run in the female side of the family. After monitoring her for a few months, he said he would give me more of an idea of how things may progress with her. So, now we wait.

I wanted to verify the neurologist's statement about running heavily on the female side of the family. I found this on the Alzheimer's Association site: "research shows that those who have a parent or sibling with Alzheimer's are more likely to develop the disease than those who do not have a first-degree relative with Alzheimer's." (Is Alzheimer's Genetic, n.d.) I found another article that shared this: "If your mother has Alzheimer's, you are more likely to develop the disease than if your father has Alzheimer's, according to a study published today in the journal *Neurology*." (Agnvall, 2011) One last site shared various studies that share why they believe women have a higher chance of developing Alzheimer's. Research shows women have a 1 in 5 chance of developing Alzheimer's over the age of 65. Statistics show that out of the 5 million people living with Alzheimer's, 3.2 million are women. Another study showed that women in their 60s are twice as likely to develop the disease than develop breast cancer. (Sauer, 2019)

As you can imagine, this concerns my sister and me greatly. We can implement some ideas like diet and exercise to help mitigate it as much as possible, but there is no guarantee that we can avoid it altogether. At least she and I now know things we need to have in place BEFORE we possibly get to that stage in our lives. Some of this involves having some heartfelt conversations with our families to be all on the same page.

To determine the level of dementia, neurologists and family doctors can run a simple mental health test. The most common mental health test for diagnosing the severity of dementia is the Mini-Mental State Examination (MMSE) test. It's a short test that can be taken at a doctor's office or home. You can do an internet search and find many sites that offer this test for free and how to "score" it. It tests the person's ability to:

- share where she is at the moment (like city, state, country, office building, hospital, etc.);
- name the current season of the year or day of the week;
- name the current president;
- recall something from short-term memory (tell the person three common objects and then ask the person to repeat those same objects a minute or so later);
- solve problems like a simple math problem or to spell a word backward;
- identify everyday objects by name;
- and comprehend and use motor skills by drawing a slightly complicated shape.

I also remember that the neurologist asked Mom to draw a clock with the hands drawn to a specific time.

The scores can be broken down into the following ranges:

24 - higher	No dementia
19 - 23	Mild dementia
10 - 18	Moderate dementia
9 and lower	Severe dementia

It's important to note that the MMSE score is not the sole determinant of diagnosing dementia or Alzheimer's. Doctors will look at medical history and other medical tests. I will explain this further in some of the posts I share after Mom's appointments with her neurologists.

Later, I learned about another memory test called the Rowland Universal Dementia Assessment Scale (RUDAS) test. It is a good test for patients with cultural barriers, low education levels, or when English is not the primary language. Mom never took this test. It was one I found out about later in our journey.

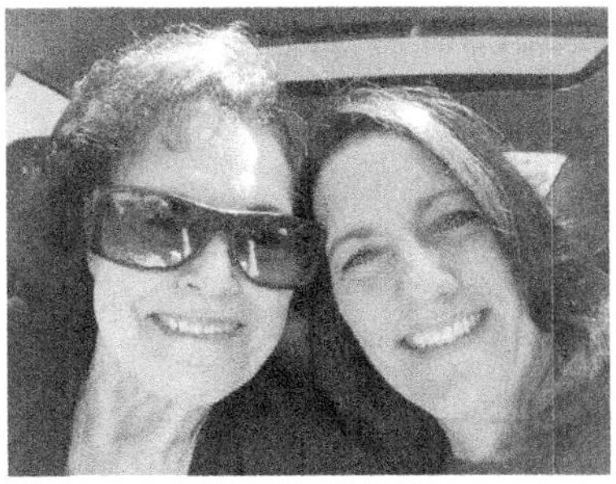

March 28, 2015

I hate selfies but love my mom. We just had our hair done. She looks beautiful!

♥

Because Mom could still function partially on her own in most activities, I would monitor Mom through the webcam throughout the day while I worked. She only had a caregiver with her for a few hours a day in the beginning. As the days and months passed, we saw that simple activities started to become problematic. For example, she couldn't remember how to operate the TV remote control. At this point, I started pulling in my dear neighbors to help if we weren't home with Mom to help her. We were all an extremely tight-knit group, so many of them came to our aid over the years with Mom.

March 30, 2015 (post to our neighborhood group page)
Our caregiver for my mom is already gone for the day. I hate to ask this, but is there anyone home right now who has time to try and help my mom get the TV back on? She tried to change channels (she has trouble with this) and clicked something that somehow made it go to the settings. I tried explaining to her to turn it off and back on to "reset" it, but it didn't work. I have a feeling that we are going to be calling on our neighbors a lot over the next few years!

♥

Our neighbors always pulled through for us. We couldn't have helped Mom as much as we did the first few years without them. We will forever be grateful that God placed us in that neighborhood on that specific block when we decided to purchase a home in Wylie.

The next thing on our plate to help her with was the pain level in her hips. Bless her heart (yes-I'm a southern gal who uses this phrase a lot!); Mom always experienced pain in her life. From a severe neck injury in a car wreck we were in during the early 1970s to knee replacements and arthritis, she dealt with pain her whole life. She was also a hypochondriac. If she stumped her toe, she immediately thought she broke it. If she had a twinge of pain in her chest - which could have simply been heartburn - she thought she was having a heart attack. So, as you can imagine, it was hard to determine sometimes if it was something serious or just normal aches and pains we all deal with from time to time. Now that her ability to communicate was diminishing, we had to look for physical signs of pain. We could see she was physically hurting because she would shift a lot in her seat and have difficulty walking. We could also hear her bones popping loudly in her hips whenever she moved. Over the next few years, we tried visiting several orthopedic doctors and pain control doctors to help her as much as possible.

April 2, 2015
We are at the orthopedic surgeon's office for Mom's hip pain. X-rays show it is bone on bone, but they don't recommend hip replacement because it tends to worsen dementia. So, they will give her a shot in her hip and want her to start using a walker. I feel bad that we aren't going to be able to lessen the pain, but there isn't another option. I don't want to see her go downhill any faster.

♥

Another thing we did during the first few months of Mom living with us was to sell her car. We knew this was going to cause a fight and be extremely stressful. I followed an Alzheimer's blogger who suggested getting a doctor's prescription stating, "No driving for six months." You don't want to say "No driving ever again" because that makes them lose all hope. You always want to give them something to hope for in the future. Let me repeat that, **you always want to give them something to hope for in the future**. They are losing their independence, and it is scaring them. By saying "6 months", you can pull that prescription note out repeatedly until it no longer is an issue.

If you can't sell the car, you can disable the car by unplugging cables, etc. I'm sure a mechanic friend can help with this. As expected, Mom was upset, but after a few months, it was no longer an issue. Once we sold the car and it was out of her sight, she forgot about it. And trust me, that little "doctor's prescription" idea becomes extremely helpful in all kinds of situations like bathing, eating, etc.

Moving on in the story, my mom's younger brother retired and moved from Massachusetts to Colorado. He doesn't travel to Texas much, but in 2015, he drove down and visited with us for a few days to have some quality time with Mom before she progressed to a point where she didn't remember him. I'm so glad he had this opportunity because the next time he visited, it was questionable whether she knew him or not.

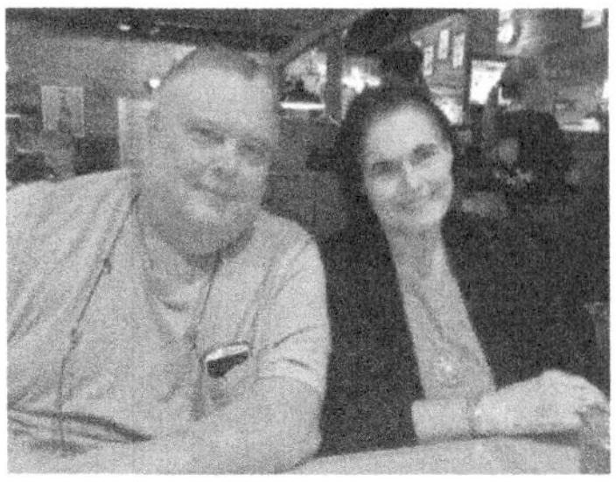

April 10, 2015
We enjoyed our visit with Uncle Quinton! Love you, Unc!!

♥

Our neighborhood had a pond with many ducks and geese. Mom loved wildlife. I wanted her to get out of the house as much as possible to get fresh air and experience the environment. She loved our walks and feeding the geese and ducks. She had a walker and a cane that she used in the beginning. Later on, we transitioned to a scooter as her mobility decreased.

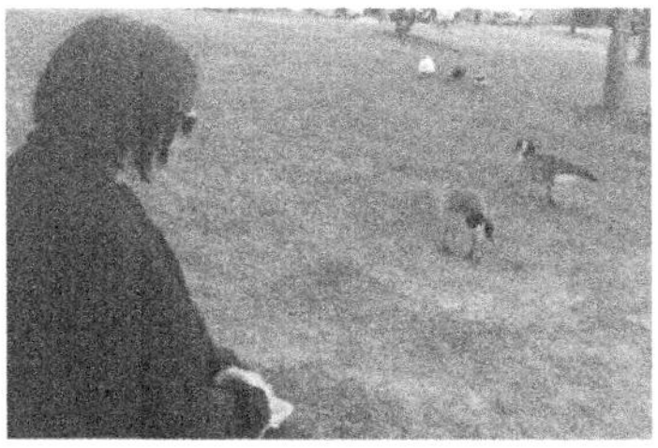

April 11, 2015
Mom loves feeding the ducks and geese. We learned that bread is bad for ducks and geese, so we buy food that is good for fowl from a local feed store.

♥

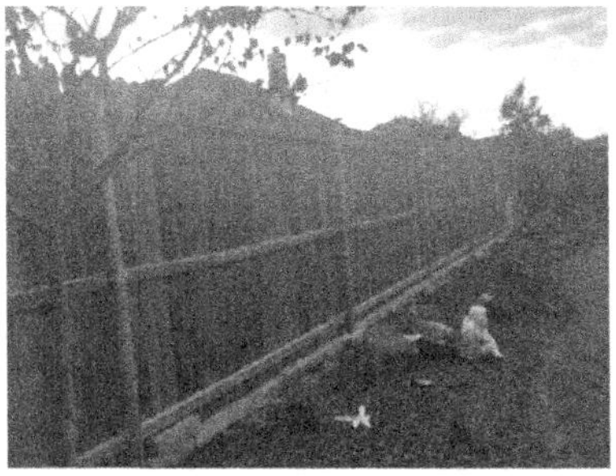

We tried different things to help keep her active and happy. Mom had a green thumb and loved to garden. I have vivid memories of banana trees and tons of roses at my childhood home in Houston. Out in California, she had beautiful flowers and fruit trees growing in her yard. Because she loved gardening so much, we had a landscaping company come in and add a small garden to our backyard. We incorporated some of her little yard statues into the garden so that she would feel at home. She would go out there often to look at the flowers and garden statues. She wasn't physically able to plant flowers anymore, but she loved to look at everything, especially as the flowers and bushes started growing.

April 29, 2015
We installed a new flower garden for Mom to enjoy. I can hardly wait until the flowers start blooming!

♥

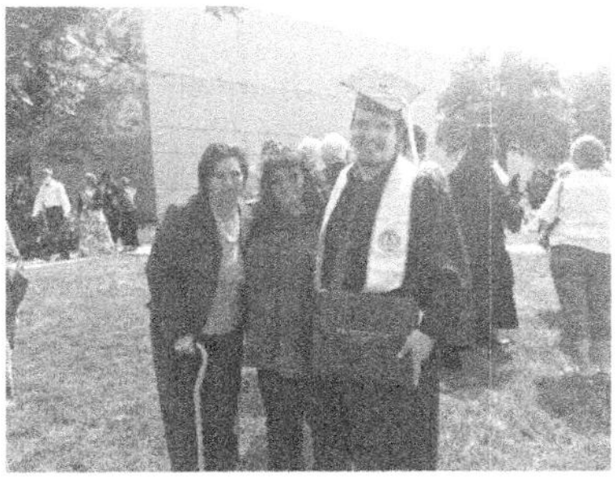

Mom was still walking during her first year of living with us. Our son, Joshua, had just graduated from college. Mom was able to walk to the ceremony on campus with her cane. She was so proud of him, as we all were!

May 14, 2015
Graduation day! I'm so happy Mom was here to witness this joyous occasion!

♥

For a graduation present, Bruce and I took Josh and a friend of his on a cruise. We needed a little break from Mom, but she needed to be taken care of that week, so Sheila took Mom on a separate cruise. One of the memorable things Sheila told me about was that Mom had a pimple come up on the inside of her nose. Remember when I said she was a hypochondriac? Since she doesn't clearly think things through now, she tried calling the ship's doctor to get help. For her pimple!! Luckily, Sheila overheard this and was able to stop her. This doctor visit would have been one heck of an expensive medical bill on vacation!

Bruce and I got a much-needed break from caregiving while celebrating Josh's accomplishment, and Sheila got a cherished memory of her last vacation with Mom. Even though it was challenging for her, she told me she was so glad she had the opportunity to spend that time with Mom before the disease progressed further.

Let's transition to another physical piece of the dementia puzzle - hearing. During all my research learning about dementia, I have learned that hearing loss can mimic dementia. If someone can't hear, just think about all the conversations they miss out on with friends and family. It is understandable to think someone is forgetful when in actuality, they just didn't hear the conversation.

Remember, I'm not a medical doctor. I'm just sharing information I have found in my research that may be helpful for folks out there who need ideas on how to help their loved ones. Researchers believe there is a link between hearing loss and Alzheimer's. They believe there is a correlation because of:

- Changes in brain function - Alzheimer's is slowly diminishing the brain, so the part of the brain that manages the auditory function could be damaged or dying.
- Cognitive load - the brain is struggling to make sense of what is being heard. The correlation could be that it just can't keep up with what is coming in through the auditory system.
- Social isolation - when one can't hear, it's hard to participate in social activities. As we experienced during the COVID pandemic isolation, we have seen a serious health decline in our elderly because they were isolated. Hearing loss can mimic this if people aren't able to compensate with hearing aids. (Albert, 2014)

We took Mom to get her hearing tested and learned she definitely had hearing loss in both ears and needed hearing aids. The aids helped for a short while until keeping up with the hearing aids became a challenge.

June 11, 2015
Hearing aids - 1, Mom - 0. After only 2 1/2 weeks with her hearing aids, she has already lost 1. This is a pretty expensive lesson to learn. Hopefully, we'll find the rogue hearing aid soon. I imagine it fell out, and Simi found it, thus enjoying a new chew toy. Who knows!!!

June 17, 2015
The most expensive game of hide-and-seek that we have ever played is now over. Woohoo! Joshua found Mom's lost hearing aid!!! Yay!!!!!!!!!!!!!!!!

July 22, 2015
We are at the ER... Mom is having a hard time breathing. Wylie EMS brought her here. I'm waiting to see when I can go back there to be with her. I think she is just having a panic attack because the medics said her heart rhythm is ok. We have fantastic medics in Wylie. Unfortunately, my live-in paramedic was working tonight and not here to help. It's funny, though, from all the years of listening to Bruce share stories of calls he experienced, I was telling dispatch that I have a 73-year-old female having a hard time breathing instead of simply saying "my Mom." Say a little prayer, please. Thanks!

♥

This was the first of MANY panic attacks through the years. I don't know if Mom suffered from these while she lived in California. After this one, we got a prescription from the doctor for anxiety medication for future attacks, and we also learned some strategies on how to calm her down. One strategy included redirection - which is something I didn't understand at the time. Redirection consists of any activity that takes her mind off what is happening at the time. Redirection examples include playing music and showing photo albums.

Besides learning all the ins and outs of taking care of Mom, we also still wanted her to stay connected to Ted and his family somehow. They had their phones and would call each other several times a day, but we also made it a point to get them together every few months. On long weekends, we would drive to Tomball, where Ted lived in an assisted living center. Mom and Ted loved seeing each other for a few hours each visit. We would go out for lunch and then go back to the assisted living center to let Ted play the guitar and sing for Mom. He also loved to introduce her as his beautiful wife to all his friends and nursing staff. You could always see the love these two still had for each other.

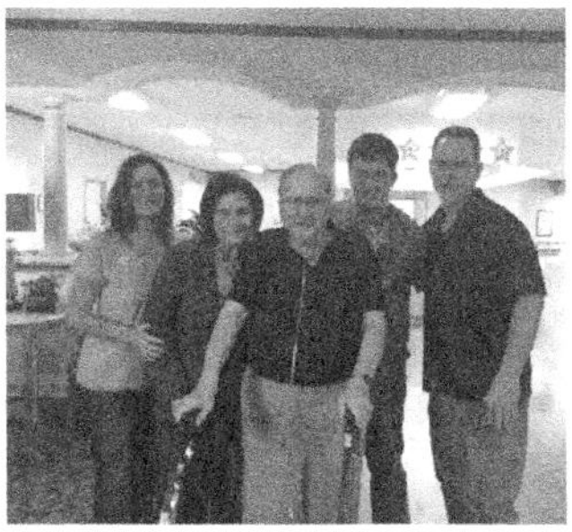

July 25, 2015
We took Mom to visit Ted today. I love seeing her smile when she sees him.

July 30, 2015
In the Aden household, we affectionately call dementia/Alzheimer's "Mad Cow Disease" (an old throwback to the TV series "Boston Legal"). So, to keep me from getting "Mad Cow Disease" too soon ('cause let's face it, it's not looking too good for my sister and me with both our mom and grandma having it), I have learned that I need to exercise my brain with puzzles, etc.
[In this post, I shared a puzzle for my friends to solve.]

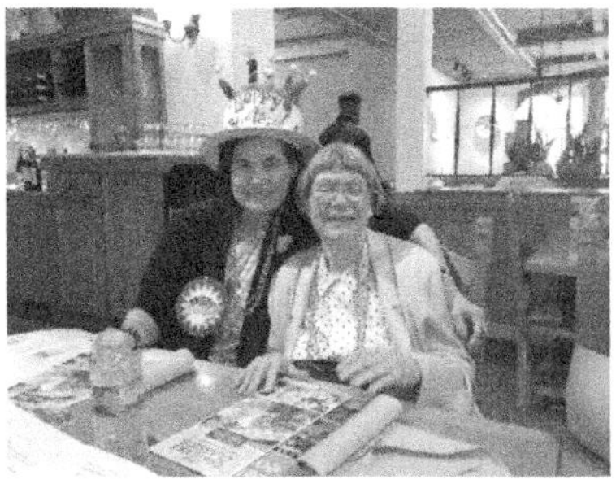

August 15, 2015
We took Mom to a restaurant tonight to celebrate her birthday a little early. I got a rare picture of her acting silly. Thanks, Cathy Randles, for bringing your mom Janet to help celebrate. My mom simply adores her!!

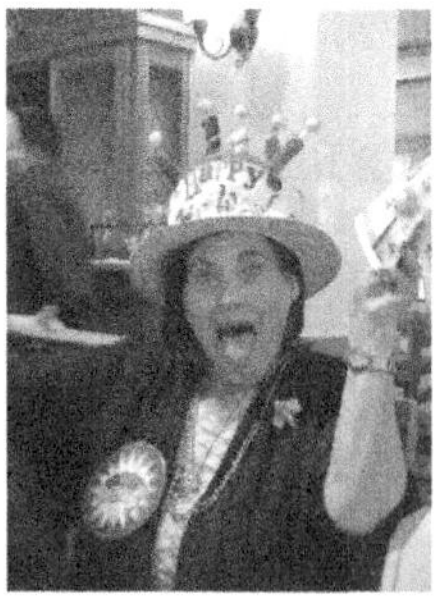

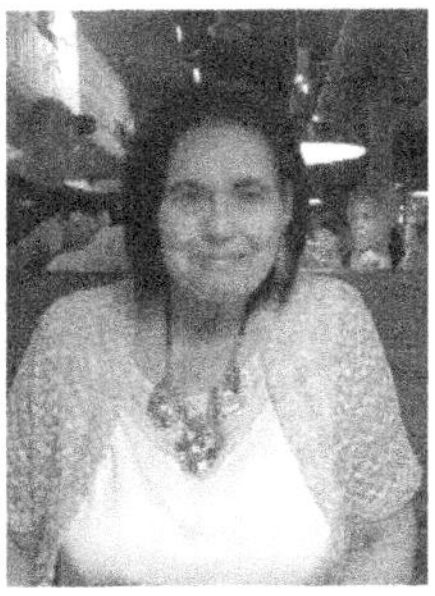

August 20, 2015
Today is Mom's actual birthday, so I am treating her to dinner at another restaurant. Happy birthday, Mom! After her birthday dinner, I took her for a walk down to the duck pond to feed the ducks.

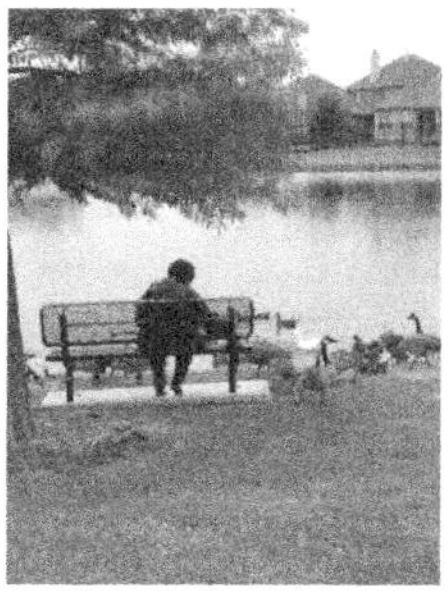

August 29, 2015
Josh is driving my mom down to Tomball to visit Ted today. It's going to be a long day for them. Prayers for safe travels, please!

September 3, 2015
Mom is having her stress test this morning. Prayers for no panic attacks, please! She is back there now for the first part, and the nurse said she would come to get me if she starts going into an attack.

September 15, 2015
Simi is getting some lovin' from Mom. Just disregard the news story going on in the background. *[Remember – the QR codes will open short video clips. Use your smartphone's camera feature or QR code reader to open the video clip.]*

September 22, 2015
This is an update on Mom. She had a couple of cardiac tests a few weeks ago, and the "test-readers" called me back then and said nothing was wrong. Soooo, imagine my surprise when we went to Mom's follow-up today with the cardiac doctor, and she said that the test results showed that Mom needs a heart valve either repaired or replaced. This is what's causing her to get out of breath and go into panic attacks. We now need to set up a couple more tests with a specialist and then go back to the doctor on November 3 to determine the next step. The bad thing is that the doctor told us that anytime she goes under anesthesia from here on out may cause her dementia to worsen. We'll just take this whole experience day-by-day and see where it leads us.

September 30, 2015
Thanks for the prayers, everyone! The doctor just came out and said Mom's mitral valve is moderately damaged but not severe. They don't do surgeries on anything except severe cases. We will just have to monitor with the cardiologist. Whew. No surgery!

November 5, 2015
Mom had a rough night last night, so I'm hanging out with her today to make sure we don't have another spell. Her back started having muscle spasms.

December 3, 2015
We had to take Mom to the ER a little while ago... We are back home now, and all is well. I just wanted to be safe rather than sorry. Thanks to my friend and neighbor Kara Adams-Sharum for taking good care of her at the ER. (It's fantastic having a nurse as a neighbor!) She's feeling much better.

December 15, 2015
Wish us luck today. We will see a new neurologist recommended to us by my friend Cathy to get a better handle on Mom's prognosis. I have to admit I've had a rough couple of days letting something she did get to me, but my loved ones are trying to help me remember it's just the disease, and I need to let it go. Bruce has started telling me a new phrase to get me to smile. He tells me to think of a box full of puppies. It actually helps!

♥

My lovely family and friends on Facebook started showering me with images of puppies after this post. I loved how they all stepped up to help my family and me through this journey, even if it was just a simple photo. It helped bring smiles to our faces.

December 15, 2015
Mom update... We went to a new neurologist today, and he is way better than our first one. He said she definitely has Alzheimer's and that she is in the "moderate" stage. Her first memory test score back at the beginning of the year with the other doctor was a "21". She is now a "16". He said a "10" is when the loved one will need long-term care. He will put her on two cognition medications and take her off another medicine that would interfere with them. We go back in 2 months for a follow-up. I am hoping the new meds will slow it down. He mentioned that the other doctor could have recommended an experimental treatment back in the spring when she was at the "mild" stage, but now it is too late since she has progressed. I'm just a little peeved. I was trying to give the other doctor the benefit of the doubt and was hoping he knew what he was doing. I'm so thankful for Cathy Randles, who recommended this new doctor. I wish I had listened sooner and got Mom in much faster than this. I will have to say that after listening to her struggle to answer questions today, I have calmed myself down from the stressor from the other day and truly remembered that she can't help herself. We will take this one day at a time, and with the help of the Good Lord, my family, and friends, and pictures and pictures of boxes full of puppies - we'll make it through this.

♥

As a caregiver, it is always important to remember to take care of yourself. Your health is just as important because if you aren't healthy, you can't take care of your loved one. Mom was having an issue in her bedroom, so I hopped up to take care of her. Before I got to her room, I started getting dizzy and dropped to the floor before I passed out. This scared my hubby and son. Josh took care of Mom's problem, and Bruce took me to the urgent care to get checked out. It wasn't anything serious, but I learned that I needed to take better care of myself.

December 17, 2015
Last night was a rough night health-wise for both Mom and me, but we both are doing better now. Lesson learned - I need to take better care of myself!

♥

Signs and symptoms in the seven stages of Alzheimer's can overlap. Sometimes she has a combination of symptoms from various stages. At this point in the journey, she started to overlap between stage 4, stage 5, and even into stage 6. She started having trouble with bowel and bladder control. An unpleasant part of caregiving is cleaning up after an accident. We pretty much gave up on trying to keep our carpet in her bedroom from being stained. I cleaned it as best as I could and just resigned to the fact that once she was no longer with us, I would just replace the carpet. It is also hard on the loved ones at this stage because they are very embarrassed and ashamed that they can't control their bodily functions anymore. There were many times Mom would cry and be upset because of the accident. I just had to reassure her as much as I could that it was an accident.

January 25, 2016
My husband is the best! He is home sick today, but my mom is having issues, and he is stepping up to take care of it since I'm at work. The next stage is finally hitting us. Caregiving is not easy - my heart goes out to my friends and family that do this or have done this for much longer than we have.

♥

Words are harder for Mom to find now. I'm in the education field but not in a specialty area where kids can't communicate verbally. As I posted our experiences with Mom on Facebook, I had friends send me ideas to try. Here is one example. It was a brilliant idea to help someone who is struggling with their words!

February 11, 2016
One of my dearest friends from junior high just recommended a "feelings chart" that I can use with my mom when she can't find the words. I just Googled that, and there were quite a few listed. By printing out a feelings chart, your loved one can look at a facial expression and point to it to help describe what she is feeling at the moment. Absolutely brilliant idea!

♥

If you remember back to the beginning of the book, Mom got lost driving to get her nails done at the salon. Mom LOVED getting her mani/pedis, so I tried to keep this up for her regularly. It wasn't just a joy for her - she also brought joy to the ladies who helped her at each appointment. Later in the Chronicles, you will see these ladies give her costume jewelry during most visits because they just loved her.

February 12, 2016
Mom is getting her pedicure done.

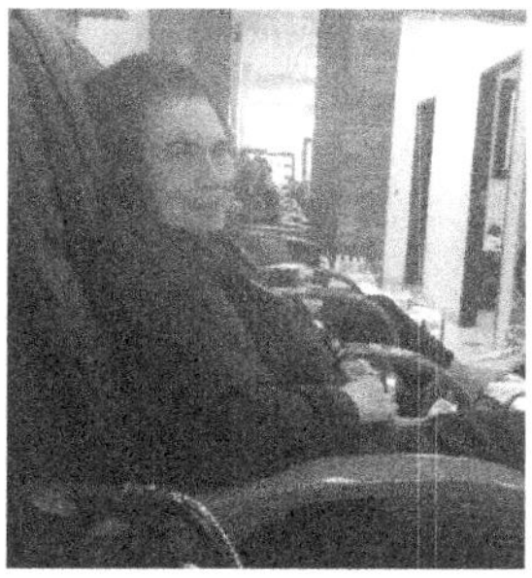

♥

Health issues will start to pile on during these middle stages. I don't remember Mom's exact problem on this ER visit (I think it was breathing issues), but you will see that I had to take her to the ER or urgent care quite often.

February 23, 2016
We are back in the ER again with Mom. It is for the same reason as last week. I'm hoping we can figure something out to help her. It's not urgent or life-threatening, but we could use some prayers that the doctors can figure something out.

February 23, 2016
Mom is back home resting. I'm about to make a medicine run. We are hoping we can figure out what to do soon to help her feel better. We have one specialist appointment Friday and will work on getting a pulmonologist appointment ASAP. Thanks for all the good vibes going her way.

February 26, 2016
Mom had another rough night. We almost had another ER visit, but we made it through. Sheila was here to help this time and will stay with her today. She has a doctor's appointment today, so hopefully, we can get some answers on how to help her. Say a little prayer for her, please.

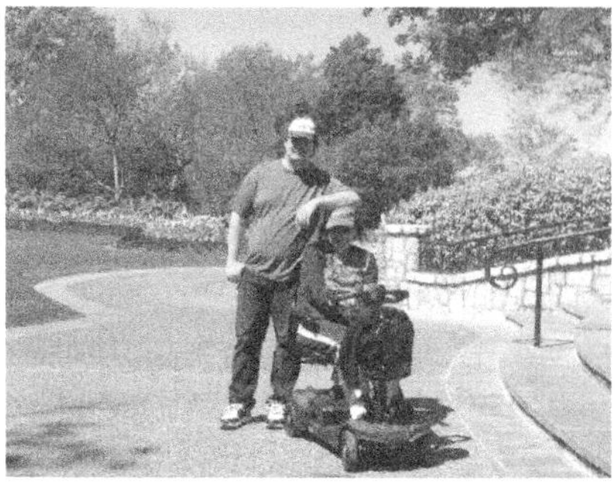

March 16, 2016
We took Mom to the Dallas Arboretum today. We brought the scooter for her to handle long distances. Her walking is much worse now. She enjoyed being around the flowers. Gardening was one of her passions as far back as I can remember.

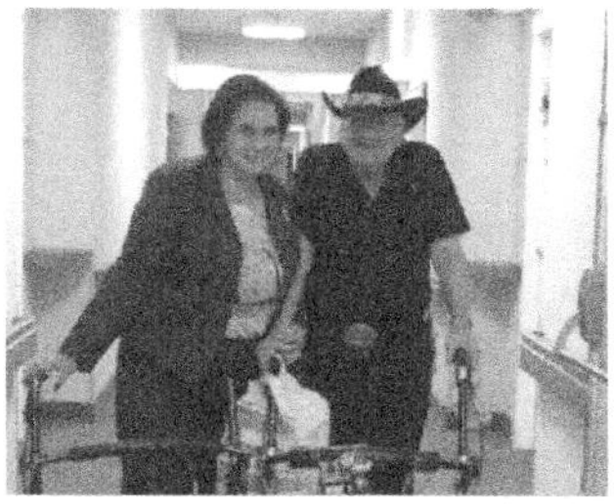

March 17, 2016
Josh and I are taking my mom to see my stepdad today. (I hadn't seen her pop out of bed that fast ever when I woke her up this morning!!) Say a little prayer to the Big Dude today for safe travels down to Tomball and back, please.

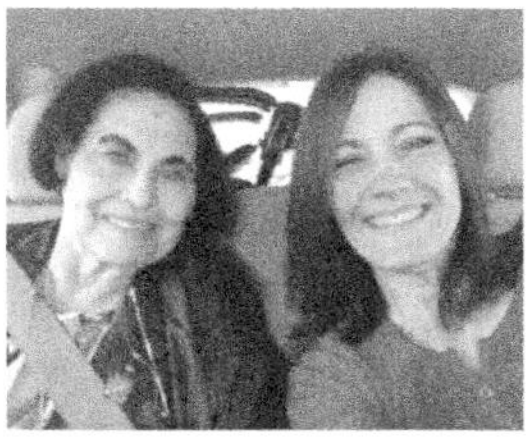

March 19, 2016
Here is Mom and I with our new "do-s"!! Mom got a lot chopped off hers. Now we are out with Bruce and Josh at the McKinney Trade Days.

April 15, 2016
Last night: Mom... I will wake you at 6:30 in the morning for your doctor's appointment.

This morning: I walked into the living room at 6:30 to head to Mom's room to wake her up. There she is, staring at me with a glower on her face, completely dressed. "You said to be ready at 6:00!"

Sigh... The day in a life with an Alzheimer's patient.

♥

As she progressed, there were never-ending doctor appointments!!! Luckily, I have a supervisor and a job that allows flexibility compared to when I was caring for my grandmother. I wasn't in danger of losing my job this time because I could make up the time that I missed in the office after hours, and I didn't have students dependent on me to teach them. It was still stressful, though, because I don't like to be late to work!

April 15, 2016
I have a million things to do at work today, but Mom has a doctor's appt at 8:00 am. We are sitting outside the office; it is past 8:00 am, and no one is here yet. I'm trying hard to be patient and understanding, but it's a struggle this morning!

April 20, 2016
A day in the life... April 20th edition. We are watching a TV show. It's a brand-new episode. She swears up and down that the network already aired this show and the game show episode we just watched. I asked her who won the challenge. "I don't remember." But she completely believes she saw these episodes today.

♥

Taking Mom to movies was always a challenge. I also just accepted that I would never watch an entire movie ever again when we took her. I would have to take her to the bathroom several times during the movie, and because her mobility was terrible, this was a very long process. I would always miss the ending of the movies, too, because she could never wait. I treasured the weekends that my sister would come up to stay with Mom so that Bruce and I could enjoy a movie all the way through.

April 22, 2016
A day in the life with Mom - April 22 edition. We just took her to see a movie, and she swears she has seen it before. I asked Sheila if she had taken her when she was up here a few weeks ago, and she said no. Same song, different verse. We just have to laugh to keep from pulling our hair out!

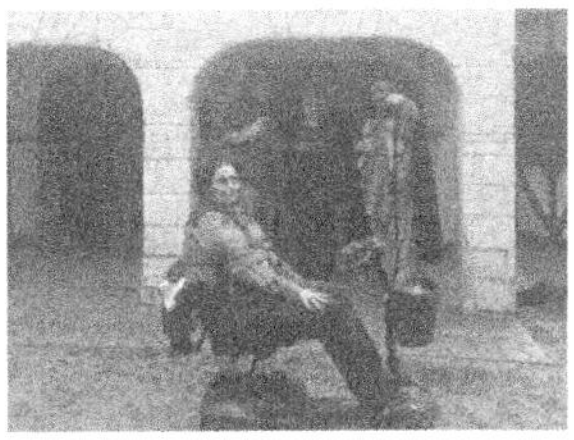

May 14, 2016
We enjoyed the day out today at Scarborough Fair. Mom's scooter got stuck in the mud a few times, but other than that, it was fun. It was great to get her out in the fresh air.

♥

Here is my first post that was officially titled "Mom Chronicles." I'm not sure why I chose that title. Maybe it was because I followed the "Chronicles of Muffin" on Facebook, or perhaps because a book series had the word "Chronicles" in it that I was reading at the time. Either way, the title stuck through the next four years.

Because words were failing her now, I had to start trying to solve the riddle or puzzle of what she was trying to say. Here is an example of how she tried to communicate with me without knowing the right words.

Mom Chronicles May 20, 2016.
I received a phone call at work this morning from Mom in a panicky voice: "Lori... The house just quit!" Translation: there was a power outage at 9:00 this morning.

Mom Chronicles May 22, 2016
Mom had one of her panic attacks this morning and couldn't breathe. She's resting and is all better now. I always feel sorry for her when she feels like she can't catch her breath. I think we have finally figured out the magic combination of what works to pull her out of these attacks. [For us, it was the panic attack medicine and over-the-counter sinus medicine to keep her from feeling like she was choking.]

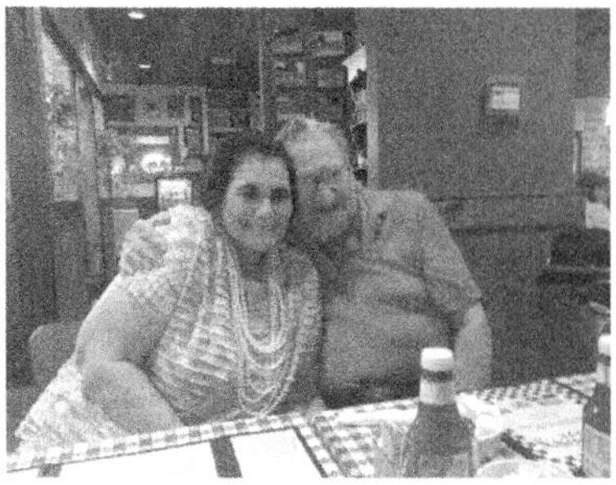

Mom Chronicles May 28, 2016
Yesterday was an adventure. We left at 8:00 am for normally a 4-hour drive to Tomball to see my stepdad. It took 6 hours to get there because of the heavy rain. We only stayed a couple of hours this time because I was getting worried about the roads. It turns out the roads we had just driven over were now flooded during that two-hour visit. Luckily, I was in the SUV instead of Bruce's car. We would have been stuck! It took an hour to figure out a way to get out of Tomball. We almost went back to Ted's assisted living center to take them up on their offer to let us stay in one of their extra rooms for the night. It took 7 hours to get home finally. Yes, in hindsight, I should have turned around and canceled the trip, as a dear friend suggested. But if you knew how much Mom and Ted were looking forward to the visit and how often Mom asks me when she will get to see Ted, I had to try. The next opportunity for a drive down there was going to be July. The smile on their faces was worth it. Knuckle biting, muscle-tensing, exhausting, but worth it.

Mom Chronicles June 2, 2016.
We are watching an episode of a cooking show, and the theme is the 1950s. I thought that it would be great to have Mom pull up some long-term memories. Nope. She couldn't get them right. She couldn't remember her first husband, who is my older brother's dad. She just seems to be going downhill faster than I thought it would happen. We will make the best out of this experience!!

Mom Chronicles June 4, 2016
My sweet neighbor was with my mom while we were helping Josh move to an apartment this morning. Mom decided to get a piece of her hearing aid stuck in her ear. And just like a child, while Lynda had her back turned just one second, Mom found a screwdriver and tried to get the piece out. Now it's down further in the ear canal, and we are up at Urgent Care, seeing if they can get it out. Lynda... Thank you so much for hanging with Mom, and I'm soooo sorry you had to deal with this while we were gone!!!

Life's an Adventure!!! Smile peeps!!!

Mom Chronicles June 6, 2016
I'm a little slow sometimes, but I finally get it eventually!! My grandmother's evil parrot Jane has come back and is haunting my mother! "Squawk... How was your day? Squawk... How was your day? How was your day? How was your day?" 😊 This isn't to make fun of Alzheimer's but to make the best out of this experience! So far, we are at four times being asked how my day was this evening. Gotta love her (but NOT Jane! She bit me when I was little, so I never liked that dang bird!)

Mom Chronicles June 11, 2016
We are going to start receiving some home health services for Mom. A nurse, physical therapist, and cognition therapist are going to start coming out weekly. Today, the nurse came out for the initial visit, and she asked Mom what her full name was. Mom couldn't remember anything past her first name for a few minutes, and then it came to her, but she "slurred" the names. She couldn't pronounce them clearly. Last week, she couldn't remember my dad's name when she looked at photo albums and saw his pictures. It's so surreal watching this unfold each week.

Mom Chronicles July 1, 2016.
After getting home after work today, Mom has asked me no less than 5 or 6 times if I had a good time on my trip since I haven't seen her since Tuesday night. Some of these came rapid-fire, one after another, within a couple of minutes of each other. Is it wrong of me to answer her differently each time??? I need to make this fun somehow!!

"Did you have a good time?" It was okay.
"Did you have a good time?" Yes, it was good.
"Did you have a good time?" No, it was awful.
"Did you have a good time?" It was great.
"Did you have a good time?" The training was boring, but the hotel room by the airport runway was cool.

I'm trying to figure out my next answer when I get asked how my trip was again in a few minutes. I really, really do love my Mom, and I'm NOT making fun of her; I PROMISE!!

Mom Chronicles July 3, 2016
We are taking Mom to see Ted today. At least the weather is way better this time, and we won't have to deal with flooded streets. They are always so happy to see each other.

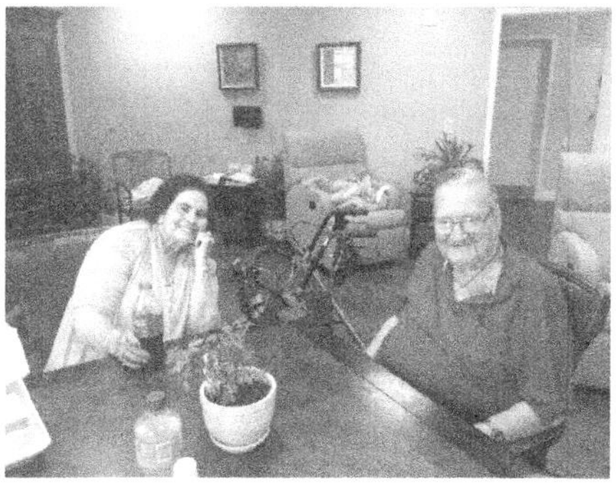

Mom Chronicles July 13, 2016
Mom went to her room, and I could hear her rummaging through things for about 10 minutes. Finally, she came back out to the living room, almost in tears. I asked what was wrong and she said she couldn't find her phone. Keep in mind that her phone is her lifeline to my stepdad. Whenever this happens, I call it from my phone so that we can find it. It ended up being in her bra, which is commonly where she puts it. She was soooo relieved. It was hard to see her almost in tears, but I'm glad we were able to avert the crisis tonight. Every day is a new day!

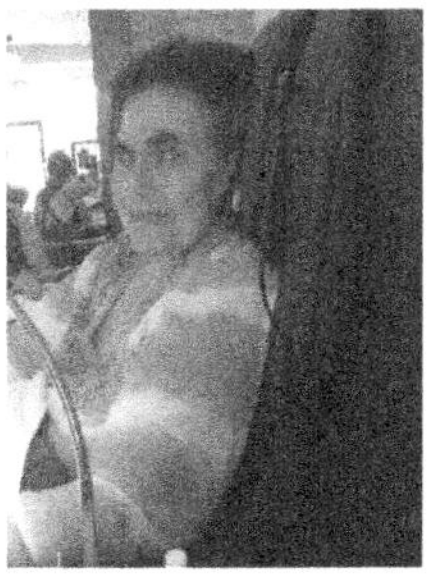

Mom Chronicles July 29, 2016
Mom and I are getting our pampering on today. Mom decided on fire engine red nails today!!

Mom Chronicles August 12, 2016
We've got a nice little thunderstorm going and the satellite is out, so that means no TV. Trying to have a conversation with Mom is an experience in itself. She was upset that her phone wasn't working (all I had to do was turn it on). What does she say? "Well, I'll be damned." Satellite... Please come back on soon!

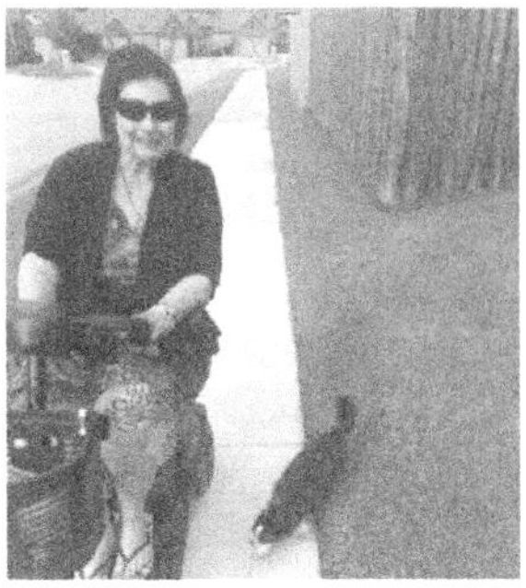

Mom Chronicles August 14, 2016
Simi and I are getting Mom out of the house for a little walk around the block.

♥

We had an artist's easel set up in the living room by a window so that she could "paint" the black velvet poster art that we had bought her. She has tubs and tubs of colored markers to paint her artwork. As she "painted," she would throw out a question about her art that we just couldn't answer for her.

Mom Chronicles August 17, 2016
Mom is "painting" her black velvet poster. She just asked me: "Is orange purple?"

♥

Huh? What the heck does that mean???? Remember the riddles I mentioned a few pages ago? I couldn't solve that one at all.

Mom Chronicles August 21, 2016
We had a fabulous birthday party for Mom at a restaurant last night. She had her sweet, beautiful friend Janet by her side, and we had the rest of the clan!!

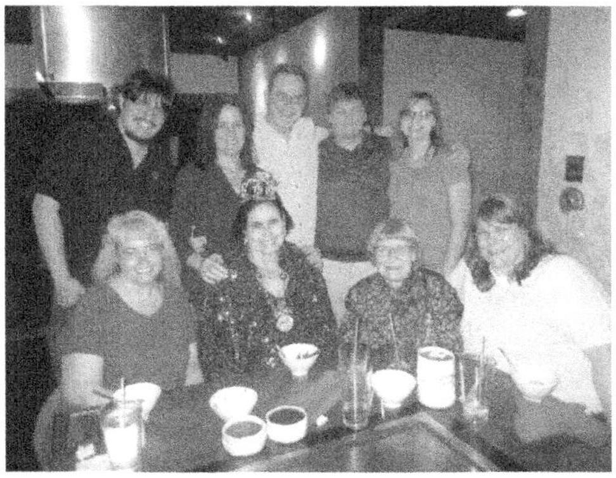

Mom Chronicles August 25, 2016
She is slowly reverting to her childhood. She just finished dinner, and I look over to see her licking her plate. She's had a very rough day, so I'm glad to see her finding something to help her feel better today!!

Mom Chronicles September 3, 2016
We took Mom to Tomball today to let the two lovebirds see each other. It's so cute to watch them both using their walkers down the hallway.

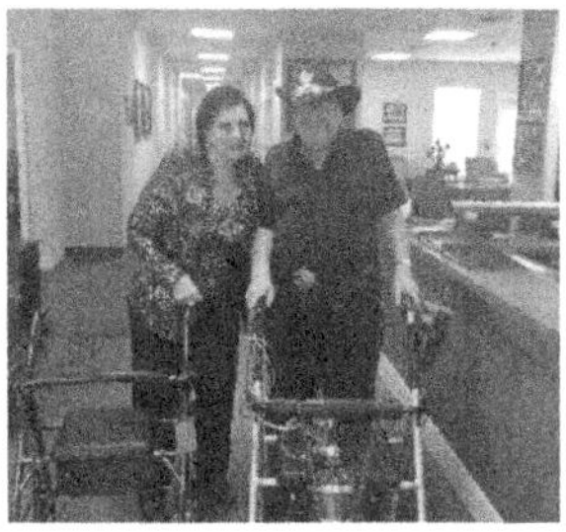

♥

Final Thoughts of Stages 1-4

The early stages of Alzheimer's are challenging. Still, if you are lucky enough to be near this person for most of these four stages, you will have an opportunity to have conversations about the disease and determine ways to help your loved one while she can still communicate with you. I highly recommend that you look at the Alzheimer's Association (Alz.org) website that lists many things you can do as caregivers or care partners. Currently, you can find the website at https://www.alz.org/help-support/caregiving. They have curated resources and suggestions for learning your new role as a care partner, helping the person with dementia live well, finding a new balance, taking care of yourself, maximizing independence, getting empowered, and understanding the emotions for both the loved one with Alzheimer's and the caregiver.

By the time we moved Mom in with us, we were past the stage of her understanding that she had a memory issue. She didn't believe anything was wrong with her - she was in complete denial. With my grandmother, we were with her early enough in her Alzheimer's journey, and she knew she was having trouble with her memory. Bruce remembers a very vivid conversation with her when she asked him if she was losing her mind. But with Mom, she had no idea this was happening to her. We had to find a new balance in our relationship and how best to care for her and keep her safe. Our familial roles were reversing. I was no longer the daughter - I became the parent.

CHAPTER 2: STAGE 5 ♥ THE MIDDLE STAGE

There never really is a clear-cut "day" of when someone moves into the next stage of Alzheimer's. They just seem to blend through several stages - at least, this was the case in our experience. At this point in our journey, I believe we had moved into Stage 5.

According to a system developed by Dr. Barry Reisberg, Stage 5 is where patients are starting to show signs of needing help with many day-to-day activities. They can no longer live alone. Patients may experience some of these signs:

- Behavioral problems like anger and suspiciousness
- Difficulty with math problems like counting backward from 20 by 2s
- Difficulty dressing appropriately; may wear the same outfit day after day until someone reminds them to change
- Difficulty recalling simple details such as a phone number or the address of where they live; they may can recall it sometimes but not always
- Significant confusion and disorientation - not knowing day/date/season or city/state/country
- Wandering risk
- Increased sleepiness

(VISN 21 MIRECC, n.d.)

We believed we were starting to move into the next phase where dementia patients forget simple processes like using utensils or cutting up food. Following is the first post we had about Mom not knowing how to eat a specific type of meal she has eaten all her life.

Mom Chronicles September 9, 2016
I made pancakes for dinner. Mom asked me for directions on how to eat them. The only good thing about this is that she LOVES them!!

Mom Chronicles September 30, 2016
The ladies at the nail salon know Mom very well and tipping well goes a long way. They just gave her TWO necklaces as a belated birthday gift. It's so cute- they call her "Mom" whenever they see her. She is HAPPY!!

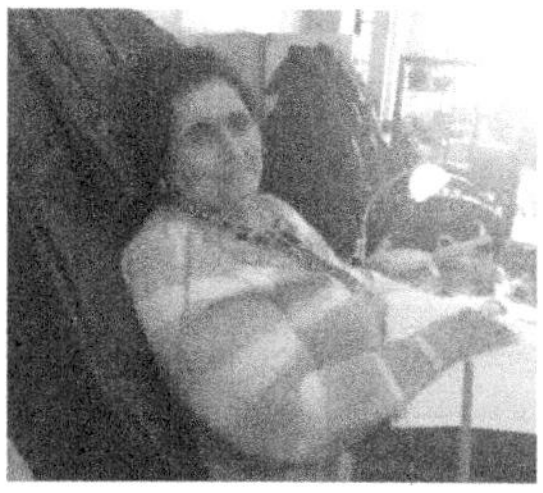

Mom Chronicles October 22, 2016
Mom Chronicles 6:00 AM (let me repeat that... 6:00 AM) on a Saturday morning.

She came to our bedroom and asked me if I'm okay. I said yes, I'm just sleeping in since it's a Saturday morning. I asked her if she's okay. She said yes, but she hasn't eaten anything. I asked if she wants breakfast, and she said no, she would just go back to bed.

Bless her heart; she hasn't felt well all week and spent a lot of time in bed this week. I think she just woke up confused and was thinking it was 6:00 at night.

Mom Chronicles November 2, 2016
We were watching a game show this evening, and the prize puzzle was about Maui. Mom piped up and said that she had been there a long time ago. She's never been there, but she could tell me it was very beautiful. I think she's getting confused with a honeymoon she had in Rio once, but we just went with it.

I asked if she saw hula dancers... she said yes.
I asked if she received a lei flower... she said yes.
I asked if she saw a volcano... she said yes.
I asked if she saw surfers... she said yes.

I'm going to say that this is probably one of the best things that can come from Alzheimer's. She has been on fantastic trips and has lovely memories… *in her mind!!*

Now, Uncle Quinton or Sheila, do you ever remember her going to Hawaii??? I know she's been to Egypt and Rio de Janeiro, but that's it.

Mom Chronicles November 12, 2016
I just attended an Alzheimer's seminar at church. Most of the information we already knew, but I did learn a couple of new things. For example, dark floors or dark spots in wood floors can affect Alzheimer's patients. They think they are holes that they need to walk around. And if they talk about a vacation they went on (like Mom was talking about last week), just go with it. That is their reality. Also, the counselor suggested printing up a few cards [business card size] that explain she has Alzheimer's so that if she is acting strangely out in public, you can discreetly show the card to the waiter or clerk that explains what is going on. *[You can purchase business card templates at any office supply store.]*

Mom Chronicles - November 14, 2016
She had a rough day but came out of her bedroom once I got home from work. After dinner, she went to her room and brought out a dress that I had given her after losing all that weight. She said it's too long for her.

I said that I had given it to her last year and it's long because I'm taller than her. Then, not even 60 seconds later, she said, "I can't remember where I got this dress. Oh, now I remember. I bought it for a party several years ago."

I opened my mouth to say, "no, I gave it to you," but remembered the seminar I went to on Saturday. So I just said, oh, okay." This is her reality, and we just have to go with it!!

Never a dull moment!! Gotta love it!!

Mom Chronicles November 15, 2016 [This story is one of my favorite memories of our journey!!]
Her daytime caregiver left a book about Michelle Obama on our coffee table. Mom just told me that she was wracking her brain to remember where she knew her from. Then she said she finally remembered that she went to school with her in Ennis when she was little and they played together all the time. Mom said she was very sweet. She said she remembers her mom and dad coming over to pick her up from the house. She also recalled that they had a large backyard with weeds they picked *(she meant crops)*. She said she's not sure Michelle would remember her now. She went on and on about how they played together.

I just went along with this and asked her to tell me more.

Keep in mind - Mom is 75. Michelle is 52 - just two years older than me.

Also, keep in mind that before Mom's Alzheimer's kicked in, she was a Republican and was not happy during the Obama presidency.

As I've said before, there is something different every day in this journey!!!

♥

If there is a silver lining about this disease, I believe it can help someone forget negative thoughts and feelings about people, places, things, or events. For example, she didn't remember that she had negative thoughts and feelings about the Obamas. There will be a story later about how she was able to forget a negative relationship with my brother as well.

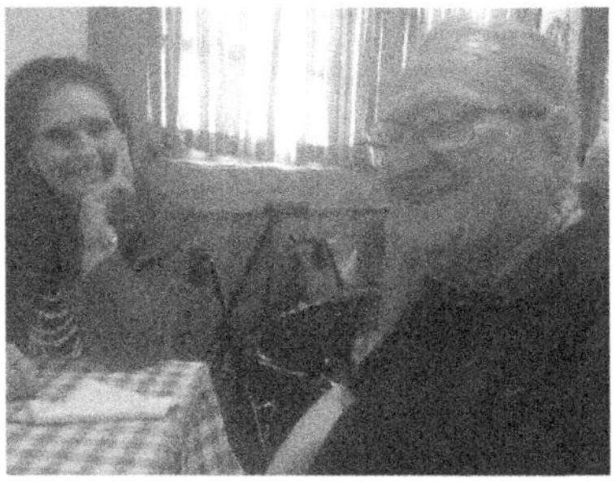

Mom Chronicles November 22, 2016
We are in Tomball today visiting Ted. First, I took them out to eat at a local café, and then when we got back to the assisted living center, we went to the common room where they were playing music and dancing. Here is a short clip of Mom and Ted dancing.

Mom Chronicles November 25, 2016
Mom found an old membership card for a flight club she and Ted were members of in California. They enjoyed flying and watching the Ultralights (basically flying go-karts). Anyways, the card's picture has a real plane (kind of looks like an old bomber plane) on the front of the card. She came out of her room so excited that she found the card and used to fly planes like that. As we have learned, we just went with it and asked her all about it. The joy on her face was worth it because she has had a rough few weeks.

Mom Chronicles November 26, 2016
I'm in the ER with Mom. She has had a rough week with an infection, and it wasn't getting any better with antibiotics. They are administering a strong IV antibiotic and doing a cat scan to see how big the infection is. Her treatment will be determined after that.

In the meantime, Sheila is cooking our Thanksgiving meal for the first time, and Josh is giving her a hand. Bruce is headed back to the house to start throwing Christmas up everywhere. We must get our inflatable dinosaurs up asap. There are neighborhood kids we need to please!!! This is just another fun day of multitasking while caregiving!!

Mom Chronicles November 27, 2016

Mom is doing MUCH better tonight!! The infection is finally getting zapped with the stronger antibiotic. So I think she will finally get a good night's sleep, which selfishly means that I will get a good night's sleep.

Mom Chronicles November 29, 2016

I'm at work, and I just got a call from Mom. She was panicking and asking where I was. She thought I was taking her to see Ted today. She had gotten up (which is great because she stayed in bed all day yesterday) and dressed up in her Sunday finest to see him. She was upset that she was confused about all of this. It's times like this I truly wished I worked from home. Unfortunately, her caregiver doesn't get there until 11:00 am.

Mom Chronicles December 2, 2016

I have many wonderful neighbors, but Lynda Hart is one of the best and is always my first one to call on when I need someone to help. For example, I just got a call from Mom saying she was having trouble breathing. Lynda hopped right over and is staying with her until I get home. We love you, Lynda!!

Mom Chronicles December 6, 2016

Hi everyone, I just learned this morning that Mom's caregiver is retiring this Friday. The caregiving agency is looking for someone to replace her, but I thought I would throw this out there in case you know someone good with the elderly AND Alzheimer's patients who may be looking for a part-time job. Right now, the hours are 11-3 Mon-Fri. The hours will probably increase as Mom gets worse. She must have lots of patience and be willing to interact with Mom to keep her mind stimulated as much as possible. If you know anyone who may be interested, please have them contact me.

Mom Chronicles December 6, 2016

This woman cooked spaghetti for us during our entire childhood and even during visits as adults. Tonight, I made spaghetti. What does she do? She scrapes the spaghetti sauce off and says she doesn't like the "purple sauce." (For those of you thinking that I did something to the sauce to make it purple, no. It's regular ole spaghetti sauce in a jar, which I have used for years and years and years!) She will probably love it next week, but tonight it was a no-go! Life's an adventure! And so is cooking around this household!! *[Side note – We could not get her to eat spaghetti sauce ever again!]*

Mom Chronicles December 12, 2016

Day 1 with the new caregiver seemed to go well. I stayed home to let her in and show her the ropes. A little young, but she seemed very nice. Mom wasn't feeling very well, so the nanny cam didn't show much interaction between the two. I will peep in from time to time this week to see how it goes. I'm not sure if she is the permanent replacement or not. The agency may send someone else after the holidays. We will see.

Mom Chronicles December 19, 2016

Today, I checked out an "adult day care" service for Alzheimer's patients called *Friend's Place*. A friend from work told me about it. It is about 15 minutes from work. It looks very impressive and is only $20 more per full day than what I'm paying for 4 hours for a part-time caregiver to be with my mom. So, we are going to try it out in the next three days while I'm off. If it works out, I will start driving Mom in with me when I go back to work on the 2nd and drop her off for the day. They serve breakfast and lunch and have tons of activities for all levels of dementia. They don't allow wheelchairs, so I'm praying we can keep Mom mobile with her walker for as long as possible. Wish us luck!! There are a few other logistical things we must figure out, but I have a great support system. We will get the challenges figured out.

♥

At *Friend's Place*, they had physical, cognitive, and musical activities scheduled all day long. I also loved that they had two "memory rooms": one for women and one for men. They were full of clothing and objects from the mid-century era when these folks would have been young. This is a time period that they will most likely remember the most. They also had quiet rooms for folks who were being overstimulated cognitively during the day and needed a break from the activities. They truly thought of everything in the design of the building and the activities for this level of care.

Mom Chronicles December 20, 2016
This adult daycare center is going to be good for her!! I am at the center to pick Mom up, and they are playing music. She is singing, and one of the workers stood her up with her walker and danced with her!!!

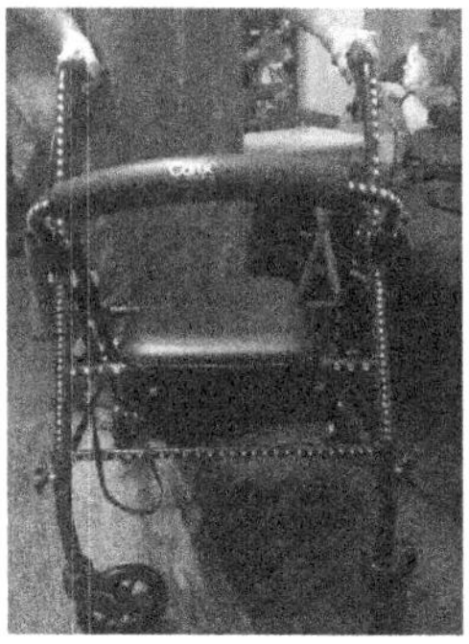

Mom Chronicles December 23, 2016
We had to buy Mom a new walker yesterday. Of course, we had to bling it up for her!!

Mom Chronicles December 27, 2016
I'm taking Mom to see Ted today. Luckily, we only have to drive halfway this time. Robin is bringing him to Fairfield to meet us. She is wearing the new purple dress that Sheila bought her for Christmas.

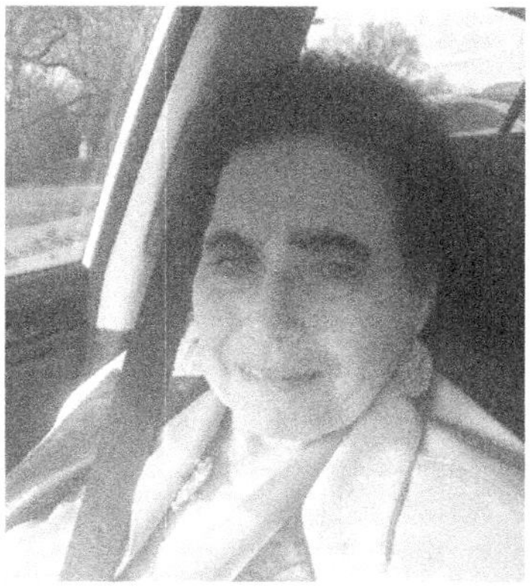

Mom Chronicles January 2, 2017
Wish us luck today! Mom starts going to *Friend's Place* for the entire day. She woke up easily at 5:30 this morning and was excited about going.

Mom Chronicles January 2, 2017
Mom had a fantastic day! She couldn't remember what she did, but she knew she enjoyed the day. I'm guessing the folks that own the place knew what they were doing when they created a daily sheet that shows the meal and activities during the day so that we would know what our parents did that day!!

♥

At this point, we believe Mom was somewhere in the middle of stages 5 and 6. She could still dress herself, but her choices were not always the best, as you will see in this next post.

Mom Chronicles January 4, 2017
Maroon top. Purple pants. Maybe my fashion sense is off, but I don't think those two colors go together. Oh well, Mom likes the way she looks, and I'm picking my battles. This battle isn't one worth fighting.

Mom Chronicles January 4, 2017
Mom had another great day! When I picked her up, they were "exercising" with short pool noodles to music. She was just laughing away! One of the staff members said that everyone loves her because she is so friendly and talks to everyone. She is getting up easily at 5:30 in the morning to get ready to go. So far, this has been a huge success!

Mom Chronicles January 8, 2017
I just had to cut my mother's meat at dinner for the first time. We have a pot roast, and she couldn't figure out how to cut it. This is just another step in this journey. I hope you guys don't think I'm posting these "Chronicles " as a "woe is me" deal. These posts are mainly for my friends going through similar situations with their loved ones and me. I will be able to look back on my memories with my mother and see the progression of this disease.

Mom Chronicles January 9, 2017
Conversation on the way home... we were at a red light (I promise I didn't take the photos while moving!!)

Mom: "Hmmm... I see a big ball of light in the thing" (She was pointing to the passenger rearview mirror).

Me: "That's the sun."

Mom: "Oh... well, what is that?" (She was pointing to the sky in front of us.)

Me: "That's the moon."

Mom: "Oh... I was getting worried. I didn't know what that was."

I can't make this stuff up. I do hate that it was worrying her, though. I don't want Mom to be afraid of anything. I did get her to smile right after, though, so crisis averted!

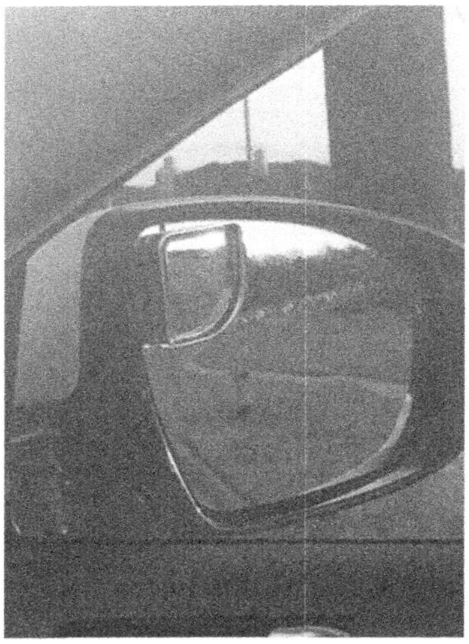
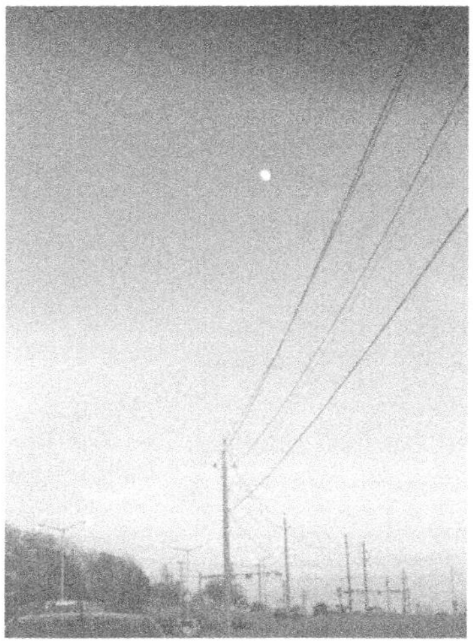
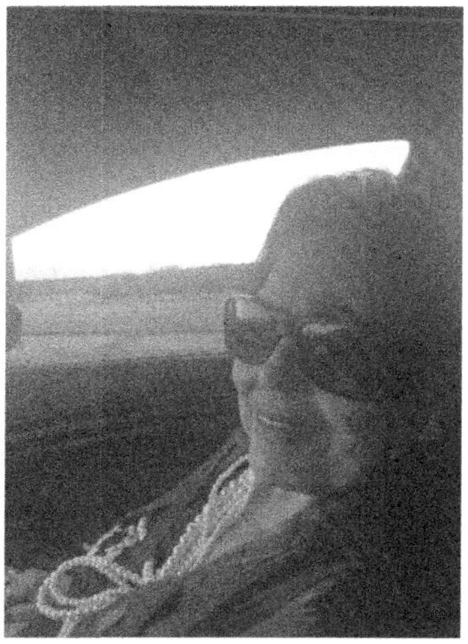

Mom Chronicles January 16, 2017

I'm with Mom getting her nails done. We found the place that her favorite nail ladies had moved to in Wylie. They gave us both big hugs when we walked in!! Mom is very happy!! Thanks, Queenie Montgomery, for letting me know about our favorite nail stylists!!

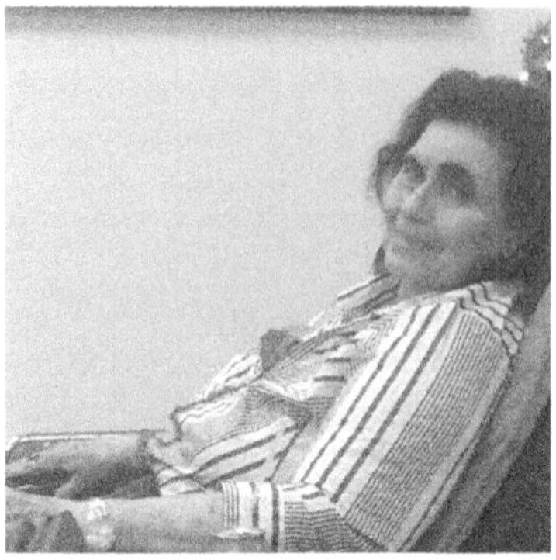

Mom Chronicles January 21, 2017 (Saturday)

To get to work on time, I have to get Mom to the adult day care center by 7:30 am when it opens. That means I wake her up at 5:30 because it takes her FOREVER to get ready and even longer to walk to the car.

She wakes up easily, but because she wakes up so early and has a full day of activities, she goes to bed early at night. (Bonus for me, I must admit!!)

Last night she was so tired that she went to bed at 7:00 pm! She is just now waking up (10:00 am). I do believe this week wore her out!!

Mom Chronicles January 21, 2017

Bless her heart. She is STILL exhausted!! I asked her if she wanted to take a nap, but she said no, she was fine.

And the picture doesn't show it, but she IS breathing!!

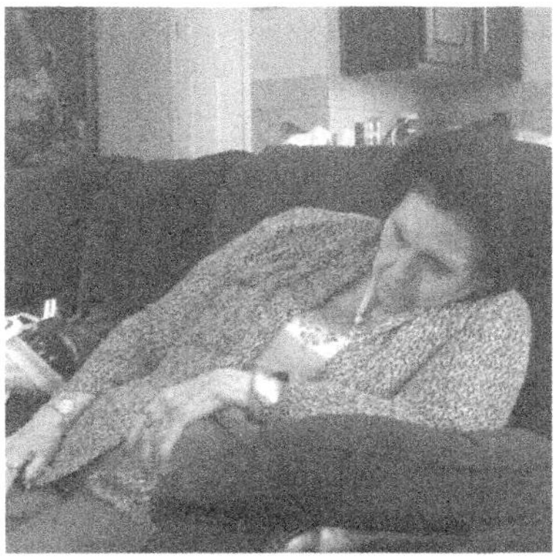

Mom Chronicles January 25, 2017

Mom is not feeling well this morning.

Mom Chronicles January 28, 2017

I heard Mom coughing and sneezing this morning in her room, so I went in there to give her some cold medicine. Simi always follows me everywhere I go. As I was walking out, she said, "The cat is still in here."

I think the majority of you know this, but Simi is a doggie.

And before I sign off on this post, would you say a little prayer for Mom to get over this cold soon, please? Catching bugs is probably one of the downsides of being in "daycare." I made sure that she got her flu and pneumonia shots a few months ago.

Mom Chronicles January 31, 2017
They were drumming today when I picked her up.

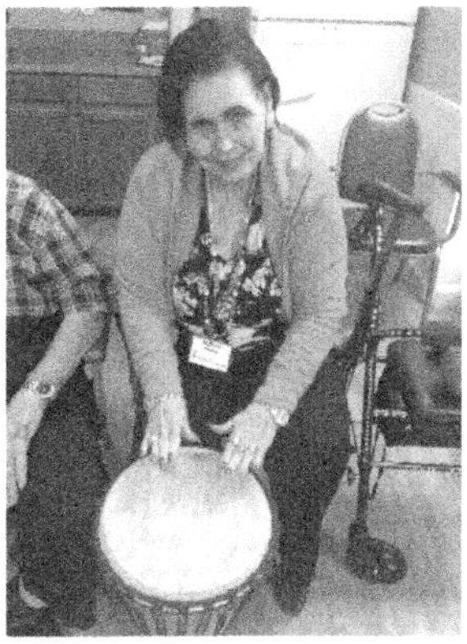

Mom Chronicles February 3, 2017
I'm here picking Mom up from the center. She's eating jello and introducing me as her "mother" to the ladies at her table. I'm not the daughter anymore.

Mom Chronicles February 6, 2017
I am glad I like solving puzzles. Today's puzzle:

Mom: "Well, there's lots of stuff, but it's not butt to butt."

My puzzle solve: the traffic is light today.

Mom Chronicles February 8, 2017
Mom and I had a short conversation about what she did today at the Adult Day Care Center on the way home. This was a fun video with her! (I was stopped at a red light, so safe driving practices were adhered to, I promise!)

Mom Chronicles February 8, 2017
I picked up fried chicken for dinner tonight. Mom looked over at me and asked, "how do I eat that?" (She was pointing at the chicken breast.) I had to explain to her to pick it up with her hands and take a bite.

Some days are good, and she knows how to eat. Some days are a mystery.

Oh, and the surprise from the video earlier is a Valentine's Day card she made for me. I saw it when I put the walker in the trunk of the car. When she gives it to me (if she remembers to!! Ha!), I'll take a picture of it.

Mom Chronicles February 8, 2017
Here is the card she made me today. She was so proud in telling me that it was blank and that she got to choose all the pieces on it. Personally, I think it is more appropriate for Ted, but she was determined to give it to me. She wuvs me.

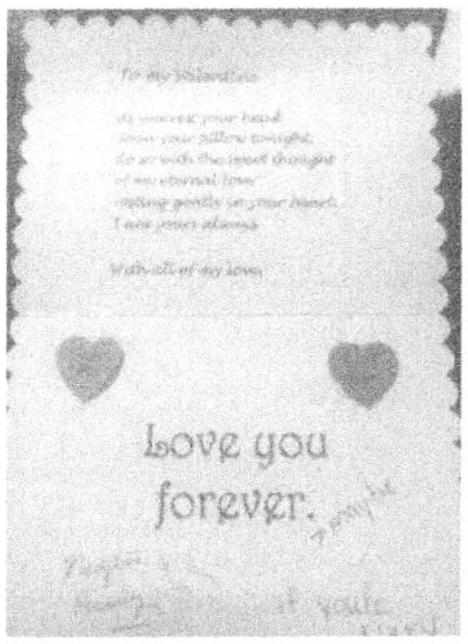

Mom Chronicles February 15, 2017
Today's post isn't so much about Mom, but about some resources shared with me by a co-worker today. Thank you, Myra Scrabeck, for your care and concern! I love getting to know my co-workers more and more through social media!

- www.onpluto.org
- The 36-Hour Day: A Family Guide to Caring for People Who Have Alzheimer Disease, Related Dementias, and Memory Loss (This book has been recommended to me by several friends in the past).

The more I share here, the more I hear of other friends going through this same journey in some form or another. These friends just aren't as vocal about it, and that's okay. I use Facebook as my "journal." It's my "therapy." Love you guys! Have a fantastic evening!

Mom Chronicles February 16, 2017
[In the post, I had shared an image of about 100 alternative curse words such as crapola, shut your piehole, and crud muffin.]
This is perfect!! Now, if I could just get my mom to quit saying "sh-t," especially in church!! ("Sh-t" is her favorite word, especially when she gets frustrated!)

Mom Chronicles February 17, 2017
Mom just talked to Ted on the phone. She learned he moved to a different assisted living center in Tomball. She said he sounds soooo happy and that he lives closer to his "mom and dad." Ummmm.... his mom and dad passed away many years ago, so I think she meant his daughter, Robin. I just love the stories that her brain kicks out now. It's quite entertaining sometimes!

Mom Chronicles February 19, 2017
A friend told me about this fantastic resource for Alzheimer's Caregivers: www.alzheimersweekly.com. Today's reading is about repetitive questions. The main takeaways I got from this one are:
1) Short answers. Simple responses.
2) Give her a hug or touch of her hand to offer reassurance because she needs to know that she's safe.
3) Not knowing the season of the year, month, or date has got to be terrifying for her to some degree, but she doesn't know how to communicate that fear.
4) Repetitive questions drive us crazy, BUT Mom CAN'T change. We, however, CAN change and adapt and not allow her behavior to drive us nuts. WE need to be the ones to adapt.

Mom Chronicles February 20, 2017
Today's puzzle:

Mom: "That's a good one."
Me: "What's good, Mom?"
Mom: She points her finger towards the front of the car and says, "zoom."

Translation: We didn't have a red light at the intersection, so we can just go through without stopping.

Mom Chronicles February 22, 2017
I'm at home today. The Momster is not feeling well, and the hubster is fighting a migraine. I am thankful for the little things, like the fact that they both are ill on the same day. I hate not going to work (sounds crazy, I know), but I'm only missing one day (hopefully) instead of two.

♥

This next post will serve as a reminder that simple words for everyday objects can fail a loved one at this stage of dementia. For example, Mom couldn't figure out the word for "seeds," so she called them "nails."

Mom Chronicles February 22, 2017
I'm home with Mom (and Bruce) today since neither is feeling well. I just gave Mom a piece of watermelon for a snack. She asked me how to eat it. She was concerned about the "nails" (seeds) inside of it.

Lesson learned: I need to remove all the "nails" before feeding her watermelon again. (I also need to cut it up into bite-size pieces.)

Mom Chronicles February 24, 2017
We keep a lot of past episodes of our favorite shows on DVR. Well, the problem with that is some of the recordings could have past weather alerts. We are watching one now, and Mom is convinced that we are going to have bad weather. There is NOTHING I can say to convince her otherwise. So now she's mad at me because I won't believe her.

♥

Later in our journey, I learned how important it is to let them know you believe them. Mom couldn't understand the concept of a TV recording from a different day, so I should have turned it off and watched it later when she wasn't watching. It would have eased her fears of the thought that we were about to have bad weather. As I mentioned at the beginning of the book, I made many mistakes in my caregiving journey!

Mom Chronicles February 28, 2017
They celebrated Mardi Gras at the Alzheimer's daycare center today. They crowned Mom "Queen."

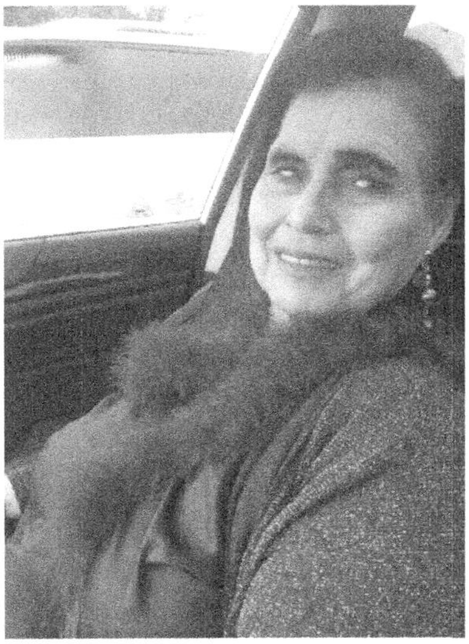

When we were leaving, they wanted to take back the crown and beads for next year, but she pouted big time. When they tried to take away the purple boa, she wouldn't let them. I whispered to the worker that I would sneak it back to them, but he said not to worry about it. They have all given up on "arguing" with any of them.

I'm going to see if I can find some on sale tomorrow to help replenish their decorations for next year.

She was a happy camper, errr "Queen" today!!

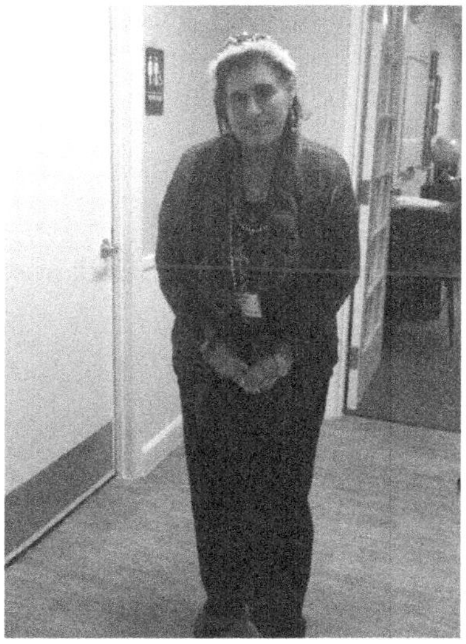

Mom Chronicles March 1, 2017
Today is Ash Wednesday. We usually go to church to reflect on the meaning of this, but this year, we didn't go, nor will we be going to the Lenten services. The main reason is that people who have dementia or Alzheimer's need a solid routine. So whenever we do something out of the norm, like go to church in the middle of the week AND at night, it throws her completely off mentally. For example, I helped her get

another shower in tonight. Up to this point, I have only been able to get her to shower once a week on Saturday nights. I know - YUCK!

I had the doctor write me a prescription to show her that she needs to take at least two showers a week to control infections.

She went willingly at first, but as the shower progressed, she got more agitated. And then, when I was styling her hair, she thought tomorrow was a church day because Saturday night usually is our shower night to get ready for church the next day. So now her "routine" is off. I'm hoping that we get this routine down soon.

I have a feeling she will wake up in the morning and think it's Sunday instead of Thursday.

Mom Chronicles March 2, 2017
Well, the Momster is not feeling well today. I need to start packing my work computer and bringing it home with me every night since this is a day-by-day deal with her.

Mom Chronicles March 2, 2017
Mom has a bug. I'm glad I didn't force her to go to daycare.

Mom Chronicles March 4, 2017
Mom is feeling better today, thank goodness. We are off to wash that gray out! It's kind of funny-she sees her gray line and doesn't know where it came from! Oh, to have that naivety again.

Mom Chronicles March 5, 2017
At church today, one of the songs had a final verse from "How Great Thou Art." With the other songs, Mom can't keep up. But when she heard the words from this song, her voice was loud and clear. She could remember those verses from her childhood/early years.

So, thank you, Ricky Dillinger and the worship team, for including a verse from a timeless hymn. You perked my Mom right up!

♥

If you wondered about the title of this book, "I Remember Me," this next post is where it originated. March 10 became a special day for my mom and me. During our conversation, the phrase she uttered became a "mantra" to help us get through this journey. "I remember me."

Mom Chronicles March 10, 2017
Driving home from the nail salon, we drove by a dilapidated old home. Mom said, "that place is horrible." Trying to persuade her not to judge, I said, "do you remember us living in a place like that one summer?" She looked horrified and said no. I told her about the summer she was married to one of her ex-husbands named *[name withheld]*. We lived in a place very similar to the old home we drove by for one summer. I asked if she remembered *[name withheld]*. (This was the husband that was mean and awful to her.) She said a little bit. I asked her if she remembers that she has been married eight times. (She gave Elizabeth Taylor a run for the record!!) She looked at me shocked and then replied in softly spoken words: "I remember me."

She remembers my dad a little bit but remembers Ted the most. I'm thankful for that because Ted has been wonderful to her. So, with the conversation we had today, I will keep her phrase in my heart: **"I remember me."**

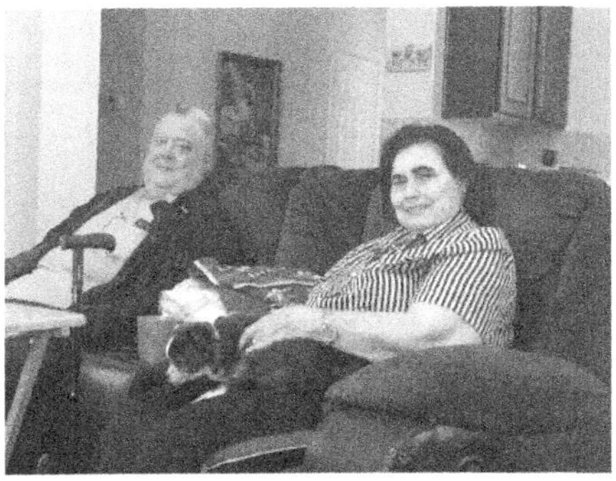

Mom Chronicles March 14, 2017
My uncle, Quinton Clark, just came in for a visit. Mom remembers him, so that's fantastic!! Love ya, Unc!

Mom Chronicles March 14, 2017
I just had to get one more pic of Mom and Uncle Quinton holding hands before he heads back to Colorado.

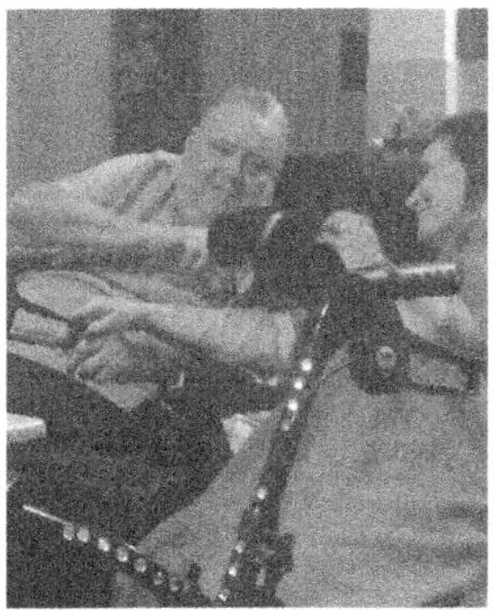

Mom Chronicles March 15, 2017
We made it to Tomball. Ted wanted to play the guitar and sing her a song as soon as we got here. They are so cute together!

Mom Chronicles March 15, 2017
Ted chose a Chinese buffet restaurant for lunch. He and Mom would eat at one in California all the time. It was their favorite place. Unfortunately, mom can't handle all the choices anymore, so I must try and pick soft foods that she doesn't need to figure out how to eat. Finger foods tend to work the best.

Mom Chronicles March 15, 2017
I always give them a few minutes alone to kiss when we visit because they are old, not dead. 😊 I like to give them a little privacy.

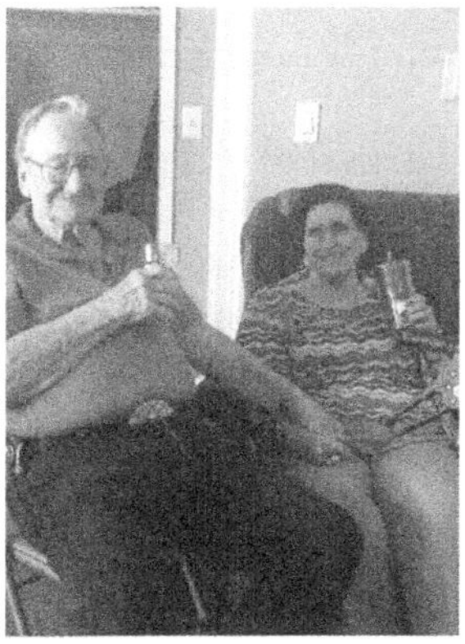

While I'm waiting for them to get their smooching over with, I will share about the drive down here today. I had my playlist going, and Charley Pride's "Kiss an Angel Good Morning" came on. She started singing and tapping her hands and feet. Loved it! Next song: "Bodies" by Disturbed. If I hadn't been driving, I would have taken a picture of the shock on her face. I busted out laughing. But you know what? She was tapping her fingernails on the car door to the beat of the song. Enrique Iglesias got her dancing again after "Bodies" was over. Time to go split up the lovebirds. We are about to work our way back to Dallas. Ciao!!

Mom Chronicles March 18, 2017
We took Mom to the Arboretum today with our friends Cathy and Janet. We all enjoyed the fresh air and beautiful flowers.

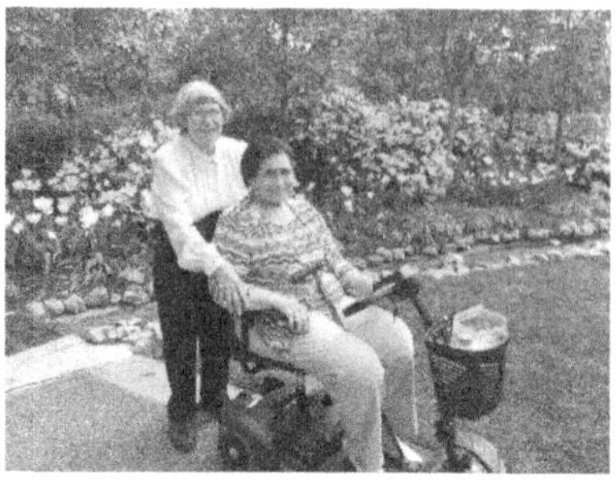

Mom Chronicles March 20, 2017
Mom has been away from the daycare for over a week because of being ill and my spring break. She went back today for the first time and had a great time. The bad thing is I got a letter in the mail on Saturday saying they are raising the daily rate. I understand why they need to do this, but this stretches my budget too much. I will need to go back to hiring someone to come in and stay with her at home for a few hours a day and then maybe just have her go to the center a few days a month for the social aspect. Soooo... if anyone has a friend that has a lot of patience and is great with Alzheimer's patients and is looking for a part-time job in the Wylie area, have them contact me. I will be reaching back out to the caregiving agency again, but I thought I would put the word out here too.

Mom Chronicles March 21, 2017
Mom had another rough night, so I'm home with her again today. Bruce and I think we have a solution to our daycare situation. I'm hoping to have an answer today.

Mom Chronicles March 22, 2017
To Lynda - Thank you so much for taking care of my mom today. You are one of the best neighbors and friends ever!!

Mom Chronicles March 23, 2017
Today's puzzle solve:

Mom: "Wow!"
Me: "What?"
Mom: "Zoom-Zoom"

Today's interpretation of "zoom-zoom": we were able to get three green lights in a row on Campbell Rd this morning. No stopping at red lights. Make it a great day, peeps!! And may you get plenty of zoom zooms on your commute!

Mom Chronicles March 26, 2017
Because Mom is having more and more difficult nights due to the disease, we have decided to change her care options during the day. Bruce is moving his work schedule to nights (with a special thank you to his boss for allowing this) so that he can be home during the day with Mom. He will go into "paramedic" mode and help Mom as a patient instead of a "momster-in-law." Because she is not sleeping well at night anymore, she tends to sleep very late, so Bruce will be able to get most of his sleep while she is still asleep. Our wonderful neighbor, Lynda, is going to help this first week by helping Mom with lunch while Bruce gets used to his new work/sleep schedule. I'm going to miss having him by my side at night, but this is only four nights a week, so we will make this work. This is only temporary. Also, this week I'm heading to Galveston

for a conference, so Joshua will be staying at the house at night while Bruce is working. Thank you, Josh, for being here for us this week. We love you!

♥

We started seeing more and more infections affect Mom. As the disease progresses, someone with Alzheimer's will start moving less and less. They also don't practice good hygiene as well as before. This makes them more vulnerable to infections. According to Alz.org, it is important to:

- Keep the teeth and mouth clean (dentures - remove them and clean them every night); bacteria from the mouth can lead to pneumonia. Use a soft toothbrush or moistened gauze pad with mouthwash to clean the gums, tongue, and cheeks.
- Treat any cuts or scrapes immediately. Clean wounds with warm soapy water and apply an antibiotic ointment. If it is a deep cut, please seek professional help.
- Flu and pneumonia can be deadly. Please get the flu vaccine every year to reduce the risk. A pneumonia vaccine can be given every five years. (Check with your doctor to ask for current requirements or advice on vaccines.)
- With COVID as a health threat now, especially for the elderly, please consult with your primary care doctor for guidance on vaccines for this virus. (Late-Stage Caregiving: Infections and Pneumonia, n.d.)

Mom Chronicles April 2, 2017
I'm taking Mom to the hospital. The left side of her face is swollen. It started as a small area yesterday, so we tried warm compresses. It obviously didn't work. I will keep you all posted.

Mom Chronicles April 2, 2017
There are no updates on Mom yet. They are running blood cultures and a CT scan. They are waiting on results before they can decide on treatment. She is having a hard time because her face hurts from the swelling, and she can't get comfortable on the hospital bed. They are pretty busy today, too, so things are taking a little while to get done.

Mom Chronicles April 2, 2017
As noted earlier, we are at the hospital. The doctor admitted Mom so they can treat her for an infection. They haven't told us what it is yet or what the CT scan showed. Soooo... she's on IV antibiotics and is staying overnight. She's in good spirits but confused as expected. Every so often, she tells me her face is swollen, so I repeat why we are in the hospital and that we are getting medicine to treat it.

I ran home a short while ago to grab some things, and then Lynda followed me back up here to take Bruce home. That way, he can drive back and forth, and I will have a car up here too. (Thank you, Miss Lynda, for always being a rock star!)

Mom Chronicles April 2, 2017
The nurse was testing Mom on her memory. She asked where she was now, and she said "church." The nurse asked her what my name was, and she got that correct, but when asked what her other kids' names were, she couldn't remember. I know it's easier for her to remember my name since I'm with her the most, but it just makes me want to cry, and I know it's going to upset Sheila. I know Sheila hates not being up here to be with her more. I also know it's worse right now because we are not at home in her normal environment.

Mom Chronicles April 3, 2017
4:45 am. Somehow, the nurse accidentally pushed a button, and we heard an entire conversation with another employee. I pushed the call button to let her know, but it took her a while to answer me. Once she did, she

didn't understand what I was trying to tell her. She thought we needed something, so she said she would be right there. Did she come right away? Nope... she just kept talking. I had to walk down to the nurse's station to let her know that I could hear her entire conversation. The light bulb finally went off, and she understood. It was just a conversation about their new charting system at the hospital. If it had been juicy gossip, I might have wanted to listen a little while longer for the entertainment value.

Mom Chronicles April 3, 2017
We are still in the hospital, and I imagine we will be for at least another day or two. The swelling has not gone down, and her white blood cell has gone up. They are treating her with a couple of antibiotics. Their latest guess on this is cellulitis, but they are not sure. She's in a lot of pain this afternoon and very confused. She's always been great with stating her birthdate, but she's had trouble telling the nurse the last couple of times. Lunch was just delivered, so I'm hoping it will take her mind off the pain. Plus, the nurse just gave her another pain pill to try and help. The nurse also marked the borders of the swelling, so now we can monitor the swelling. The doctor assigned to her never came by today.

Mom Chronicles April 3, 2017, 2:45 pm
The infectious disease doctor said she would be in the hospital for at least 2-3 more days for IV antibiotics. She said it takes about two days to check the blood for infection, so that's another reason why she needs to stay here. Then she will be on a pill form of antibiotics for two weeks. The doctor is testing Mom for a couple of other issues, but that's the latest.

Mom Chronicles April 4, 2017, wee hours
I'm sure this is because she's way out of her routine and not feeling well, but now whenever the nurse asks her for her name and birthday, she can only remember her first name. She can't remember her last name nor her birthdate. She looks over at me with confusion on her face wanting me to help her.

Mom Chronicles April 4, 2017
Her swelling is coming down, but her confusion is still high. She's had a couple of meltdowns when she was hurting (understandable) and just wanted me to take her home. She's good right now. The nurse gave her some pain meds that have finally kicked in.

We will probably be here one or two more days, and then she will be going to a rehabilitation center for at least 20 days. They will continue the antibiotics and give her some physical therapy. I know she isn't going to understand, but since it's close to home, I will stop by there every evening after work to check on her.

Sheila is coming up tomorrow night to step in for me. I have a couple of important meetings at work Thursday and Friday that I really can't miss unless it is an absolute emergency.

Mom Chronicles April 4, 2017, 7:30 pm
She's feeling better tonight and is acting a little spunky with me. She fell asleep twice mid-bite with her dinner. The 2nd time was with a spoon of pudding. It fell on the napkin. When I went to take it away from her to throw it away, she cut me with those eyes!!! (This look is also known as the "Go to H-E-Double-Hockey-Sticks" stare that Sheila inherited!!). That blob of pudding was still good enough to lick up, and I dare not take it away from her!

The swelling is going down, but with the outline drawn on her face, the rock band KISS has been on my mind since the nurse drew it.

Mom Chronicles April 5, 2017
Mom was able to get a better night's sleep, thank goodness (which selfishly means I did too)!

Mom Chronicles April 5, 2017
Mom will be in the hospital for at least one more night. It looks like she will be released tomorrow to the rehab center. The doctor said the infection was probably caused by her scratching her face (which is a constant, nervous tick that she experiences, and I have read that this is common for Alzheimer's patients) and from not washing her hands well. She has long nails, which keep bacteria under her nails.

So, I may need to be the mean daughter and have the fake nails removed even though she loves them. Maybe I can still get them painted to make her a little happy. I will probably have to do the "prescription trick" that I've learned and have a doctor "prescribe" no long fingernails so that I can show her that over and over.

On another note, the housekeeper is in here changing the linens. Mom told her she was a nurse too. Ummmm... nope. Mom was a real estate agent.

Mom Chronicles April 5, 2017
Thank you, PK (Pastor Ken), for coming by the hospital to visit Mom and praying with her. It meant the world to her (and me). Bruce and I will call you and Pam during our 3-week break from the momster while she is at the rehab center so that we can visit and catch up.

Mom Chronicles April 6, 2017
My sis, Sheila, has been with Mom since 11:00 last night. They had a rough night. I won't go into details, but they didn't sleep well.

The Infectious Disease doctor said Mom has a skin staph infection. She's off IV meds and on tablet meds that need to be taken four times a day. Any dosage can't be missed, so I'm glad she will be in rehab. The wheelchair van will be here to pick her up at 3:00 pm.

Mom Chronicles April 6, 2017, 9:00 pm update
We are at the rehab center. So far, Mom is adjusting well. She doesn't seem to be stressed and upset. She is still very confused, but that's to be expected. The administrator told us we are approved for 100 days of care with her supplemental insurance, so if all goes well here, we may take advantage of that if the level of care is going well. This place seems to be very nice. The nurses we have met so far have been great.

Sheila and I will be back over here in the morning when they do all of their assessments. Mom won't be able to answer their questions, and Sheila may not know everything since she's only up here a few days a month. Soooo... let's all say a little prayer that this place works for her for the next 100 days and that we are led on the right path of care for her.

Mom Chronicles April 7, 2017
I struggle with how much to share to retain Mom's dignity, but I also know that many others are going through this or will be going through this at some point with their loved ones. In the later stages of Alzheimer's, a very common problem is incontinence. Over the past few months, this has become more and more of an issue with my mom. She has had several accidents during the day and especially at night. I found a great website from the Bladder and Bowel Foundation that explains why and has suggestions for helping prevent accidents.

https://www.bladderandbowelfoundation.org/bladder/bladder-conditions-and-symptoms/alzheimers-and-incontinence/

I got here to the rehab center this morning, and it was apparent she had about 5-6 accidents last night. She does wear incontinence garments, but that doesn't always help.

She's resting at the moment, and we are waiting for the physical therapy folks to assess her. They just took her room partner for therapy, so I'm hoping they will be evaluating her next.

I brought Simi up here to visit this morning, and Mom loved that. Bruce dropped by after his night shift to say hi and to take Simi home. I'm thankful the center allows pet visits!

So, right now, Mom is still confused and exhausted. We are praying the nursing staff gets her into a routine that will reduce the accidents.

Mom Chronicles April 7, 2017, 2:00 pm
You know how a car never shows the problem it's experiencing when you take it to the car repair shop? Well, Mom decided to show a decent day when showing her mobility to the physical therapist (PT) during her PT assessment. Generally, at home, she can barely move. The PT said we might not be able to get the full 100 days. We may only get 30.

We will take what we can get. On a good note, she got up and dressed in one of her sparkly outfits and put on makeup.

Mom Chronicles April 8, 2017
We are visiting Mom. She's still confused, and she's hurting. I asked them to give her a pain pill.

We have permission to put in a webcam on her side of the room, so Bruce is working on this. I will be able to monitor her and make sure she hasn't fallen and that she is getting the care she needs.

Mom Chronicles April 8, 2017
It's the little things we take for granted. Bruce and I are getting out of the house for a little bit to grab a shake and ice cream sundae. It's so nice just to leave the house and do something "fun" for a few minutes.

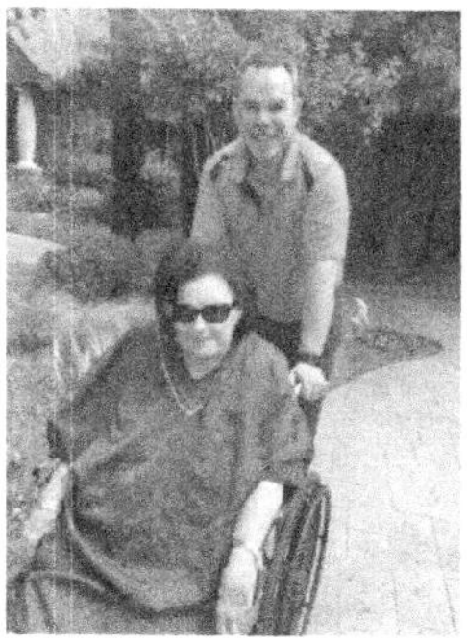

Mom Chronicles April 9, 2017
Mom is staying in bed constantly, so we are getting her outside to enjoy the fresh air. Hopefully, this will give her a good boost to get out of bed more.

Mom Chronicles April 10, 2017
Mom played the piano when she was a teenager. I sat her down in front of the piano in the lobby. She was nervous to touch it at first, but she finally started tapping the keys. It's not a song, but she enjoyed it. She wants her old music books, so I told her I would find a book at a bookstore. She may not be able to read it anymore, but who knows.

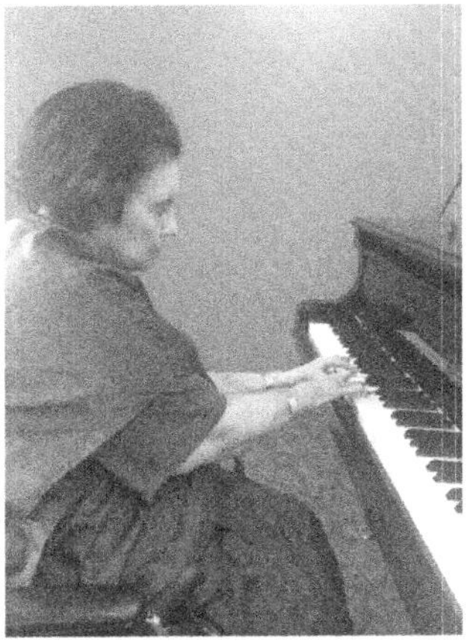

Mom Chronicles April 13, 2017
I need to take the bad with the good. She had a great day yesterday but not today. I popped in on the webcam throughout the day, and she never got out of bed. The nurses checked on her all the time, though, so she was taken care of all day.

I'm here visiting her now, and she just doesn't feel good. So I brought her a strawberry shake to try and raise her spirits some.

And on another note, I contacted Larry Graves for assistance in getting a plot set up for her near my dad and Bruce's parents at a cemetery in Coldspring. Larry is amazing as usual! He is one of the best funeral directors around! I don't like thinking about the end of Mom's life, but I would rather start planning now to make all the hard decisions before I'm too emotional to deal with them.

Mom Chronicles April 13, 2017
I wanted to go to the Maundy Thursday service tonight, but she's depressed and crying a little. I couldn't leave her in this shape. She wants to come home. Maybe she will be better tomorrow so that I can go to the Good Friday service. I'm going to get her out of her room for a little bit to try and cheer her up. It's nice outside, so maybe the garden will work. Wish me luck!

Mom Chronicles April 14, 2017
Bruce and I had a nice breakfast at the cafe in downtown Wylie this morning.

Once Simi is finished with her grooming appointment, we will pick her up and take her to see Mom. The webcam shows she's having another rough day.

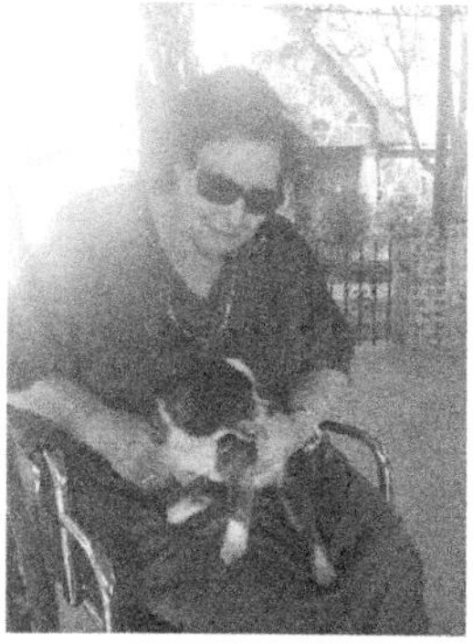

Mom Chronicles April 14, 2017
Simi works her magic!

Mom Chronicles April 18, 2017
The infection is way better, but she is staying depressed at the rehab center. She's not getting out of bed to go eat in the dining hall or participate in any activities. So when I arrive after work each day, I get her up and take her outside to get some fresh air (except yesterday because of the rain) and to call Ted so that she can talk to him for a few minutes. She tells me she misses me and wants to come home.

There is a care plan meeting on Thursday that Bruce is going to attend for me. We should know a little more about when they will release her.

I hate seeing her depressed, so as much as I like having the time alone at home for a while, I will be glad to have her home so that she can perk up.

Mom Chronicles April 19, 2017
I talked to the cemetery caretaker in Coldspring and reserved a gravesite next to my dad for my mom. I don't like even thinking about this outcome, but unless the Good Lord comes again before she passes, it's a fact of life. I'm glad she will be next to my dad. Even though they were only married about ten years, they loved each other dearly. Unfortunately, his alcoholism was just too much of a problem for her to stay with him.

Poor Mr. [name withheld]-he thought Mom had already passed or was about to pass away in the next few days, so he already had it staked out for the funeral home to dig. I had to tell him she is still very much alive and well, and this purchase was just a planning step for the future.

Mom Chronicles April 19, 2017
I brought her a strawberry shake to cheer her up a little. She started eating it with a spoon, and she dropped some on her blouse (yay for the fact that she got up and got dressed today!!) I told her it might be easier to drink it with the straw. She looked around on her tray and picked up the straw, and asked, "this"? I said, yep!

Then she came across a chunk of strawberry and said, "there is meat in here." I explained it was just a piece of strawberry. She said "oh" and tasted it then when "mmmmmm." Strawberry shake for the win!

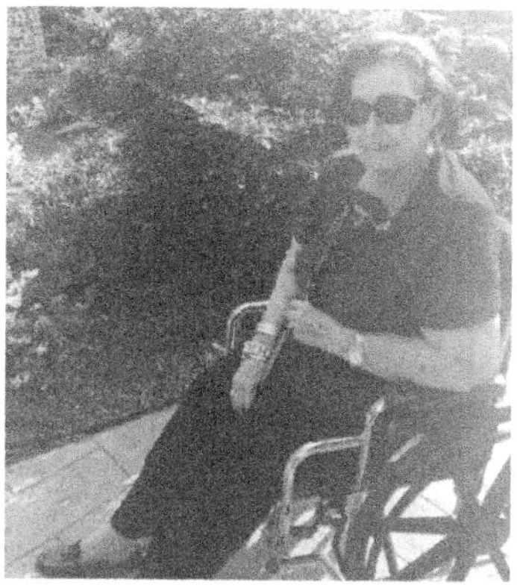

Mom Chronicles April 21, 2017
I'm helping her fly from the coop for a few hours and hoping this will cheer her up a little. Red sparkly nail polish should do the trick. These little ladies just love Mom! This is the 2nd time they have bought her jewelry and given it to her when we show up. To heck with red sparkly nail polish; the jewelry wins hands down!!

Mom Chronicles April 23, 2017
We went to visit Mom today. We left a letter for the administration to make sure they follow through with getting her out of bed and down to the activities that they promised us in the meeting last Thursday. So far, they haven't. She's staying in bed all day, and that's not good for her.

Bruce will go by there for me and have a little chat face to face with them. The nurses and aides are all extremely nice, but I want them to take just a few minutes to help encourage her to get up and out of her room every day for things other than therapy.

I checked her skin, and luckily there is no breakdown. She just needed some lotion because it was so dry.

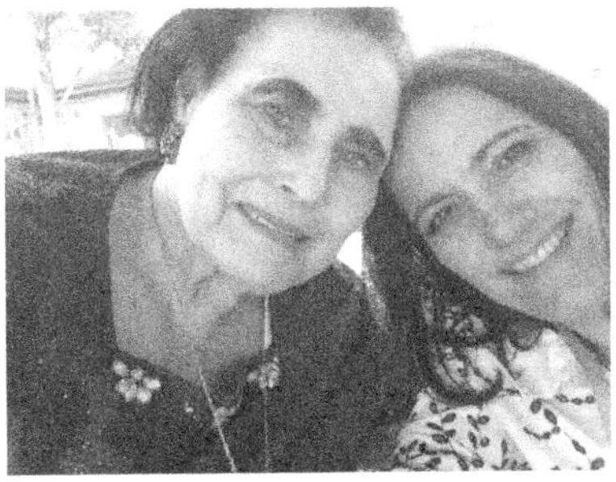

Mom Chronicles April 25, 2017
They helped encourage Mom to get up, and she was out of her room most of the day. She's soooo much happier today!!

Mom Chronicles April 26, 2017
We are at the piano again today since it's cold outside.

There is a hymnal beside the piano, but she couldn't read the notes, so I told her just to put her hands on the keys and see what happens. This is what happened. I think it was pretty good! I almost turned the camera around so that you could see the smile on my face, but I didn't want to take it away from her!!

Mom Chronicles April 27, 2017
Back in March, I posted about a conversation that Mom and I had on the way home from the daycare center. I was asking her if she remembered some various events in her life, but she couldn't. She could only respond with "I Remember Me." That phrase really hit home for me. So much so that when a friend posted that we could use that phrase in a business, I couldn't sleep that night thinking about it. I believe that was God whispering through her.

Bruce, Sheila, and I started brainstorming. We are getting the details worked about, but today, the 2nd phase of our project came through. Our LLC has officially been filed with the state! Our first phase was the logo. Connie Swiderski created this logo for us, and we absolutely love it! We also have a website URL purchased: **www.irememberme.life**. It's not up yet. I hope to have it up within a week.

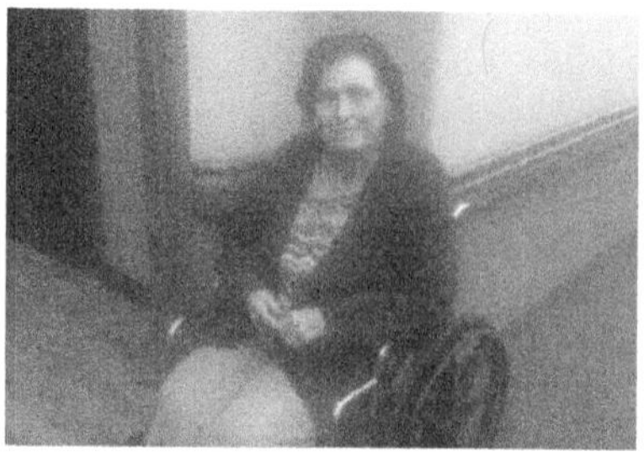

Mom Chronicles April 28, 2017
Mom was HUNGRY today!! I walked in and found her sitting by her door, watching for the food tray. I knew it would be about 30 minutes before the aide brought it, but Mom refused to go very far. I couldn't get her to go outside or to the lobby to play the piano. She wanted to stay near her room so that she could see when the food was delivered. The aide said she's been watching for it all afternoon! I'm glad she is getting her appetite back!!

Mom Chronicles April 30, 2017
We have Mom at the piano for the 3rd attempt today. Each time we place her at the piano, she has relayed a story about how she had stage fright during a recital in high school. So, I decided to record the story this time. I don't want to forget these stories. Plus, I want Sheila and Joshua to hear these too.

Mom Chronicles May 2, 2017
Yesterday was a rough one for me, so I wanted to wait to post until today when I had my emotions in check.

I had a conversation earlier in the day (yesterday) with the social worker and the physical therapist about my concern that she no longer walks with her walker but stays in the wheelchair 24/7. She is getting weaker and weaker, and I'm concerned about how that will play out when she comes home. They told me that Mom has been refusing to do physical therapy many days and that they can't force her to do it. I think they can try a little harder, but that's my opinion. I asked them to try harder because I need her to walk as much as possible when she is back home. I suggested writing the prescription down for physical therapy from the doctor and showing her. I don't know if they will try it, and I don't know if Mom will be a stubborn mule and dig her heels in.

When I arrived at the rehab center after work, I asked Mom to walk with me down to the door (about the same distance from the front to the back of our home). She didn't want to, but I tried to encourage her anyways. She fussed and kept making excuses. I got her down to the door and then had her sit to rest. After letting her rest for a few minutes, I asked her to walk back so that she could eat her dinner. The tray was just delivered. She was furious at me and did not want to walk back. She tried to just scoot herself back on her walker. I got a little firm with her and said I needed her to walk to get her strength back. She didn't understand the concept of building up her strength. She was extremely mad and yelled (YELLED) at me this time. Needless to say, I let this get to me, and I shouldn't have at all.

She walked back to her room, but she was still furious at me. So I went ahead and decided to leave because I knew I didn't have my emotions under control yet.

At first, I wasn't going to go back to visit her today, but I changed my mind and will go back after work. She probably won't have remembered that she yelled at me. I know this is just the beginning and that she will probably scream many more times at me. I just need to grow some thick skin. Poor Bruce - he didn't know how to deal with me when I got home blubbering like a big ole' baby. Sorry, sweetie!! I promise I will start handling this better!!

It looks like she will be coming home around May 12, so Josh and Sheila will help us switch Mom's room around this weekend. We will put her in the room right off the living room, which is more easily accessible with a wheelchair. I don't see her walking much anymore, unfortunately. So, today sounds like a pity party, and I don't mean for it too. It's just another one of the roller-coaster days that I will experience in this wonderful life as a caregiver. I promise I am totally fine - I just had to get past this first round of her yelling at me. Now... if I could just spank her and make her mind, we would all get along so much better! Just kidding, guys - no spank vs. non-spank war of words here!!! Just a joke about switching roles of daughter/mother to mother/daughter.

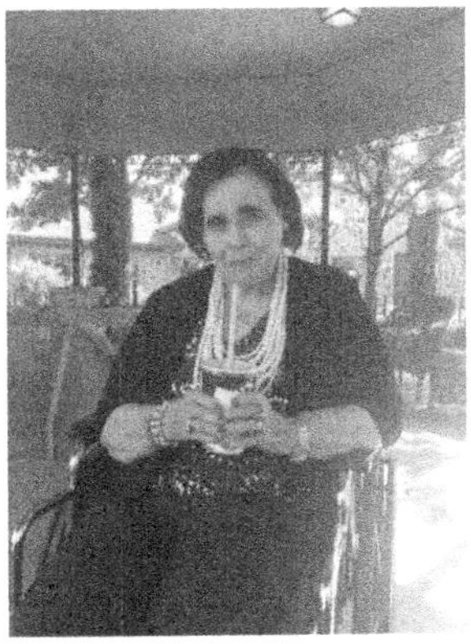

Mom Chronicles May 2, 2017

All is well with her today. Sometimes I wish I could have a clean slate with no remembrances of being mad... then again, maybe not. And yes, I'm bribing her with another strawberry shake. It works…

Mom Chronicles May 5, 2017

I received a call from the rehab center this morning. The physical therapy folks wanted to release her TODAY because Mom keeps refusing therapy. I balked at that. No warning is inexcusable. The social worker got the discharge date moved to Sunday. We still need to get her room swapped out so that she can access it easier with a wheelchair.

The social worker said she hopes this doesn't affect the chance of bringing Mom back there when it's time for long-term care. I wasn't ugly because I know she was just the messenger, but I told her we would NOT take her back to that center. She is weaker now than before we took her there, and the staff does not know how to work with Alzheimer's patients.

Soooo... Mom is coming home on Sunday. It will be interesting to see how she adapts and how far she has declined in her health. I've been told that each hospital stay makes it worse on a dementia patient. I'm going to keep positive thoughts, though!! They are giving us some home health services for a while. One person will be able to bathe her, so that is one responsibility off my plate. Hopefully.

Mom Chronicles May 7, 2017

We are at the center working on checking her out. We are just waiting on the nurse and the final paperwork.

Ted had been in the hospital this past week in serious condition (he is better now, and I just learned he is being released from the hospital today), so Mom hasn't been able to talk to him in a while. I've told her he's been in the hospital. Bless her heart; she just asked me if I saw him "when he was dead." She thought he had passed away. I had to reassure her that he is alive and well. Hopefully, they will be able to talk today on the phone.

Mom Chronicles May 7, 2017

Mom is home and happy. We got her home this afternoon. She wanted to keep riding on her walker, but we encouraged her to WALK with the walker instead. She's been doing it all afternoon and not fussing. The portable wheelchair will arrive in the middle of the week, but we will keep it hidden until she needs it. I need her to walk for as long as possible. Wish us luck!!

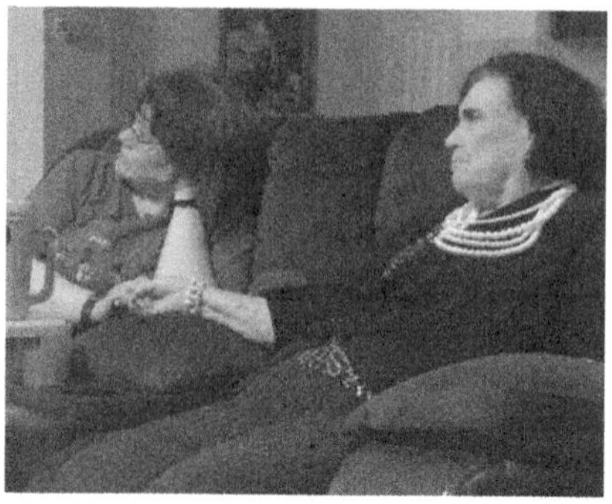

Mom Chronicles May 8, 2017

This is the first full day for Mom back home. I checked in on her through the webcam from work, and I noticed she seemed a little confused in the kitchen. Bruce had already made her a sandwich with her name on it and placed it in the refrigerator by her juice. I got in touch with Bruce (he was sleeping for his night shift tonight), so he went in there to help her. She had started trying to make another sandwich and had poured her juice into a bowl instead of a cup. Yep - she's a little more confused than before she went to the hospital.

I placed a puzzle on the kitchen table before leaving for work, so she is working on that now. Hopefully, that will keep her busy for a while.

I'm hoping I can get home health to come out for a couple of hours in the middle of the day to give her assistance when Bruce needs to sleep the most.

Mom Chronicles May 11, 2017

This is just a quick update. Things have been steady for a couple of days. She is settling back into her routine, working on a puzzle on the kitchen table, etc. So far, so good.

I read a blog from the Alzheimer's Reading room and today's message had some great tips. Mom is not a wanderer (yet), but they suggested hanging a picture of a bookshelf over your door so that your loved one won't realize it's a door and try to leave. How freaking fantastic is that idea??

I also need to work on stopping talking to her like she's a child. I need to quit that. There's soooo much to learn! (10 commandments of Alzheimer's Caregiving, n.d.) *[At the time of writing this book, the link to the blog I was reading is no longer active.]*

♥

I learned that it's against the fire code in some states to put a picture of a bookcase over a door in a long-term care facility if there is an emergency. You will see in a future post that one memory care center does this, but the other one did not because of the fire code. Another tip I learned later about preventing wandering is to remove any items associated with going outside. For example, if a jacket, purse, or car keys near a door is something your loved one will want to pick up to take outside, move it to a place out of their eyesight.

Mom Chronicles May 12, 2017

The nurse aide came today for the first time to shower her. Bruce said Mom didn't get fussy and went willingly. Yay!! I don't pretend to believe this will be the case all the time, but we are happy with at least one successful bath time. Bruce was a sweetheart and took Mom to Wylie for lunch and ice cream - kind of a reward for going willingly with the aide to get her shower. This afternoon she worked on her jigsaw puzzle on the table and her "paintings." The "paintings" are those black velvet posters that use markers for coloring in between the felt lines. It's good to see her pick this hobby up again. (She used to paint for real when she was younger. I have a fantastic painting that she did of me holding Josh on my chest as a baby. I will treasure that painting forever.)

Tonight, I had to teach her how to close the mini blinds. She couldn't remember how. I will probably have to teach her every night, but that's okay. So... today was a good day!!

Mom Chronicles May 14, 2017
I know that this may be the last Mother's Day that Mom "knows" me, so this Mother's Day is special. She may surprise me, though, so we shall see. She doesn't understand special days. Birthdays, Christmas, etc., don't mean anything to her anymore, but she used to go all out on special days.

Mom Chronicles May 14, 2017
We are watching a movie that references the horrific events of 9-11. I asked Mom if she remembered 9-11. She didn't. She was truly shocked to hear how many died that day. It's crazy how this disease wipes away so much. But I guess it's good that life is innocent and sweet and that she doesn't remember anything bad.

Mom Chronicles May 16, 2017
Spaghetti has now become a finger food for Mom.

1) she no longer likes red sauce or purple sauce (spaghetti sauce).
2) she doesn't like cheese, but I make alfredo sauce since she won't eat red sauce. I call it "white sauce."
3) she doesn't like any sauce directly on her food anymore, BUT she doesn't know to mix or dip food in it.
4) She ate the sauce with a spoon but couldn't figure out how to eat the spaghetti. We tried to teach her to wrap her fork around it, but she didn't do that so well. Instead, she used her fingers mostly to eat the spaghetti. Too bad she no longer likes red sauce. I would love to get a picture of spaghetti sauce all over her face like a toddler!!

Mom Chronicles May 19, 2017
Mom is a little ticked at me.

We are at the nail salon, and I explained that we need to keep her fingernails short. She didn't like that one bit. I guess I need to get that prescription pad option back out for this challenge too. We will see the doctor next Friday so she will write that script for me!! The ladies here understand, so they are doing as I requested instead of what she wants. They are trying to make her feel better about it.

I will just smile through this because I realize that this is temporary. At some point, she won't even know she wants her nails done anymore. I kind of want to be a little devil and say we are doing this "because I said so!" (You know... since I'm the "mom" now!!)

Mom Chronicles May 19, 2017
Today's puzzle solve:
Let me set the context first: we drove home from downtown Wylie on Sachse road after getting her nails done.
Mom: "I see it, but it must not be well."
Puzzle answer: she noticed the road construction that was happening on Sachse Road on the way home.

Mom Chronicles May 20, 2017, 4:30 am

Well, we have hit the next progression in this disease. Mom woke up about an hour ago (3:30 am) and got completely dressed with her full makeup. She is wide awake. She thought it was morning and time to get up. We believe it was either the storm or having an accident that woke her up, but she doesn't remember. Bedding is changed, and we put her poster painting art in her room to work on since she's not sleepy. I double-checked our alarm and door locks, and now I'm going back to bed.

Mom Chronicles May 21, 2017

A few of our "I Remember Me" shirts and caps came in yesterday. Exciting!! **www.irememberme.life**

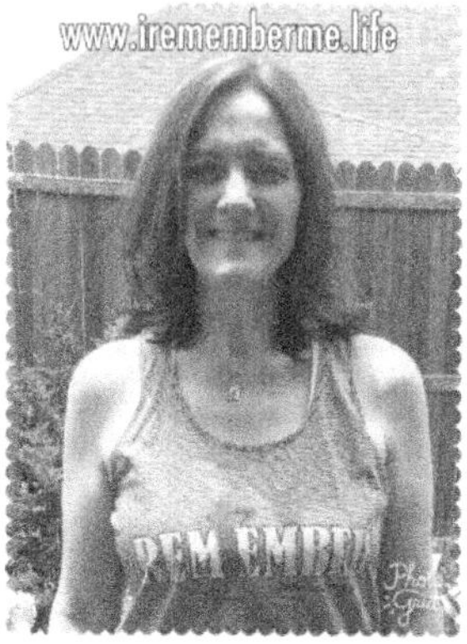

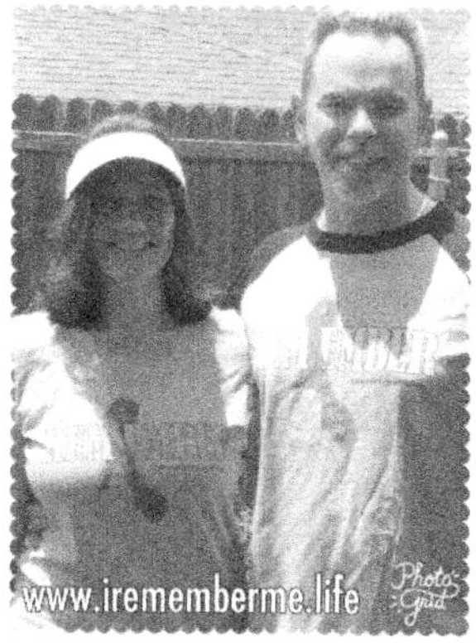

Mom Chronicles May 24, 2017

So, as you may or may not know, Bruce works nights so that he can be at home during the day while I work. I keep the nanny cam going so that if I see anything that indicates Mom needs help, all I will have to do is call Bruce and wake him up.

Today, she was having trouble with the remote on the TV. I could tell she was getting an error message. I didn't see that my neighbor was home through the outdoor webcam, so I called Bruce to wake him up to help her. Otherwise, she was about to get very aggravated. Yes - the TV is a babysitter for us. He went in there and realized she was using the wrong remote control, so he got the TV up and going in 2 seconds.

Immediately after he went back to lay down, I noticed that she started removing her gown. Completely. No clothes on. I texted Bruce to NOT go back out in the living room unless he wanted a sight that he couldn't unsee. I needed to figure out what she was trying to do first before I had him go back in there to help.

She decided she just wanted to change her clothes right there in the living room instead of her room. Luckily, Bruce didn't have to go back in there and tell her to put her clothes back on. In my mind, I just kept hearing the song "The Streak." "Ethel... get your clothes on!!!" Another day, another story to tell.

Mom Chronicles May 26, 2017

We had Mom's follow-up appointment with her primary care physician today. She said it's time to start thinking about an Advanced Directive (not that anything is imminent, it's just that we are moving to the final stage). This stage could last years, so again it's not close.

She said that the things that could happen are aspirations of her saliva or food and drink because swallowing will become harder. She also told us that infections might become more prevalent, which we experienced a couple of months ago. She could become septic. Infections will probably happen more often. Soooo... my sister and I have briefly talked about DNR (Do Not Resuscitate) in the past, but it's always been too hard for her to discuss. She is much closer to Mom than I am. It's time to make some painful decisions. And this is something EVERYONE needs to talk about with their families. Advanced Directives don't mean they won't treat something like an infection. It just means if a condition is terminal, and your quality of life would never improve, the EMTs and doctors have permission not to take extra measures to prolong life. Of course, this is a very personal decision, unique to each person, and best made when one is still capable of sharing their wishes.

Mom Chronicles May 28, 2017

Well... several things happened at church today. First, Bruce is suffering from a migraine and had to stay home from church. He is usually there to help me with Mom whenever I need it. Things usually go well, but not today.

Second, when the Friendship Register was passed down the aisle, Mom tried to sign her name. She was able to get the first three letters of her first name and then couldn't remember what was next. Finally, in frustration, she asked me to finish it.

Third, during the songs at the beginning of the service, she started having severe pain in her hip and knee. It was getting worse through the prayers before the sermon. I was scheduled to be an offering counter, so I had to get someone to step in for me to handle the counting. Then I had to get her up from the chair, which was difficult due to her pain level this time. Several friends from church were there to help me get her up and get her out to the car.

Lessons learned: whenever I can get her to church, I will need to take the Friendship Register from her to prevent her from getting frustrated, AND I will start taking her portable wheelchair. I wanted to keep her walking for as long as possible, but I think the wheelchair is the best option on church days.

Thanks to my church friends who were there to help me with Mom today. Love you guys!

Mom Chronicles May 29, 2017

When one needs a wheelchair-accessible seat at the movies, one must get to the theater early to nab them!! I'm hoping the movie is good! You can't go wrong with Johnny Depp!!

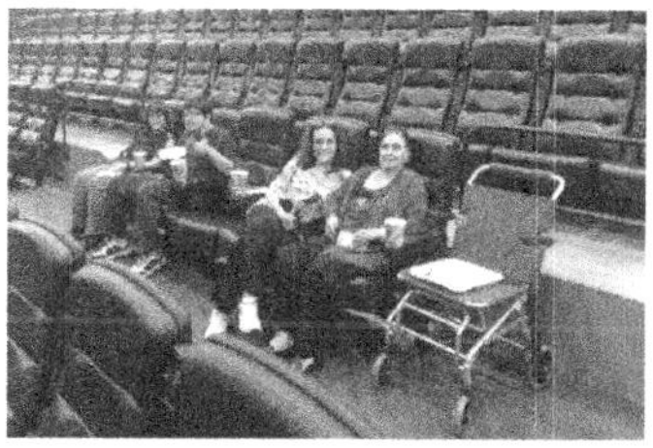

Mom Chronicles May 30, 2017

Sometimes it's the simplest of words that escape her. We had a housefly flying around during dinner. She was swiping at it and calling it a "bird."

Mom Chronicles June 3, 2017

Mom is a make-up fanatic. So much so that sometimes she puts so much color on her eyelids that we secretly nickname her "Mimi" when she does. (A Drew Carey Show reference.) I am NEVER going to tell her NOT to do that. Make-up and jewelry make her happy. Yes, she looks like a clown sometimes, but she is happy, and that's all that matters.

Today, I bought her a new base foundation compact. This woman has opened these compacts for years and years and years. It has a simple little snap, but she couldn't figure out how to open it today. Maybe tomorrow will be a little easier.

Mom Chronicles June 5, 2017

I showed Mom a bunch of the black felt art posters that she had forgotten she had. She's like a kid in a candy store. She thinks she's "painting" again and that she's sold many of these in the past. Hopefully, she will start coloring them again instead of being glued to the TV. There are only so many reruns of "Dancing with the Stars" I can take!!

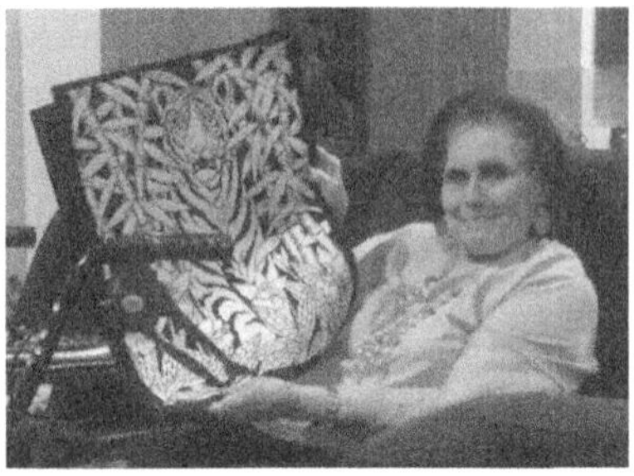

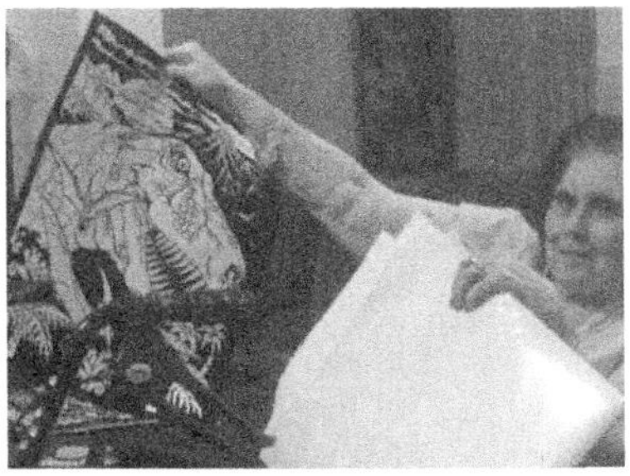

Mom Chronicles June 5, 2017

She's going through all of them saying "cute," "awww," "ohhh," and then all of a sudden, she says, "ewww... that's not cute"! So this is what she shows me... She did NOT like the dinosaur!

[For my friends who know me, they know this was my personal favorite poster since I love dinosaurs!!]

Mom Chronicles June 7, 2017

Bruce had to work the day shift Monday, Tuesday, and Wednesday this week due to several folks being out on vacation at his job. To keep me from having to take off from work, my beautiful, fantastic neighbor, Lynda, stayed with Mom during the day.

Everything went well until today. Today, Mom got snippy with her and made her cry! Miss Lynda understood why Mom did this, but it catches you by surprise when you get fussed at out of nowhere. Miss Lynda has such a sweet, kind heart. She was more upset that Mom was unhappy at the moment instead of being upset that Mom fussed at her. Of course, Mom doesn't remember this.

Mom is getting snippier lately. I sure do remember getting snippy with her when I was a teen once. She slapped my face, and I never did it again! Don't worry, folks - I won't be smacking her for talking back to me! Anyways... I'm so sorry that she raised her voice at you today, Miss Lynda! Love and hugs, and thank you soooo much for taking care of Mom the last three days!

Mom Chronicles June 9, 2017

This evening, we went to a Mexican food restaurant in Richardson to meet with my friend to plan some events for the next couple of months for our side gigs. We ordered queso and chips. I wasn't paying attention to Mom, but thankfully Bruce was. He cleared his throat and pointed with his eyes towards Mom. She had picked the spoon up out of the bowl and started to eat the queso like it was soup. I was so embarrassed because this lady is a new friend that we just met for the first time tonight, so she knew very little about Mom's condition. She handled it like a pro, though. As I was teaching Mom how to dip her chip into the queso, LeeAnne Knisley made light conversation about how it did look like a bowl of soup. I'm very thankful for people with kind hearts and compassion like she showed this evening. (LeeAnne-I enjoyed meeting you tonight and look forward to working with you!!)

On another note, I was able to finalize the DNR paperwork this afternoon with Mom's doctor just in case we need it in the future. It was not an easy piece of paper to get signed, but I believe it's for the best when the time comes.

Mom Chronicles June 11, 2017
Ricky Dillinger... Mom is humming to the "How Marvelous, How Wonderful" song you all are practicing before the service. Thank you!!

Mom Chronicles June 14, 2017
I took Mom to the back doctor today to ensure nothing is going on with her spine because of her pain level. When the doctor came in to ask Mom questions, she started going way back to when she sold real estate. He got impatient and said, "let me stop you right there because none of that matters-I need answers about your pain level right now." I had to explain that she has Alzheimer's, so he lightened up a little bit. I was about to come unglued on him. At first, I liked him because he entered the room and asked if I was her granddaughter. Yes, I LOVED that! But when he got impatient with her, that compliment and my happy feelings went right out the door. I realize they need to keep moving to the next patient, but it just irked me.

The good news is there is nothing wrong with her back or spine. We will go to the orthopedist next week. I'm hoping he can give her a cortisone injection to help alleviate some pain.

Mom Chronicles June 16, 2017
First and foremost, happy birthday to my Mom's baby brother, Uncle Quinton! If Mom could remember this, she would be calling you and telling you herself!!

Second... Fridays are half days at work. While Bruce sleeps (since he works nights for us to be home during the day), I monitor Mom through the camera and wake him up if needed. Unfortunately, I couldn't watch while driving, so when I got home, I walked in to find red juice all over the kitchen tile floor, and Mom was in the pantry pulling out a jar of alfredo sauce to put on her sandwich. Bruce usually has a sandwich ready for her in the refrigerator, but he didn't this time since he knew I would be home by lunch.

I helped her with her sandwich (since she likes mustard - not alfredo sauce) and then worked on cleaning the red juice off the floor. I can't get mad for several reasons:
1) She can't help it
2) I was the world's largest klutz and spilled lots of juice when I was little. She never got mad at me!
3) We have replacement tiles from the home builder, so when this phase of our life passes (and I don't mean for that to sound flippant), we will change out the carpet in her room and the stained tiles.
4) Pink tiles and grout are a new style, right??!!
5) I can blame my terrible housekeeping skills on Mom!!

Until our next adventure... smile, peeps!! Life is grand… and MESSY!
#pinktilemakesmesmile

Mom Chronicles June 16, 2017
The physical therapist was here with Mom for her last round of therapy. She was madder than a hornet and kept trying to quit. She doesn't like therapy!! He had her walking laps around the kitchen (across my new pink tiles), and she kept trying to veer back to the couch. I had to bribe her to do one more lap, and then I will take her to get her nails done.

And she forgot my name today when the therapist asked her what it was, but she did remember Bruce's name. This didn't sting as much as I thought it would. I'm making progress!!

Mom Chronicles June 16, 2017
I had to give a "life" lesson to my 75-year-old "child." The nail salon lady gives Mom costume jewelry pretty often, which is incredibly sweet. Mom tried to tell her she wanted the bracelet in a different color.

No, Mom... this is a gift. We should say, "Thank you"!!

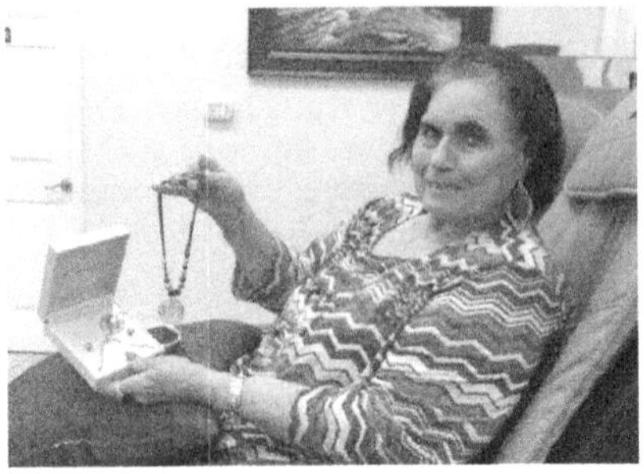

Mom Chronicles June 20, 2017
A friend of mine from work named Vickie Sullivan shared an article with me about Maria Shriver's new Alzheimer's Disease Coloring Book. The important thing I "drew" (pun intended) from this story is that I need to spend more time with her doing things that don't require conversations. She struggles for words now, so just spending quality time with her is what is important.

Coloring (or painting as Mom calls it) would be an excellent way to do this. I confess that spending quality time with her is something I need to work on. Working on simple puzzles is another way to spend time as well.

Mom Chronicles June 20, 2017
We are currently waiting at the doctor's office to see if we can get a cortisone shot in her hip. It's been hurting more lately.

We got over here a little early, so I stopped to get her an ice cream cone. When she got to the paper part of the ice cream cone, she didn't know what to do. I had to show her how to tear the paper off. I guess a little "fiber" in her diet wouldn't hurt??!! She LOVED the Cherries Jubilee flavor.

Mom Chronicles June 20, 2017
Her hip joint has gone from a slim sliver of space between the bones to NO space between the bones in the past two years. Surgery is not an option because of her age and Alzheimer's, so they will give her a cortisone shot in her hip joint. She's not going to be a happy camper. I may have to buy her another ice cream cone.

Mom Chronicles June 23, 2017
Things have been relatively calm the last few days. We have noticed that she nods off while sitting in her chair quite a bit.

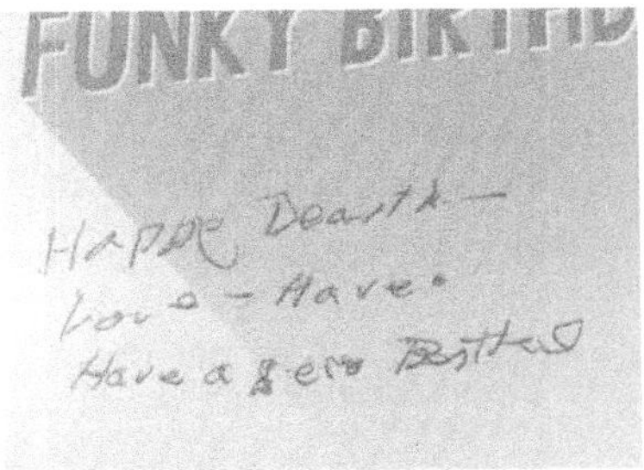

Mom Chronicles June 28, 2017
Bruce helped Mom "pick" a birthday card for me and had her sign it. I was shocked to see just how far she has declined with her writing. I'm happy she is still with us, so I will be thankful even if it comes down to signing with an "X."

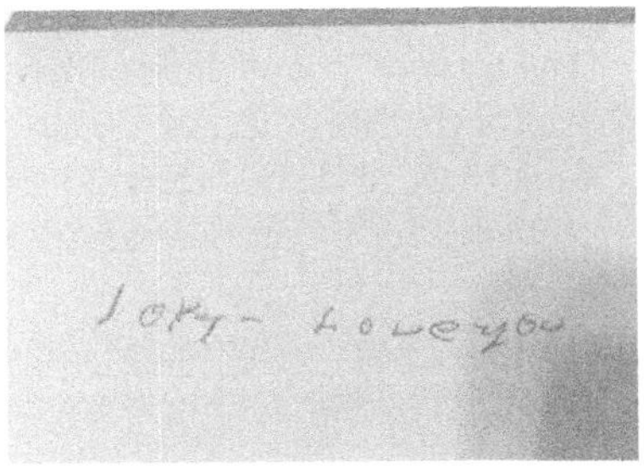

Mom Chronicles July 3, 2017
Mom found a gold glitter nail polish bottle in her room this afternoon and asked what it is used for. So Sheila and I had to explain that it is nail polish that goes on her fingernails.

Mom's "must-haves" are: jewelry, acrylic nails with sparkly polish, make-up, hairspray (lots and lots of hairspray), oh-and did I mention jewelry and pretty, sparkly nails? It was kind of weird that she forgot what nail polish is. I do have to admit that I will be glad when she forgets about some of these things!! It stretches my budget too thin!

Mom Chronicles July 4, 2017
Sheila and I drove Mom down to see Ted today. We couldn't take Ted out to eat for lunch since he fell the other day and injured his foot, so we brought lunch to him.

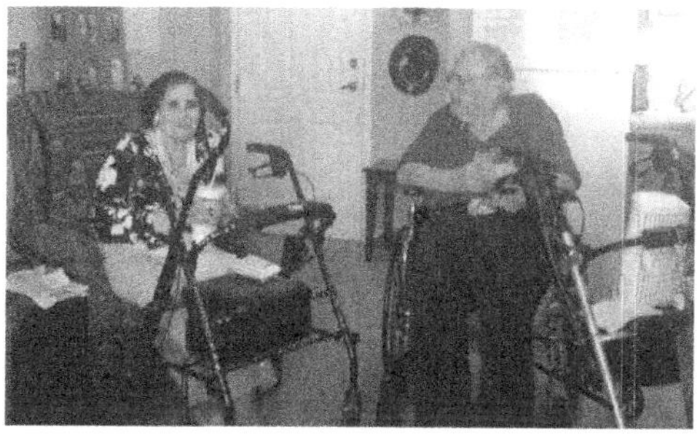

Mom Chronicles July 4, 2017
The drive down and back to Tomball was interesting. Her words are getting so limited, slurred, and even made up. "Snibbles" was one of those words. We figure it was a combination of "snack" and "nibble." She wanted to "snibble" the chocolate-covered almonds we bought at a favorite pit stop.

When we passed both Ennis and Huntsville on the way down, she got confused and thought she grew up in both places. She lived in Huntsville for a few years as an adult, so she had that in the recesses of her brain. She did grow up in Ennis, so she got that one right.

All the road construction near Corsicana had her calling it "big places." I try to figure out what she's saying, but most of the time, all I can say is yep, uh-huh, sure, how about that, or cool!

♥

The lines between the stages are not clear. At this point, I see some signs from Stage 5 and Stage 6. As mentioned in the beginning, I was constantly researching ways to understand and help Mom's disease. I found some Alzheimer's Caregivers Support Groups on Facebook. Here is a post that I added to one of these groups. This shows the extent of Mom starting to fall asleep constantly. The term "LO" stands for "Loved One."

July 11, 2017 (Post in an Alzheimer's Caregivers Support Group)
Mom (Stage 5 or 6 Alzheimer's) has started nodding off constantly. This started about a month ago. She completely falls asleep while sitting up, taking a bite to eat, etc. She will wake up for a few minutes most of the time because her head bobbed, but sometimes I have to pat her arm a few times to wake her up.

Medicines have not changed, and we haven't noticed anything different with her sleeping pattern. (We have a camera in her room so that I can check to make sure she hasn't fallen during the night.) She also has Mitral Valve Prolapse, and her feet are starting to swell a lot more. We aren't sure if this is part of the valve issue or because of Alzheimer's. I have tried doing an internet search on this but not finding a lot. Her next neurology appointment is in August. Has anyone else experienced this with your LO? *[I later learned that falling asleep throughout the day is VERY common.]*

Mom Chronicles July 14, 2017
Mom was talking to Ted a little while ago on the phone, and she asked me when I would be able to drive her back down there to see him. I told her it would be Labor Day weekend which is in September. She repeated it back to him (slurring the word "September - many words are slurred now") since apparently, he had asked her when I was going to drive her down there again.

A few minutes ago, she asked me if tomorrow was the day we are going. I asked where she wanted to go. She said "Ted" in a tone that was like, "don't you even know what we talked about a few minutes ago." I had to tell her again that we weren't going until September.

Methinks I will be having this same conversation a few more times tonight. This reminds me that I have the movie "Dejavu." I believe this is a good weekend to watch it!

Mom Chronicles July 15, 2017
Well, this morning was a "first" in our journey down Alzheimer's road. Mom slept late and came out of her room frazzled around noon because she had an incontinence accident and got her bed and floor wet. She was near tears about the mess and kept apologizing. I told her as calmly as possible that everything is okay, and I will get it cleaned right up. That in itself wasn't the "first," but I believe that her frazzled state is what led to the "first."

The "first" is this:

I had her bowl of cereal, her cup of juice, and her medicine cup with her morning vitamins/meds on her TV tray. I am still trying to have her do as much as possible on her own, so I watched her and noticed she had the meds in one hand, and in her other hand, she was trying to scoop juice out of the cup with the spoon. I went over to her and explained that the best way to take her meds is to hold the cup and take a drink. For some reason, she couldn't process that mentally this morning. I had to hold the cup and help her take a drink with each pill.

Again, I really think it was because she was frazzled this morning. We will see how she does tonight with her evening meds.

Mom Chronicles July 15, 2017
I found this article on a caregivers group page that I view daily. It has excellent information about the five love languages. "The 5 Love Languages" is a book that Bruce and I read when we had marital problems a long time ago, but this article puts a different spin on it through the caregiver's eyes. My mom's love language is definitely "receiving gifts"!
www.crhcf.org/Blog/the-five-love-languages-of-caregiving/ (Meredith Fields Lawler, 2016)

Mom Chronicles July 16, 2017
We took Mom to church this morning, and sure enough, her hip started hurting bad again. We had even given her a strong pain pill before leaving the house to try and prevent the pain.

Unfortunately, it didn't work. We had to leave right when PK (Pastor Ken) started his sermon. Since this seems to happen the most at church, the only thing we can guess is that the chairs are not soft like the sofa she sits on at home. It is probably putting more pressure on that bone-on-bone hip joint. She loves going to church (and even gets upset if we miss), so I know it's not an act just to leave. Soooo... we will try buying a super-soft cushion to bring with us to church to see if this helps. Bruce and I may have to resort to taking turns each Sunday to go to the early service to still get our worship time in. And we are incredibly thankful Concordia records PK's sermons so we can get part of the service later.

It's all about adapting and figuring out ways to solve the problem.

Mom Chronicles July 18, 2017
Here is just another way our roles have reversed. I put too much on her plate for dinner tonight. I could tell something was bothering her because she kept looking over at me and my plate. I asked what was wrong, and she finally got the words out to ask me if it was okay not to eat it all?" She was full but had the "you must clean your plate mentality" (which I remember all too well from my childhood)!!

I must admit the little red dude on my shoulder is tempting me hard to cook boiled okra (ugh) and make her eat it!! I have many yucky memories of that horrible vegetable!!

Mom Chronicles July 21, 2017
This is just a public service announcement. If you pray for patience... He, in His almighty wisdom, is going to give you something to practice patience with. Just sayin'!! Don't say I didn't warn you.

The Momster has turned into my dearly beloved grandmother. Whenever Grannie wanted something done, she wanted it done right then and there. You couldn't wait 5 minutes or however long you needed. It had to be done RIGHT THEN.

I am no longer praying for patience. I've got that under control now. I'm praying for the skills to handle wealth. It's a simple request. I would love to show HIM that I'm willing to work on these skills. A simple request, right??? Or maybe I should pray for guidance on getting these last 15 pounds back off??? That's something very important too, right???

Mom Chronicles July 22, 2017
My sister is up here this weekend to give us a little break. She mentioned this conversation that happened this morning with Mom. They talked about watching a TV show that was "live" (a regularly scheduled program) versus a recording on the DVR. Sheila was trying to explain that the TV show that was "live" was about to go off in 5 minutes, but Mom couldn't understand. She asked Mom if she understood the difference, and Mom replied that "live TV isn't dead."

We have noticed a big difference this past month in her comprehension between the two. She also can't figure out how to turn the TV on anymore.

Mom Chronicles July 23, 2017
Today PK preached a wonderful message on God's sustaining grace. He helps us through one more day, and then another, and then another. This is our mantra right now, as I'm sure it is for many of you—one day at a time.

Thank you to so many folks at church today who showed my mom love. She loves going to church. This is her only window to socialization. We love our church family!!

Bruce bought a memory foam cushion this past week, and that did the trick (at least for today!) Mom was able to make it through the service without any pain. Woohoo!!

Mom Chronicles July 25, 2017
Mom is now using the phrase she uses when watching something on the TV that she doesn't want to watch.

If it's a TV show she doesn't want to watch (and it could be a brand-new episode), she will say we have seen this already and wants us to change the channel.

Tonight, she said we have been having the same meal lately. I'm not the best cook in the world, but I haven't been serving the same dinner over and over. I offered to give her something else (although I was very tempted to tell her what she would say to me when I was little - eat it or go to bed hungry), but she just sighed and said no, she would eat it.

The joys of Alzheimer's!!

Mom Chronicles July 26, 2017
Mom still has her phone and remembers how to make calls using speed dial. I just got a phone call from her asking if we were going to church today. I had to explain that today is Wednesday, that I'm at work, and that Bruce is hanging out with her today. Bless her heart.

Mom Chronicles July 28, 2017
Today is our last summer half-workday Friday at the office. Soooo... I'm taking advantage of it by taking Mom to get her hair colored and cut. It's been a while!!

I have her dropped off securely with the hairdresser, phone # given in case she needs me back asap, and now I'm sitting in the food court area eating a sub sandwich and just decompressing for a little bit. I love watching the kiddos jump on the "bungee ride." There is so much happiness on their faces!

Mom Chronicles July 28, 2017
The Momster and me. She has a new "do."

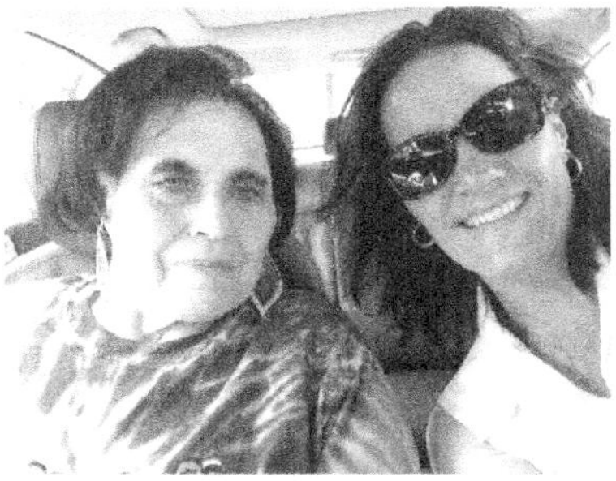

Mom Chronicles July 28, 2017
I'm not sure if she's just more tired than usual since I took her out for her hair appointment or what, but she is STRUGGLING to find the right words to say this afternoon. She got so frustrated at one point, she raised her voice and said, "well damn, I can't think straight." It took me quite a while to figure out what she was trying to tell me this time. I'm usually pretty good at solving her puzzles. This one was harder. She was trying to tell me she needed more clothes hangers and that she needed a blanket on her bed. She has her four-letter words down pat, though!!

Mom Chronicles July 30, 2017
Routine is EVERYTHING with Alzheimer's. EVERYTHING! Saturday night is shower night. (We try to do more than that, but it throws her off. She thinks any day after a shower is church day.) Soooo, we got her shower done, and I let her know we aren't going to church tomorrow because Bruce and I are driving to Huntsville for a funeral. Lynda and Jan are going to sit with her while we are gone. She was upset because

she "hasn't been to church in a long time." (We went last week and the week before.) I then told her the only option of going is to go to the early service, which means I must wake her up at 5:30 am. She said, no, she didn't want to get up that early.

Not 60 seconds later, "tomorrow is church day?" Yep. I give her the spiel again. She wants to go to the early service. I tell her, okay, we can do that.

Another 2-3 minutes later - same question. She wants to go, so I tell her I will wake her up at 5:30. "Okay." I get her to her bedroom and tell her goodnight and remind her again that I will wake her up early for church. "Okay."

About midnight, Bruce gets a call on his phone from her, but she hangs up. Of course, we both jump up to see if she is okay. She is okay. She was just trying to find someone to take her to church tomorrow. She was looking on her phone for some ladies to come to pick her up. I explain that we are taking her to the early service - again.

Bruce and I go back to bed. Fifteen minutes later, Simi starts barking because Mom has come to our bedroom asking who will pick her up from church. I explain the spiel again.

Fast forward to 5:30 am. I go in to wake her up. She asks, "we have to get up now??" Yes ma'am. She lays in bed another 15 minutes, and we are now running late.

We will need to leave before communion starts, so that will throw her off more. Oh well... if it weren't important to us to go to Pastor Wuensche's funeral, I wouldn't change her schedule like this. She will forget about it soon enough.

Mom Chronicles July 31, 2017

I'm taking a little "vacation" day (ha) today to hang with Mom while Bruce works a day shift in the office today. I'm glad I was here. She had a big "accident" this morning and needed my help cleaning everything up in her room. Have I mentioned lately that Alzheimer's sucks? I know "sucks" is not a nice word, but it's the only word that fits right now.

Mom Chronicles August 6, 2017

Today, we experienced another "first" with Mom in our Alzheimer's journey. She was already frazzled this morning when I went in to wake her up for church (she had another accident which is very common right now, but to her, it's not-she doesn't understand.) I got the room straightened up and then went to make my coffee. A few minutes later, she calls me from her room, asking for help. I walked in there and saw that she had her dress, shoes, and hose all laid out. I asked what she needed help with, and she said, "me." I asked if she needed help getting her clothes on, and she said yes.

I know this is one of the symptoms that we hadn't experienced yet. She has always been able to put her clothes on - her matching choices have not always been great, but she has always been able to dress herself so far. Soooo... I'm not sure if today was a fluke and she will be able to dress herself tomorrow or if this will be a regular deal now. If this becomes regular, I will have to go ahead and hire someone to be here in the mornings to help dress her while I'm at work because I know Bruce will not be comfortable dressing her (and she would be more at ease with a woman dressing her). Another day in our journey.

Mom Chronicles August 6, 2017
She is trying to take her vitamins using a spoon full of milk from her cereal instead of drinking from her glass of juice. She was frustrated because she couldn't swallow the pill. I explained to her about taking a drink of juice with her medicine. That worked like a charm, and she said, "oh!"

She has done this before, so this may be becoming a more commonplace deal for her.

Mom Chronicles August 8, 2017
So much happened today… this one is a little long, so feel free to just "drive on by." This is just me journaling our day.

First of all, Mom was complaining about the new sheets I had just bought for her bed. Because they were the "deep mattress" kind, they were not tight on the bed, so they bunched up some. This is something that she is kind of "OCD" about now. Her bed needs to be perfect now. I admit I got mad that she was picky about this, but I had to keep telling myself this is just the Alzheimer's talking; it's not her. That helped me calm down, and I went to the store later and bought new sheets that wouldn't upset her.

Second, I took Mom to her orthopedic appointment. There is nothing more they can do for her since she is not a candidate for surgery, so we have been referred to a pain management doctor. While we were in the waiting room, a lady was chatty and wanted to talk to Mom. She was very sweet, but there was no way I could gently tell her Mom has Alzheimer's, so when Mom would answer strangely, she would look over to me with a questioning look. I would explain the answer as best that I could. I just didn't want to blurt out Mom's condition with Mom right there. At one point, she asked how many grandchildren Mom has, and Mom answered "4". (She only has one unless she was thinking of Robin's kiddos.)

Third, on the way home, she had to go to the bathroom. With Stage 5/6, bladder functions are greatly diminished. There's no way to "hold" it. I found the first gas station I could find because I don't think Bruce would have liked me turning his car into a boat. Anyways, this particular gas station is not typically one I would have stopped at (not that I'm snooty-it just looked a little rundown.) I had to get her inside to the restroom as fast as I could. Unfortunately, this gas station/store had one bathroom at the back of the store, and it was not handicap accessible. There were two giant steps she had to climb to get into the restroom. Her mobility is soooo bad now this was almost impossible to do. The only thing that saved us was the owner or manager (I am not sure of his role, but he was in the store's office), who came over and helped me get her up the stairs and then back down once she was finished. I was so scared she would fall, and then we would have a whole new set of problems. God blessed us on this one. I tried to give the man a tip for helping, but he wouldn't take it. He was incredibly gracious and kind and said we all would be in that situation someday, and he just hopes someone helps him. (I think I will still send a little thank you note to him even though I don't know his name. I know his store, and he deserves to know I thought he was our little guardian angel today.)

Finally, at home, we were watching the 5:30 news with Lester Holt on NBC. They were doing a story on Glen Campbell because he passed away today from Alzheimer's. They talked about the last interview he had with them and that he was at Stage 6 then. Then the reporter said, "Stage 7 is the end." I lost it. I had to jump up quickly and go to my room before Mom saw me crying. Bruce understood completely and came in to just hug me for a few minutes to let me cry it out. I'm fine now. It's just that sometimes emotions jump out at me from nowhere.

I will be staying home tomorrow with a vacation day to take her to her neurology appointment. I hope to get a clearer picture of what I can expect this next year from the doctor. Wish us luck! For those of you that read to this point, thank you for loving and caring for me, my mom, and my family. Your virtual hugs and prayers mean so much to us! Remember - this is not a pity party for me. I just like to "chronicle" this crazy journey so that my sister feels included in what is happening with our Mom, and it is a simple way to help me deal with the emotions.

Mom Chronicles August 9, 2017
We are in the waiting room at the neurologist's office, so I gave her a magazine to thumb through. She is so excited to see people (celebrities) that she recognizes. She is giggling and pointing out the dancers from "Dancing with the Stars" and Princess Diana and Jennifer Anniston. She is saying, "I know him! Or I know her!" Now... I'm not sure if she thinks she knows them (like the Michelle Obama story from a while back) or if she just recognizes them. I didn't want to pursue the line of questioning I was tempted to do with all these people here. (Although they probably would completely understand, judging from the type of doctor we are all seeing today.)

Mom Chronicles August 9, 2017
I took Mom to her neurologist appointment today. The last time we went was a year ago. On the MMSE (mini-mental state exam) last time, she scored a 16. Today she scored a 10. The only questions she could answer were her name, how to spell it, and how many children she has. She didn't know the month, day, year, the president, or where she lives (town and state). On the way to the appointment, I asked Mom if she remembered her birthday. She couldn't remember it.

The doctor told me that since she is in the severe stage now, we can probably expect her to be at the stage where she will not be able to swallow in about a year. Full-time nursing home care is around the score of 10, and that I need to go ahead and start looking at getting nursing care now.

He asked if we wanted to try some non-FDA-approved trial treatments showing signs of slowing the symptoms in mild cases. I said, sure, it can't hurt. We aren't sure if Medicare will approve one of them because it is insulin. They may not approve it because it is for diabetes, but in this instance, it gets sprayed in the nostrils (so that it goes straight to the brain) twice a day. He said it is expensive if not approved, so I will find out the cost when the pharmacist calls me. The other medication is an antibiotic. Medicare should approve this one, and he said this would also help with the infections she has been getting. He said he hopes these two meds are FDA approved for Alzheimer's treatment by 2020.

He told me not to get my hopes up because of her level, but it was worth trying to see if it slowed some symptoms. Our next visit will be in 6 months. In the meantime, Bruce and I will start trying to figure out how to transition her to full-time care. This will be a challenge, but we are sure the answer will be provided to us.

I know this may sound extremely horrible to some of you, and I'm sorry if it does, but my prayer for my mother is that she passes from a heart attack before she gets to that final stage. She has a moderate case of mitral valve prolapse, which can't be treated because of her Alzheimer's, so I pray this is what she passes away with so that she doesn't suffer the end stages of Alzheimer's. I just don't want her suffering. She's oblivious to her condition right now, so we aren't there yet. As long as I can keep her happy, we are good.

♥

I wanted to interject here to remind folks that everyone's journey is unique. Notice the doctor said Mom would probably have a hard time swallowing in about a year. Now that I have the beauty of hindsight, she did have many occasions where food or drink went down the wrong pipe, which could have been from a weakening of the throat muscles. Having difficulty swallowing didn't happen until the spring/summer of 2020.

Mom Chronicles August 12, 2017
The TV is my babysitter today (I know, I know - that's not a good thing), but I need time to work on building out my adjunct college course. She loves NASCAR (which is crazy-she never did until she met Ted), and she just told me she met one of the drivers at least once or twice. I just went along with it and said that must have been really cool!

For you NASCAR lovers, please tell me what the draw is for this??? Drive fast, left turn, drive fast, left turn, drive fast, left turn. Hoping to see a crash... drive fast, left turn, drive fast, left turn... It is a fantastic metaphor for what we are going through right now with her!

Mom Chronicles August 16, 2017
I have an Elvis special on TV right now to try and help bring back some memories for Mom. She is saying her catchphrase, "Oh my God," whenever they play a song she remembers. In her mind, she met him. She said she was at a concert near the front of the stage and he came down off the stage to give her a photo.

Oh, to be in her mind-what fun experiences she has had!! At least these are good "memories" even though they aren't true. You guys should see her smile right now.

Mom Chronicles August 18, 2017
I'm off today with the Momster so that we can go to a couple of doctor appointments. The first appointment is over, so now we are at IHOP treating her for being good while getting her blood drawn this morning.

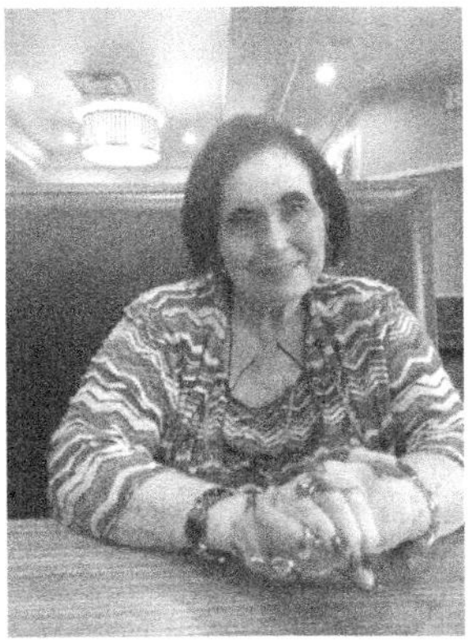

You can't go wrong with red velvet pancakes—my 75-year-old kid.

Mom Chronicles August 18, 2017
I am rethinking my decision to take her out publicly. She has no filter now. When she sees someone who doesn't look "normal" (in her mind), she makes strange faces and points at them. There is no way to teach her a lesson like we would a child about accepting people of all types. She would forget it immediately.

Mom Chronicles August 18, 2017
I like the philosophy of this pain doctor. He doesn't just throw pills at her. He prefers to treat the nerves causing the brain to think there is pain! We will try anesthetizing the nerves around her hips first next week (hopefully), and if that works, we will go back, and he will cauterize the nerves next.

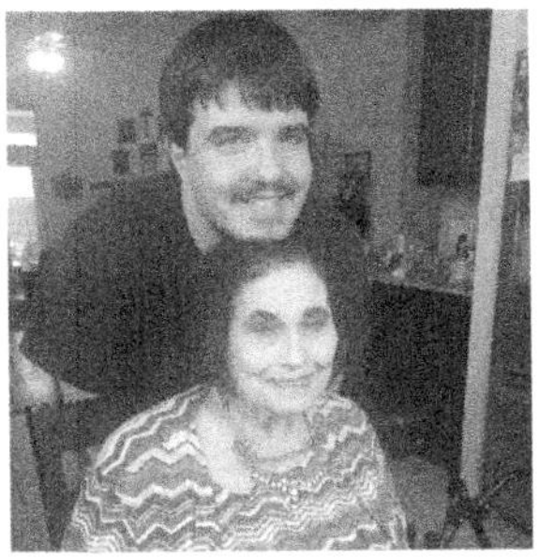

Mom Chronicles August 20, 2017
Here are some pics from today. Thank you all for the birthday wishes for my Mom. And thank you also to everyone at church who came up and hugged her today. You guys rock!! A special thank you to Carolyn Holboke for the birthday card. She was so happy to receive it!!!

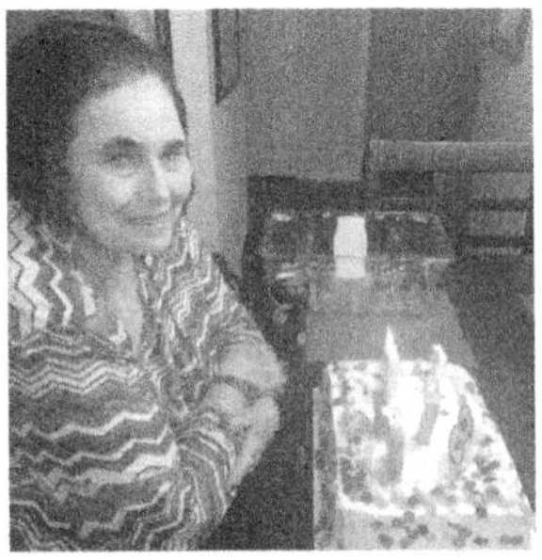

Mom Chronicles August 21, 2017
God is a sneaky dude. About a week ago, I had a severe case of feet/toe cramps. It was so bad that I was a whiney baby and called Bruce. For me, that is unusual because I have a very high pain tolerance. He talked me down and told me to eat a banana, drink a sports drink, and walk it out. I admit I am not the best at eating right and getting my vitamins. Mom, on the other hand, gets daily vitamins. I take better care of her than I do of me!!

Well... Mom just called me to come to her room. She was having severe feet/toe cramps. Like I said... God is a sneaky dude. I knew exactly what to do with her!! I played "this little piggy went to market, this little piggy stayed home...". She ate a banana, drank a sports drink, and we played piggy footsies (since walking isn't an option) for a while until the pain eased up. I got her laughing which took her mind off it for a little bit.

She is lying back down now, so hopefully, there will be no more toe cramps. I don't want to play "this little piggy" all night. Please pray the piggies are all in their blankets resting now. I know. Bad pun. It's late. I'm tired.

Mom Chronicles August 23, 2017
Mom's confusion level/communication is off the charts tonight. I am struggling to solve the "Alzheimer's secret codes" and am not doing so well!! I'm having to resort to answers like "yes ma'am" or "okay" or "that's cool" or just "hmmm."

I'm sitting on the couch making little video replies to my online college students, and that is throwing her for a loop and making it worse, I think. She doesn't understand why I'm talking to the computer and not her.

Mom Chronicles August 24, 2017
Without going into details, I'm at the ER with Mom. It's nothing serious, but we need to stay until her pain goes down and the doctor says it's okay to go home. There is a chance we will have to stay for 24 hours observation.

Mom is furious and agitated at me. She wants to go home and doesn't understand why we must stay. She just keeps repeating she wants to go home, and she's getting madder and madder. I hate Alzheimer's. Hate it. Hate it. Hate it.

Mom Chronicles August 25, 2017
We did a little more pre-planning today for Mom while my fantastic neighbor, Lynda, did some Momster-sitting for us. We stopped at a local funeral home to get info on funerals, caskets, etc. I feel better prepared now. We already have the burial site, and I know we will use Sam Houston Funeral Home in Huntsville (Larry Graves is phenomenal!) to help with the graveside service. I just needed to get information on things to do up here. I did well... I was expecting to cry when I looked at caskets, but I did great! The funeral director showed me a pretty lilac color one, and he said we could bling it up to our heart's content!!

And then Bruce and I joked about my casket someday. We want to spring-load it with silly string.

Mom Chronicles August 25, 2017
I just bought these for Mom. I hope they fit! If so, I truly expect her to wear these every single day!! Unfortunately, the picture doesn't do them justice. They are silver and very sparkly!

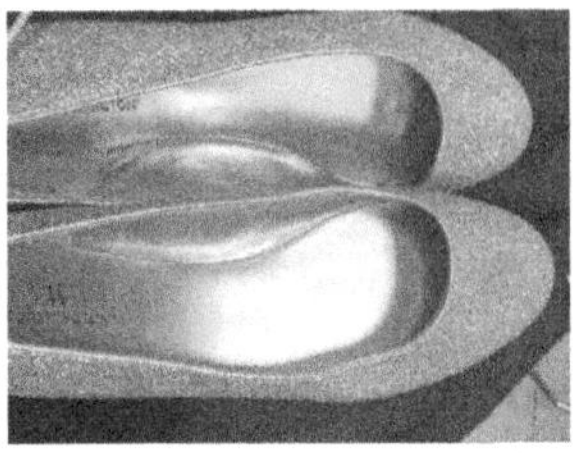

Mom Chronicles August 26, 2017
Last night was a rough one for Mom. She called me into her room around 11:00 pm with more toe cramps. Soooo, listening to suggestions from friends from the last round, I tried the pickle juice. This didn't work out so well. It solved the cramps, BUT it caused major heartburn and indigestion. She was in so much pain from that (Mom can't handle ANY kind of pain), she thought she was having a heart attack. Then she went into a panic attack and had a hard time breathing. Using a pain pill, a panic attack pill, and some heartburn chewable tablets, I was finally able to calm her down and get her to rest by 12:30 am. The hard part for me was hearing her pray to God out loud that she needs His help. She told Him she "wasn't working" anymore and she needed his help. She meant her body is having lots of problems. With Alzheimer's, she doesn't remember experiencing any of these issues before. All I could do was just sit there with her, hug and hold her and wait for the panic attack medicine to calm her down. I try hard not to use the pain or panic attack meds, but sometimes it is necessary. As my neighbor mentioned to me yesterday, if there is something to help the last year(s) of her life be more comfortable, do it. As for the toe cramps, I'll try the tonic water suggestion next. Does anyone know if this will cause heartburn too??? If so, I'm not sure if I should use it.

Mom Chronicles August 26, 2017
I just gave Mom a bowl of ice cream. I watched as she attempted to eat it. She fell asleep four times while trying to eat. She would jerk awake and look over at me, confused. I am telling her that she is falling asleep, and she replies that she is not. Then she starts laughing like she's embarrassed.

I just found this article about Alzheimer's patients' sleep patterns:
www.agingcare.com/articles/alzheimers-and-sleep-156720.htm

The article does a great job of explaining why sleeping is an issue with people who have Alzheimer's. As the author says, "if a loved one with dementia isn't sleeping, then neither is their caregiver." (Botek, 2020) That is so true. I will share a little bit more about sleep patterns and sundowning shortly.

Mom Chronicles August 27, 2017 (4:00 am)
Mom is wide awake and completely dressed, and ready to go to church. The camera shows she woke up at 2:00 am to start getting ready.

So now I'm hanging out with her in the living room while she eats some cereal. Do you know there is nothing on TV this early? I found "101 Dalmatians" with Meryl Streep, so that will have to do. Puppies. Boxes and boxes of puppies. (How many of you remember that 'Mom Chronicles' post from a while back?)

Mom Chronicles August 28, 2017
Paranoia is a symptom of Alzheimer's, and getting mean and fussy at times are symptoms. I have been calling this behavior "persnickety." Mom has been having these feelings quite a bit the last few days, and it is really, really trying our patience. She had been on a kick about her pants being too long, so I took several pairs to a neighbor to hem. Mom swears they have been stolen because they aren't hanging in her closet. She also

complained about her shoes, so I bought her new ones, including the sparkly silver ones. She liked them at first but then said they were too big. She is upset because they don't fit exactly perfectly.

A few minutes ago, she came out of her room and just spouted off in an angry voice that she should just die since she doesn't have anything. And to top it off, her sleep patterns are worse, so she wakes us up in the middle of the night, either wide awake or having health issues and wanting to go to the hospital.

Right now, I'm just exhausted, and I know we haven't even gotten to the worst part of this journey yet. Bruce and I are trying to figure out how we can get her into a memory care home. It breaks my heart because I'm concerned she won't get the care she needs, but at the same time, we need someone to give her the care that we can't provide. I chatted with my sister for a little while this evening about this. She understands and just wishes she could be up here to help more.

Maybe things will be better in a few days, and I will be able to power through a bit longer. It's just been a difficult few days. Hopefully, I will be able to post something lighthearted soon. Have I mentioned lately that Alzheimer's sucks? And in just the few minutes that I have been typing this post, she looked over at me and smiled after seeing a funny commercial. Oy!!

Mom Chronicles August 30, 2017
Mom had a rough night and then again this morning. We are taking her to the ER to see if they can give her some relief. After that, we will go ahead and find a facility that can take care of her. After last night/this morning, I realize I just can't physically do this. She was pretty much dead weight, and I can't lift her anymore. Prayers for guidance because there are a lot of decisions to be made over the next few days.

Mom Chronicles August 30, 2017
She is being admitted to the hospital for observation. We are praying for three days of care in the hospital so that Medicare will cover some possible rehab time. This will give me more time to find the perfect memory care facility for her. I have met a new neighbor (virtually - not face to face yet) who highly recommended a place in Mesquite. I will check there, a place in Sachse, and another site that is located a block away from my office.

And I just realized that today is my dad's birthday. Happy birthday in heaven, Dad. You will have the love of your life back in your arms again soon. And before tears start falling, let me add a little humor here. Mom is on her 8th marriage (common law sort of with Ted), so all the hubbies will have to fight over her when she gets there!!

Mom Chronicles August 30, 2017
My hubby is the best! He bought Mom a teddy bear from the gift shop, and she hasn't let it go at all.

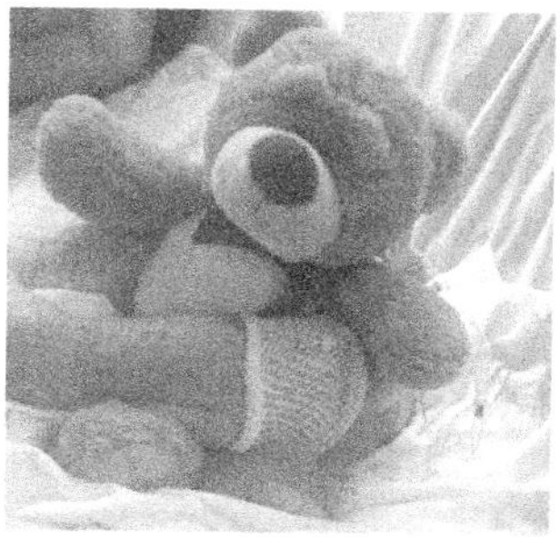

Mom Chronicles September 1, 2017
We are still in the hospital and probably will be until Saturday. She is currently experiencing "sundowning" and hospital psychosis. She doesn't understand she is in the hospital and is madder than a hornet. She ripped

out her IV and took off her heart monitor leads while I had my eyes closed. Thankfully, they had the bed alarm set. She was trying to get up so that she could leave.

They had given her something to help her rest, but it has done the opposite tonight. She's very, very agitated and giving ALL of us the "go to hell" look. If looks could kill, we would all be 6 feet under.

Anything out of a routine is soooo bad for the elderly, but especially for Alzheimer's patients.

She will be going to a rehab facility (my guess is Saturday). After a stint there, we are going to place her in a memory care center in Sachse. The good Lord is providing us with a way to pay for this, and they are running a special with reduced rates through the end of October. The timing has been perfect.

I am past the crazy part of the year with my job, so it's a little easier to be away. My co-workers have been "holding down the fort." HIS timing is perfect. For those of you awake right now, say a little prayer that she can get some rest.

Mom Chronicles September 1, 2017
Nada Zero Zilch
No sleep even though they tried something to help her sleep.

There should be a stronger phrase than "madder than a hornet" because she is way madder than that. She removed her IV and her telemetry unit again when I dozed. The techs monitoring her heart were concerned because she was showing v-tach. I have no idea what that is. But finally, I overheard the nurse talking to the doctor on the phone, and because she is DNR (Do Not Resuscitate), they decided not to put the unit back on her. They are still determining if the IV is going to go back in. They are probably going to wait until shift change and let the next group handle it. I can't say that I blame them.

Her confusion level is off the charts. I even recorded one of her rants so that Sheila and Bruce could hear it later. It made absolutely no sense whatsoever.

She cussed the nurses a little bit ago. I feel bad, but I know they understand. That's another group that needs our utmost appreciation.

Sheila will be hanging with her today. If Mom gives her the stink eye, Sheila will give it right back. She's a tough cookie!!

Mom Chronicles September 1, 2017
And just like that, the sun is out, the blinds are open in the room, and breakfast has been eaten (but not before I glanced over and saw her drinking the syrup out of the packet). She is smiling and laughing. It is a complete personality change. Sundowners is relatively new to us. We have noticed slight changes in her personality over the last few weeks, especially in the evenings. Last night was just one of the worst, which I can only assume was heightened by being in the hospital.

♥

What exactly is sundowning? Pulling information from alz.org, sundowning increases confusion, anxiety, agitation, and disorientation, beginning at dusk and continuing during the nighttime. Patients might pace back and forth during this time frame. There are several reasons why Alzheimer's patients may be experiencing this. Some possible reasons are:

- Mental and physical exhaustion
- A biological switch where the body can't distinguish between day and night.
- Reduced lighting may increase shadows that may cause Alzheimer's patients to get confused about what they are seeing.

The alz.org site suggests these tips that may help with sundowning:

- Schedule activities like doctor appointments, trips, and bathing in the morning or early afternoon hours.
- Encourage a consistent routine of waking up, mealtimes, and bedtime. (Remember-Mom's routine was out of whack while being in the hospital, so sundowning hit her very hard.)
- When possible, try to get your loved one outside in the sunlight.
- Make notes about specific things happening before sundowning events to help you determine the "triggers."
- Reduce stimulation during the evening hours like TV, doing chores, and loud music to reduce confusion levels.
- Offer a larger meal at lunch and keep the evening meal a light meal.
- Keep the home well-lit in the evening.
- Do not physically restrain the person; allow him to pace back and forth with supervision.
- Try calming activities in the evening, such as viewing photo albums, listening to calming music, or watching a favorite movie.
- Take a walk with your loved one if she is restless.
- Talk to your loved one's physician to determine the best times to take medications (some may interfere with sleep and are best taken in the morning).
- Reduce or avoid alcohol, caffeine, and nicotine.
- Always approach your loved one calmly.
- Try to determine if she needs anything.
- Gently remind him of the time.
- Avoid arguing.
- Always offer reassurance that everything is okay.
- Finally, if the behavior interventions and environmental changes do not help your loved one, talk to your loved one's doctor. (Sleep Issues and Sundowning, n.d.)

Luckily, my mother never had the pacing part of sundowning. She just had agitation and confusion. When we finally moved Mom into a memory care center, so many of the patients walked and walked in their safe area of the center. It was a big adjustment for us to see this side of Alzheimer's and other dementias.

As we close out the chapter of Stage 5, here are some more tips for caregiving at this stage from the Alzheimer's Association (Middle Stage Caregiving, n.d.):

- Understand the changes in behavior. I believe we have covered many of these behaviors that Mom experienced in this chapter. However, if your loved one is experiencing something different, don't hesitate to contact a doctor.
- Communication is more complicated. They struggle to find the right words, express clear thoughts, and have difficulty following conversations. I watched a Teepa Snow video once where she explained that an Alzheimer's patient is hearing us talk with jumbled words instead of clear sentences, so it's no wonder they can't follow a conversation. They have trouble finding the right words, repeating questions, losing their train of thought, relying on non-verbal language, and if they are bi-lingual, they may revert to their native language. For us as caregivers, we can speak slowly in a gentle tone and use short sentences. Jenni Knutson also taught me to repeat the same sentence if Mom did not understand because it takes time for that sentence to make it to the brain. If you keep changing the sentence, she will have a more challenging time trying to decode what you are asking. I also remember that it was better to ask yes/no questions so that Mom didn't have to come up with an answer filled with words.
- Daily care needs become more difficult. Your loved one is losing independence and privacy, so it's important to be patient and sensitive. Allow the person to do as much as possible to maintain dignity and

some sense of independence. For example, when it's time to get dressed, help that person nonverbally by laying out the clothing in the order the item is put on.

- Provide activities that have meaning. This will enhance their quality of life and can reduce unwanted behaviors like wandering and agitation. Remember not to treat him like a child. Activities can safely be provided that are age-appropriate. Consider making dinner together, gardening, listening to music, or going for a walk. I once saw a video of an assisted living center putting up Christmas trees scattered around a room without the ornaments, and they had someone dress up in a reindeer costume and allowed the residents to "hunt" with Nerf guns. Be creative. Yes, this is a touch on the childish side, BUT who doesn't like to shoot Nerf guns at any age? What did they want to do in the past that can be modified safely for them to do now?
- Driving is a big challenge in this stage. It will clearly be time for a person with Alzheimer's to stop driving. Remember, my mom got lost going to a place she visited every week. The Alzheimer's Association believes you should try to involve the person in the decision to stop driving as much as possible. They suggest explaining your concerns by giving specific examples. It's important that your loved one knows that you will be doing everything possible to make sure they have transportation wherever they need to go. They are fearful of losing their independence. Also, remember the example of what we did to help take away driving from my mom. We used a prescription card from her doctor saying, "no driving for six months." We didn't want to take away her hope. We also heard of others disabling their loved one's cars to keep them from driving. Do what you need to do in a kind, compassionate manner to keep your loved one safe.
- Other safety concerns at this stage include not leaving them alone. They don't remember how to operate stoves or other appliances safely. They may leave the house and get lost. There are many tragic stories of things that happen to a loved one at this stage. We moved Mom in with us but knew we needed some sort of care for her at all times. We used a combination of part-time caregivers, neighbors who could be called at any moment, changing shifts so that my husband was home during the day while I worked, etc. Every family's situation, resources, and the number of family members/friends who can help will be unique.

This stage can seem daunting because there are so many changes happening, and they can still communicate to some degree. It's also tough to watch your loved one "deteriorate" to the point that you may no longer be able to care for him at home. By the end of this stage, we had to make the hard decision for full-time care. The steps we were taking to make sure Mom was well-cared for all the time were not working anymore for our situation. It was time for us to move Mom to a memory care center.

CHAPTER 3: ALZHEIMER'S STAGE 6 ♥ THE MIDDLE/LATE STAGE

Stage 6… this one is a tough stage - not that any of the others aren't tough. This one is where the disease picks up steam in their bodies, and more functions start to deteriorate. At this stage, you can expect some or all of the following signs:

- Difficulty dressing: choosing wrong clothing, putting clothing on wrong, needing help putting an arm through the sleeve, etc.
- Can no longer bathe themselves or use proper hygiene, can't brush their teeth, can't remember mechanics of toileting
- Urinary and bowel incontinence
- Confusion and unawareness of environment like current address or weather conditions
- Inability to recognize people except for close friends and relatives; they might mistake someone for someone else (for example, Mom would call me her "mommy" instead of her daughter many times)
- Unable to remember personal history details and may forget many of their younger years' memories
- Difficulty with calculation tasks such as counting backward from 10
- Unable to channel their energy into productive activities; fidgeting, pacing, moving objects around; wandering
- Speech is becoming limited
- Fear, shame and frustration may lead to personality changes and potential behavior issues; may suffer from delusions; verbal and/or violent outbursts
- Fear of being left alone

(VISN 21 MIRECC, n.d.)

Recalling what the neurologist said during an office visit, loved ones usually need full-time supervision and professional care when they score around a ten on the MMSE test. Mom had this score during a recent visit, and with the level of care we had been progressing to, it definitely turned out to be true in our case.

I was not ready for Mom to go to a nursing home yet. I wanted her to go to a memory care center where they would work with her and keep her active, engaged, and safe in an environment suited directly for dementia patients. Unfortunately, at this time, memory care is not paid for with Medicare or Medicaid. Some folks use partial funding from military service, and others can use a long-term care insurance policy to help pay for this level of care. Mom did not qualify for my dad's military service since she divorced him and remarried several times over the years. She also did not have long-term care insurance.

Memory care centers are EXPENSIVE. The range at the care centers I visited (at the time of my mom's care) was \$4,000 - \$10,000, depending on the center and the level of care in the Dallas area. Some centers just use one all-inclusive fee. Others use a graduated fee depending on the level of care. This means as the patient's physical needs increase, the price gets higher. We also still had to provide incontinence supplies like diapers for Mom and gloves for the nursing aides, which added more to the expense.

When investigating memory care centers, consider asking several questions. I've compiled a few of these questions to ask the administrator of the facility:

- What is the staff to resident ratio?
- Is there a registered nurse (RN) on duty, and if so, how often?
- Is there a doctor assigned to the facility?
- Are there activities available for the different stages of dementia, and if so, how often? What kinds of activities? Art therapy? Music therapy? Pet therapy? Outdoor gardening? Puzzles? Games?
- Are residents assisted with daily activities, if needed, for bathing, toileting, feeding, etc.?
- What happens if my loved one has behavior issues?
- Are outer doors locked so that residents can't escape?
- Are bedroom doors locked? My opinion of this is that they shouldn't be locked, depending on the disease stage. My mother didn't remember how to operate a lock.
- What are the visiting hours? Do family members have access to the keycodes to get into the facility?
- Can my loved one have personal belongings? ***From personal experience, please don't allow your loved one to bring valuables. For example, mom lost an expensive ring. In hindsight, I should have told her I needed to take the ring home to get it cleaned.*** Keep in mind that dementia patients are constantly walking into other resident's rooms and will pick something up that catches their eye. Label as much as you can with your loved one's name so that staff members can help get the item back to the correct resident.
- Are nutritious meals provided? Snacks? Are drinks encouraged since dementia patients, especially later in the disease, don't realize they are thirsty?
- Are fitness and wellness programs offered and encouraged?
- What kind of training does the nursing staff receive specifically for dementia patients?
- Do they conduct training in how to bathe/shower a dementia patient?. If they are a well-run facility with experts in dementia care, they should be able to explain everything to you that will happen with their loved one.
- Does the facility provide incontinence supplies like diapers and gloves, or does the family? What other supplies does the family provide?
- Are family members allowed to participate in care plan meetings?
- Are there current resident family members available to give you a review of the facility and staff?

This is not an exhaustive list, but it's a good start. A well-established memory care center will have these answers prepared for you, plus more.

We were able to find a center that answered many of our questions satisfactorily, and they were running a special at the time of our decision to move Mom into a memory care center. But to do this, we had to do some creative financing. I was working three jobs (my main job plus two adjunct faculty teaching jobs), my hubby was working his main job, we had a small home-based business, and we decided to sell our home during the hot housing market since our equity had gone up over the past five years. We hated leaving our beautiful home and wonderful neighbors, but we believed family comes first, and this is what we had to do to pay for the memory care center.

We downsized our household to an RV since it was just my husband and me. Our son was now out on his own after college graduation and had an apartment. Buying an RV was a dream of ours for when we retired, but we weren't expecting to do this 15 years before retirement. We had to sell almost everything. We put important items like photo albums and some special furniture from my grandmother's home in a storage facility so that once we can buy a home again, we can pull those items back out.

We firmly believe that memory care facilities should also have a funding source that allows for Medicare/Medicaid. It is a health care service that functions as a nursing home. There is a post coming up where I spoke at a town hall meeting with our local representative. He even brought up that he would love to see studies done on how much income is lost by caregivers having to stay home to care for their loved ones versus being out in the workforce.

Bruce and I were lucky in that we have good-paying careers that allowed us this opportunity. But it did take sacrifice. We couldn't stay in our home and afford a nurse 24/7, so we figured out a different way to handle the challenge.

Here is the beginning of our big life decision to downsize to help Mom in this next stage of her Alzheimer's journey.

Mom Chronicles September 2, 2017
Today is the big day. She is being discharged from the hospital and moving into a local memory care center. Her roommate is named Marilyn!! The staff is already joking about calling them Marilyn 1 and Marylin 2. Of course, my mind immediately went to "Thing 1" and "Thing 2" from Dr. Seuss.

Bruce, Josh, and I have her room all set up. I need to get a few other little things from the store, but other than that, she is set. I am expecting the transition to be bad for a few weeks. The director said it might take 1-2 months before she settles in. Mom may beg me to come home but to try not and let it get to me.

I met "Thing 1's" son and daughter-in-law. They are lovely people. They said the place and staff are fantastic. The son is retired (retired early to take care of his parents), and he comes up here several times a week. He has my phone number and said he would contact me if he sees anything concerning my mom. That put my mind at ease.

Prayers for a fast transition. There are lots of things about to change in the Aden household over the next few weeks. We will post more on that later.

Mom Chronicles September 2, 2017
She is doing great!!! I don't expect this to continue, BUT for this first "see you tomorrow," she said, "okay." She was smiling and hugging all the staff. We got her out of the hospital gown and into her clothes. She feels normal again. We will go back tomorrow to visit. Hopefully, she will still be happy!!

♥

We visited quite a bit, but there will be many centers that advise that you don't visit for a week or two. This will help your loved one get acclimated to her new environment. Ask the memory care director what she suggests. It won't be easy, but it will be worth it if it helps them become accustomed to the new routine faster.

Mom Chronicles September 3, 2017 [Post on our neighborhood block page]
Howdy neighbors! As you may or may not know, we have moved my mother into a memory care unit. The downside to this is that we have to do some "creative financing." Soooo this means we will be selling the house and downsizing. We will be selling just about everything: furniture, TVs, dragons, and dinosaurs!! We would love the kiddos on our block to continue enjoying the inflatable holiday decorations. We will start posting soon but feel free to message me if you are interested in one or more of the inflatables. We are out running errands but will be home later this afternoon.

Mom Chronicles September 4, 2017
I know these sweet ladies didn't do it for the accolades, but I wanted to thank Carolyn Holboke and Madison for going to visit my mother today. They brought her a stuffed animal and spent some time with her. They said she was doing well, and they were able to get her to laugh.

Carolyn and Madison... thank you from the bottom of my heart for visiting my mom and showing her love. You both ROCK!

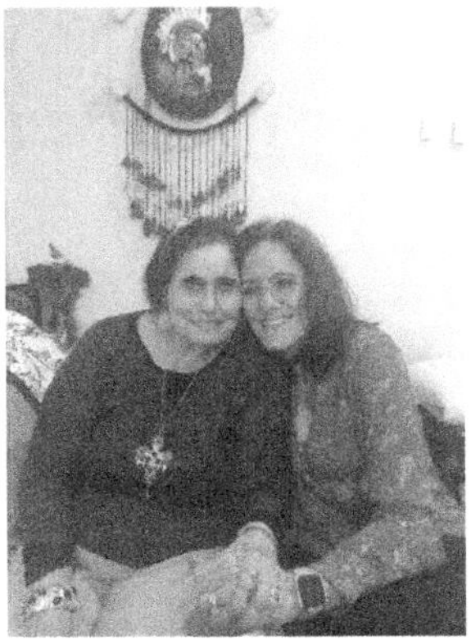

Mom Chronicles September 5, 2017

Bruce and I visited Mom this afternoon. She had a fantastic day!! We saw the Executive Director and the Social Director when we first got there to donate some art supplies, and they said all the staff just love her!! They got her to play the piano and participate in some singing today.

Mom said everyone is very sweet. She said she remembers her visit from Carolyn and Madison. She couldn't remember their names, but she said she loved visiting with them.

She did not tell me this time that she wanted to go home with me. The only thing a little upsetting to her is that she doesn't have her phone. I am telling her a little fib by saying I can't find it right now. If I give it to her, she will call me all the time, especially at night. I need the staff to handle the care for her. I promised her I would look for it and would be up there every few days to visit. That appeased her for now. So far, so good. Things are going well!!

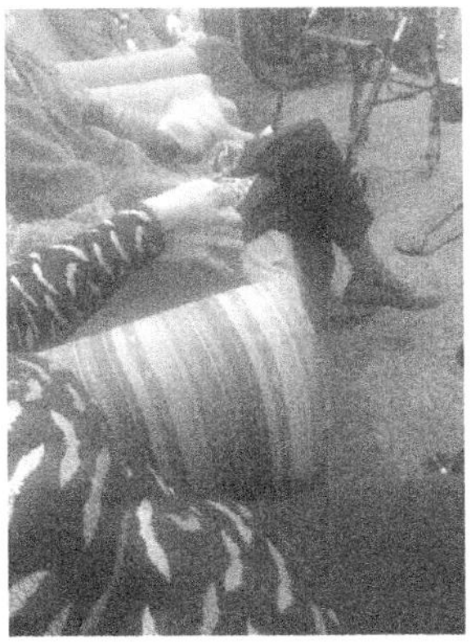

Mom Chronicles September 7, 2017

This journey with my mother has been a blessing in disguise. For a very long time, I didn't really "like" my mom. I always loved her but didn't like many of her decisions, so I distanced myself from her. Having to take care of her the last few years has helped me learn to "like" my mom again. Today really, really made me see what a caring person she is.

I went to visit her at lunchtime. She was sitting next to a lady who is a little further along in the Alzheimer's journey. Her words were even more jumbled than Mother's. Mom kept looking at me and would give me the "look" that said, "this woman is crazy!" (I had to keep from laughing!!) You could tell this other lady was very agitated. At one point, Mom reached over and put her hand over the lady's hand and said, "it's okay. You're okay." I think Mom will be in a "comforter, protector" role here until her condition gets worse.

Mom seemed well (especially since I brought her a chocolate shake!!) and didn't ask me to take her home. Another successful day and visit with no tears!!

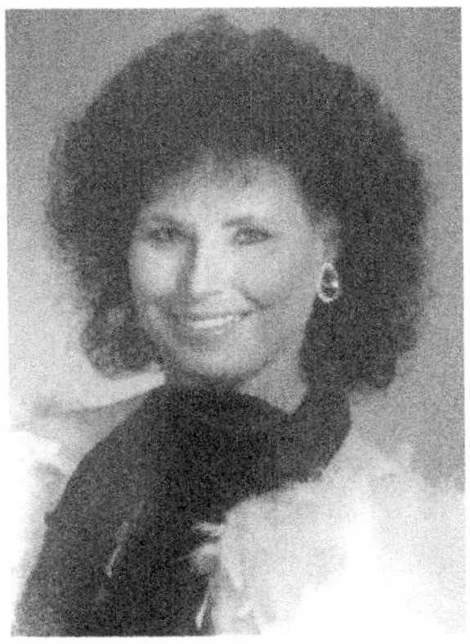

Mom Chronicles September 8, 2017

As I'm working on packing the house, I came across this one of Mom during the height of the glamor shot's years and another one that shows how much braver (or self-assured) she is than me!!! I'm very self-conscious if I have cleavage showing. But mom had no problem with this!

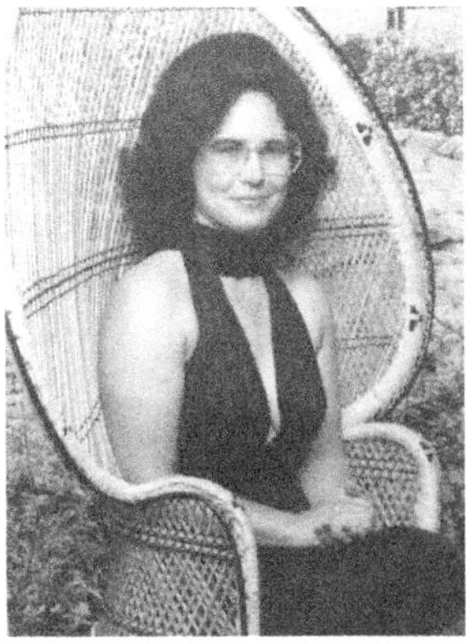

Mom Chronicles September 9, 2017

Here is another shout-out to some amazing friends for bringing smiles to my mother's face today!! Thank you, Carolyn, Madison, Cathy, and Janet! You ladies are fantastic for visiting her and spending some quality time with her!!! And I'm sure she LOVED the milkshake and cupcake!!!!!! I'm sending the biggest hugs to each of you!!!

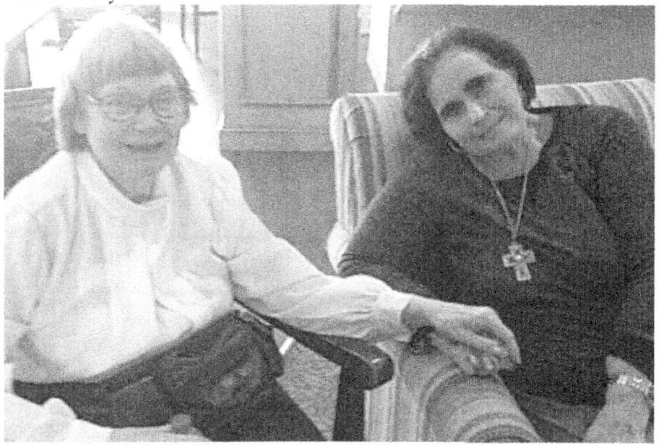

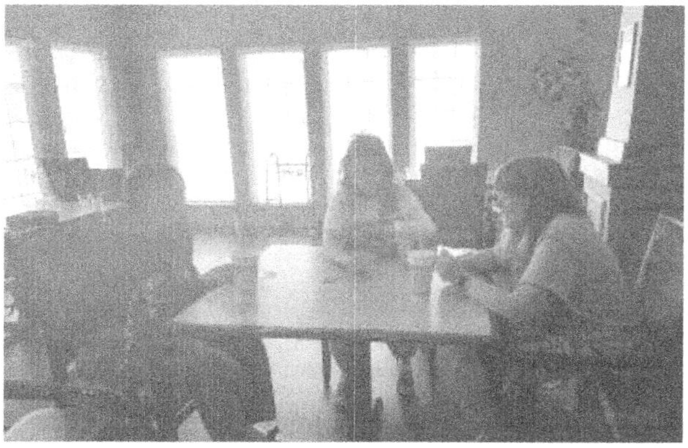

Mom Chronicles September 10, 2017

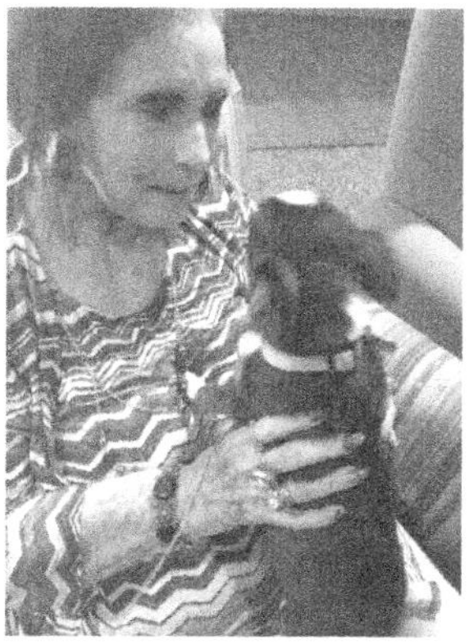

I finally was able to get over to see Mom around 6:30 this evening. She is doing well but told me she misses me. And then she said that a man came to visit her and told her she didn't belong there. So I think that is her way of trying to tell me to take her home.

And then the "crazy lady" was sitting beside Mom again tonight. Mom was looking at me hard and rolling her eyes. She wasn't very nurturing to her tonight like she was the other night. This might get a little interesting. I had to keep from laughing and telling Mom that she does the same thing, just not as bad.

I did bring Simi up to see her, and she loved that. At one point, I had four ladies standing/sitting around me wanting to pet Simi. Poor Simi. She was freaking out, but she did very well and didn't snap at any of them. One lady asked to hold her. I said we could try, but Simi is a "momma's girl" and may not like it. Sure enough, as soon as she picked Simi up, Simi practically jumped out of her arms to get back to me. So, it was a good visit: no tears, but this time she hinted at wanting to come home.

Mom Chronicles September 11, 2017

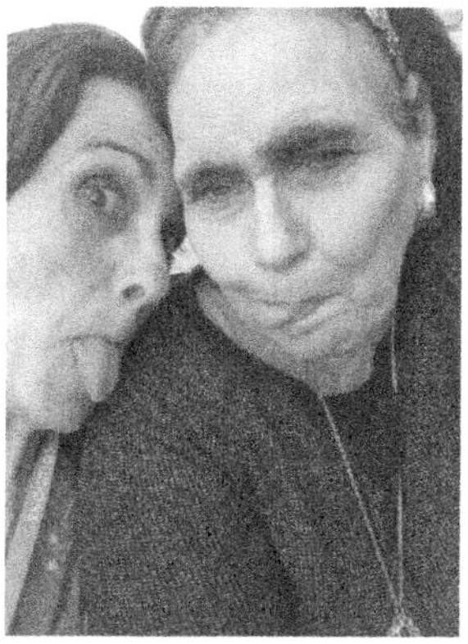

I left work a little early today, so I stopped by to visit Mom at a better time during the day. She was fantastic! We called Ted so that she could talk to her honey, and then the aides had all the residents go outside in the shade to enjoy the beautiful weather. I had her acting silly so that I could hear her laugh. She got a kick out of it. These are NOT the most flattering pics, but that's okay. She was laughing!!

I chatted with the social director for a few minutes, and she said Mom is adjusting well. She is going to post some pics of her on the center's Facebook page. I will share them when I find them. And the notes from the nighttime aides show that Mom is sleeping well. So far, so good!!

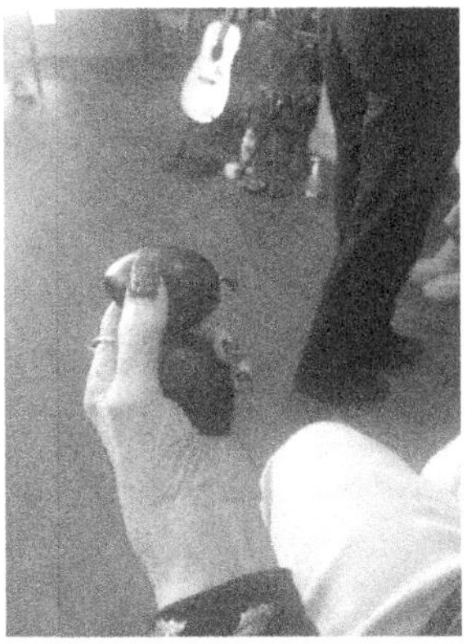

Mom Chronicles September 14, 2017
I left work a little early today to surprise Mom with a strawberry shake. They are playing a guessing game about songs and using shakers to fun music. I'm soooo happy that they are keeping her engaged!!!

Mom Chronicles September 15, 2017
"Sh*t-a&$". That is the term Mom not-so-affectionately called the pain doctor this morning amidst screaming bloody murder and scratching him. Thank the good Lord above; he was extremely kind and gracious and understanding. He had never heard that particular term before, and his team had to explain that it was a "southern-thang"!! He did a nerve block on her left hip, and she was in full-blown panic attack mode. She did not want that procedure done at all!!

Afterward, I started taking her back "home." She saw the George Bush turnpike sign and told me she had dinner with him and several other people and that he gave her something but couldn't remember what it was. I asked if it was Bush Jr or Sr. She couldn't remember.

Then, I bought her a burger and a soda. I knew that would help her forget the traumatic experience she just experienced, and yep, it worked.

Finally, I got her back to the memory care center. When we drove up, she asked me where we were going. I told her this is where she is living right now. She asked if she could come home with me. I told her not yet. We needed her to stay here a little longer. Once I got her inside the center, sitting at the table to eat her burger, she was fine again. This was a very eventful few hours!! Whew!!

So, for those of you not familiar with southern sayings, if you get told you are a "Sh*t-a&$," somebody is MAD at you!! Oh... and don't Google that term for some cute images to use on a post like I just did. You will just get all kinds of icky stuff showing up!! I can't unsee those images! Ugh!

Mom Chronicles September 19, 2017

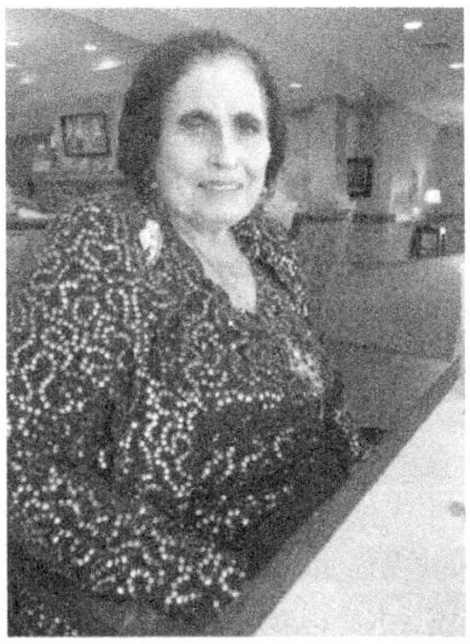

I'm a little behind on posting about Mom. Friday night after midnight, I received a call from the memory care home. They called the paramedics because Mom was having one of her panic attacks. Basically, she has a lot of sinus drainage and starts going into panic attack mode, thinking she can't breathe. The medics got on the phone with me, and I told them this is normal; the memory care staff just had never experienced it before. Her vitals were fine, so I told them not to take her to the hospital. The problem was they didn't have the medicine that I had left for them (long story, but that was resolved today).

Luckily, Sheila had just arrived here from Huntsville and is a night owl, so she went up there to help calm her down. Mom was a little patooty, but hey, 1-2 in the morning after a panic attack, she had a right to be. Sheila said the staff was being good with her. Those ladies deserve halos!! Then today, I visited Mom right after work. Every time she sees me now, she acts like she hasn't seen me in years - which I guess is probably true in her mind. I sat with her while she ate her dinner, and she whispered to me that many people there "aren't right." All I could do was grin and nod my head.

There is a sweet resident there who has a daughter named "Lori Ann." So, every time I visit, she asks Mom who I am, and every single time we talk about how my name is the same as her daughter. I feel like I'm in an episode of "Groundhog Day" every time. It's cute.

Mom didn't ask me to take her home, but she did say she missed me a lot. I hear she is adjusting well, so that's good. I'm hoping to take her to get her nails done on Friday. That should give us a little bit of quality time.

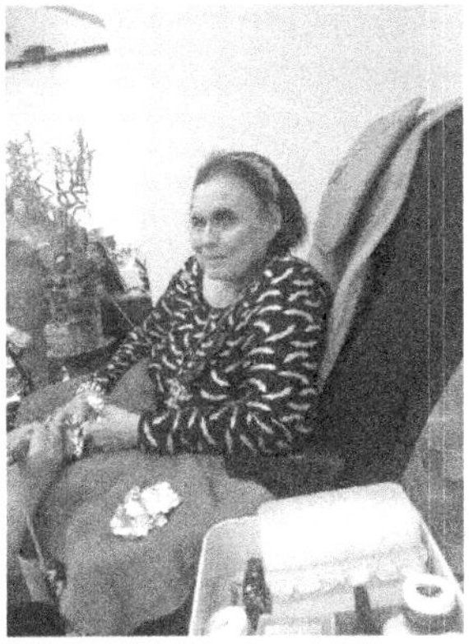

Mom Chronicles September 22, 2017
I helped Mom fly the coop this afternoon to buy some new shoes and get her nails done. First off, I want to say thank you to the sales clerk at the shoe store. She let me take several pairs of shoes out to Mom to try on so that she wouldn't need to get out of the car and walk into the store. That was a huge blessing!!

Now we are at the nail salon, and Mom is acting persnickety. She didn't want her pants legs rolled up for the pedicure. She is yelping at every little thing the ladies are doing (trimming toenails, etc.). She doesn't understand (remember) the process of getting her nails done.

I think I will need to try and hire someone to come in and do her nails at the center personally. They have someone who will do the basic nail service, but Mom is adamant about having the fake nails. So that may be a challenge.

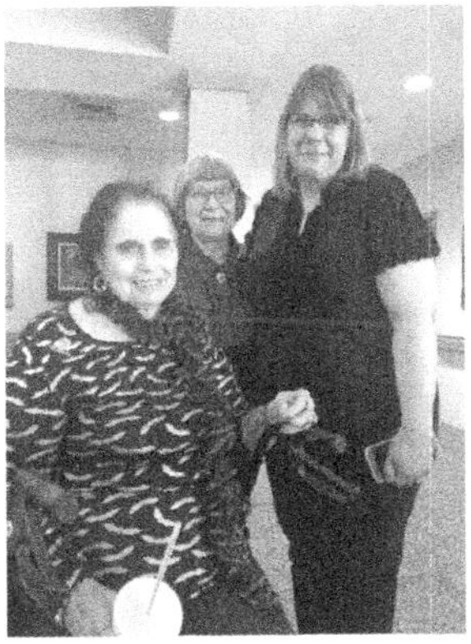

Mom Chronicles October 3, 2017
Bruce, Simi, and I went to see Mom Sunday afternoon. When I first got there, she was crying and saying she can barely walk anymore. She said she was "scared." She was also in pain at the moment, so the nurse gave her a pain pill.

Cathy and Miss Janet showed up, and we were all able to get Mom's mind off everything and laugh. Miss Janet brought Mom two scarves, so Mom was absolutely thrilled.

She did ask me to take her home, but I changed the subject quickly and diverted her attention to something else.

Today, the nurse called me to tell me about the doctor's visit. The doctor has removed her from a 2nd blood pressure medicine (she was on three), so I asked if they would monitor that very closely. She assured me they would. However, she also told me that the doctor took away the hydrocodone for as-needed pain and replaced it with Tylenol. This concerned me, so I talked it over with my medic hubby to determine my rights as her daughter and medical POA. After talking to him, I called the nurse back and said I am very uncomfortable with that decision. I know how much pain she can be in at times, and although I don't believe in popping a pill every time, I do believe in making sure the last few years of her life aren't unbearable. She told me that was a good call and that she was hoping I would tell her that. Apparently, she's not allowed to tell the doctor her opinion, but she can relay my concerns to him. As caregivers of someone who can't speak for herself, I thoroughly believe we must be her advocates and speak for her on her behalf. I just want her happy and as pain-free as possible.

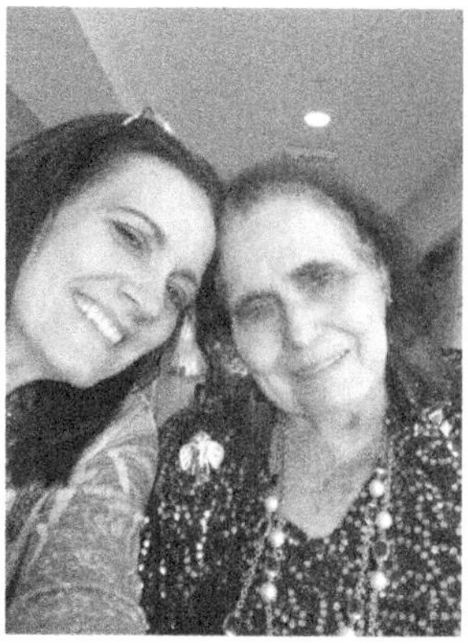

Mom Chronicles October 6, 2017
I sure hope she adjusts to this place soon. It's so hard to hear her ask me if she can come home now. It's like she thinks I'm punishing her.

I was hoping that coming here a little earlier in the day than normal would help (I get off work at 3:00 pm on Fridays), but nope… that was the first thing she asked me. I bought a strawberry shortcake ice cream sundae to try and get her mind off that topic. She loved that!!

Mom Chronicles October 6, 2017
Sheila's Post: Mom sang happy birthday to me.
[We treasure these video clips where she could communicate clearly.]

Mom Chronicles October 11, 2017
I received a call from the nurse at the memory care center today. I always get a twinge in my stomach when I do, especially when she starts with, "I need to report what happened today."

They are trying to get her to accept a wheelchair (which I am totally fine with now since her mobility is bad and pain level is high). But, she wants to keep using her walker, and she wants to sit on the walker (which isn't safe - I remember the adult daycare center wouldn't allow that). The nurse and staff here don't want her to do that either for safety. She blew up and cussed them out and slammed her hand on the table. So, they did what they are trained to do and redirected her by letting her have her way for the time being. I asked if they were going to kick her out, and they put my mind at ease and said no, this is common behavior. But if she ever hits anyone or tries to harm herself, they may have her admitted into a behavior unit to get her meds adjusted.

We are going to have to convince her soon to use the wheelchair. It's so strange that we couldn't get her out of the wheelchair when she was in the rehabilitation center. Now she doesn't want to get into one. The director helped me understand that she thinks she is forfeiting her independence if she does this. I also learned that because she is not using a wheelchair, they can't convince her to go to many activities because it's too far to walk. That makes me sad because she would be so much happier if she would participate.

She is also obsessing over the fact that she only has seven pairs of pants. She doesn't believe the staff washes her clothes - (they do every day). So, I went to pick up a few more pairs this afternoon to ease her mind on this current obsession. I will drop them off tomorrow.

The final thing I learned is that the staff has noticed that the days she "blings out" more than usual are the days her memory is the worst. They believe she is using bling to cover up her insecurity. I love that they have team meetings to discuss each patient and have started learning details about each one.

So, I always try to use humor in my posts as much as possible. The "funny" today is that the director had me laughing at the end of our little meeting this afternoon by saying that when the nurse calls her in the evenings, she always starts the call with "nothing is wrong, no one is hurt but…". She said that the phone calls to me will always start with "we aren't kicking your mom out but here is what happened."

Mom Chronicles October 13, 2017

She is having a good day!! She is having her first hair appointment here and is in a good mood. I mentioned we would work on getting her a wheelchair to make it easier for her to move around, and she said, "oh good!" All I can do is just shake my head. Tomorrow may be a different story... heck - a few minutes from now may be a different story. So, I will take this good day and let it propel us into the weekend!! *Edit-finished hairdo, and of course, I needed to show you her sparkly silver shoes.

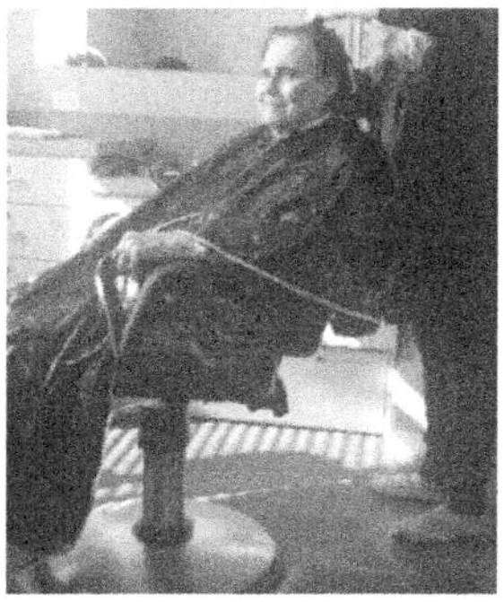

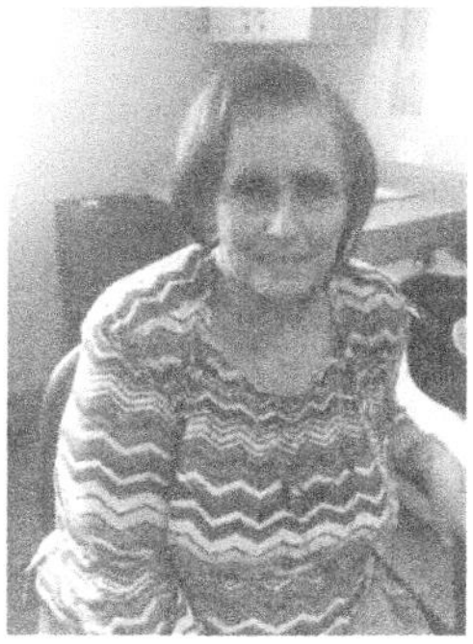

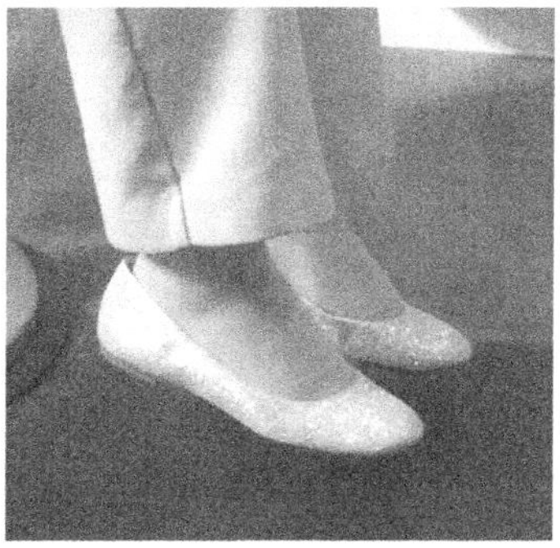

Mom Chronicles October 16, 2017

I stopped to see Mom after work today. She was blinged out so that cued me in to expect more confusion - since I learned that little tidbit from the director. When I got there, she was sound asleep in a chair in the living area. Once I got her awake, she was happy to see me. She kept saying over and over how much she missed me and that it has been so long since I saw her. She also introduces me as her daughter to everyone every time I visit her. Today, I was her "mommy" when she introduced me. The good thing is she didn't ask me to take her home. She just wanted me to stay longer to visit.

Also, when I got there, two of the women had a little fight that had to be broken up. Thank goodness it wasn't my mom!! The caregiver on duty had to step in to stop it, and she was so calm and handled it very well. Methinks at least one of them may be going to a behavior unit soon! Soooo, other than introducing me as her "mommy," it was a good visit. We are making progress!!

Mom Chronicles October 22, 2017

Sheila had a nice little visit with Mom today. Mom was showing off her favorite charm bracelet.

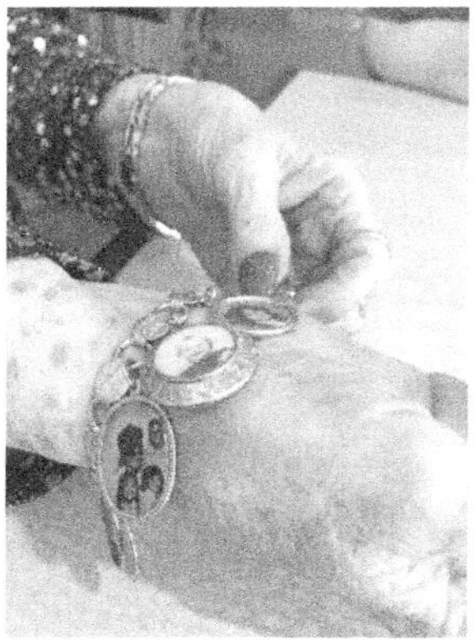

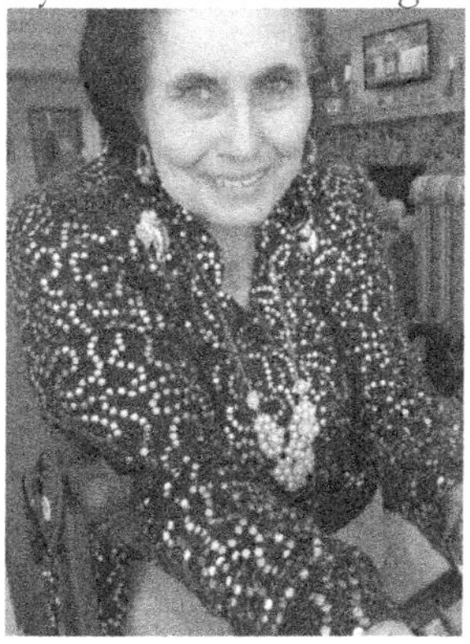

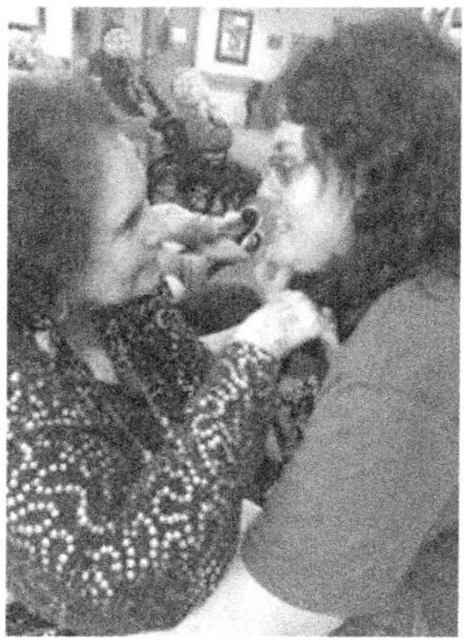

Mom Chronicles October 24, 2017

Well, today was a rough one. I got a phone call from the nurse this morning saying the wheelchair was finally delivered. She sat in it, but it was kind of small, so they tried to get her in the larger one. She refused, so the delivery person could not leave the larger chair. Mom wasn't being very nice again and had a few choice words for them.

I got a call from the nurse later in the afternoon, and she told me that they were able to get her in the chair by saying that it was from me. That made her happy, so she got in the chair. Soooo, when she refuses the chair, they are going to use that phrase. They do what they do best - try other staff members, try different times, and redirect, redirect, redirect!! The nurse said that we are just going to use the smaller chair. She said I could bling it out to make it appealing to her.

So, I went up there this evening. When I got there, she was sitting on her walker, and she just started crying when she saw me. She said they were mean to her, and they cuss her, and she can't stand it there a minute longer. They were killing her, but I've learned from the best. So, I redirected her by trying to get to the root of the problems. She was upset that there were some necklaces on the bottom shelf (they had broken, and she couldn't hang them up); the bed wasn't made up neatly-the bed cushion wasn't lined up perfectly, and then, of course, there was the wheelchair issue.

Step 1 - I told her I would take her necklaces home and fix them - problem solved; I laid them on the bed so that I wouldn't forget to take them home, but she kept asking about them. I told her several times I was taking them home to fix them. Finally, I put the necklaces in my pocket. Problem solved - again! (I CAN be taught!! - I always use Robin Williams' Genie's voice from "Aladdin" when I say that!!)

Step 2 – I fixed her bed and made sure it was nice and neat - problem solved.

Step 3 - I put on my best acting skills (ha!) and got super darn excited about the wheelchair and how it was going to help her move around so much easier. I learned one of the main problems with this - she was afraid she wasn't going to be able to move once she sits in it. Soooo, I taught her how to use the side wheels to move herself. She was like a kid in the candy store once she realized she could move herself. I had to show her several times, so she will probably need taught several times this week before it sinks in. I will go back tomorrow with some rhinestones to put on the frames. The only other issue that I need to solve is to add some kind of pouch to hide her "treasures" (napkins, forks, spoons, popcorn kernels, straws, forks, spoons – oh - already said that, and earrings that she takes off during the day, etc.). I bought one, but it goes on the back, which won't do any good. I did buy a cup holder, so that will hold some of it, but I will look at other accessories to see what can be used for this purpose.

By the end of the visit, she was smiling and laughing. Several crises averted today. (I had to look up the plural spelling of crisis since I hardly use that word!!)

Mom Chronicles October 25, 2017

I made an extra visit this week to bling out her chair. I am thanking the geniuses who created sparkly duct tape!!! I'm not the best decorator, but it's pink and gold and sparkly. That's all that matters!! I think the other ladies are a little jealous, so I may be picking out some different colors and working on their chairs too!!

And thanks to Pastor Ken, who was there when I arrived. It did my heart good to walk in on prayer time and see that he had given her communion. She's happy today, and that's all that matters in the world!!

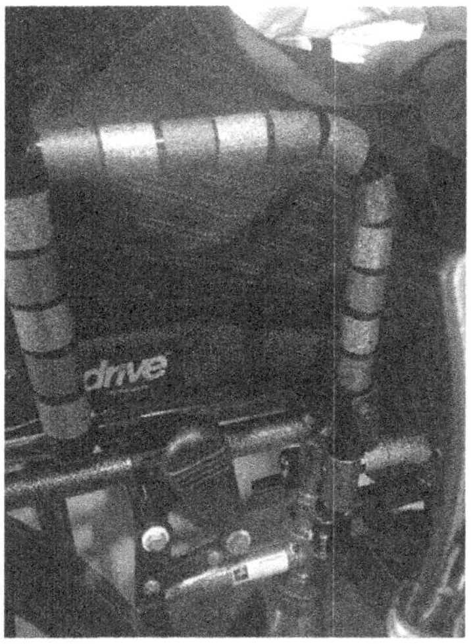

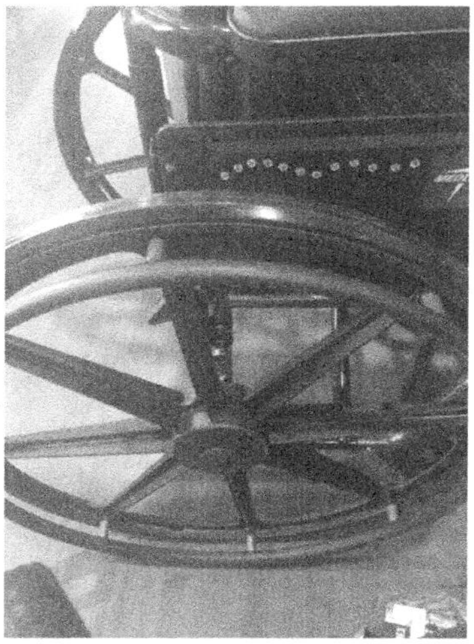

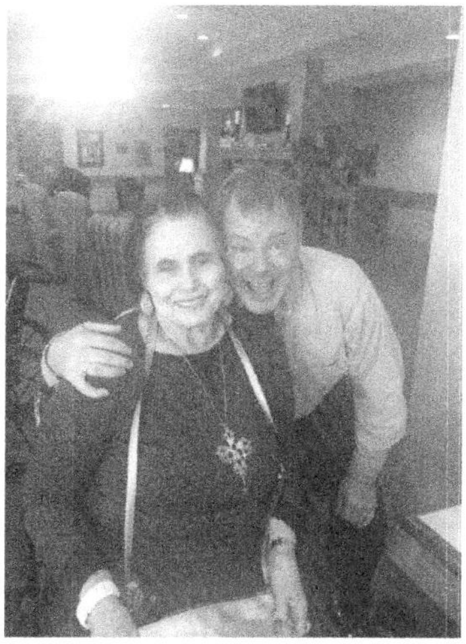

Mom Chronicles October 28, 2017
Today was a mixture of good and bad. We stopped by at lunchtime because 1) we needed to be out of the house for a showing, and 2) we needed to deliver a product to Mom for her to start trying. We had a great visit and worked on a puzzle. She was sitting on her walker instead of her wheelchair, though. We helped her into the wheelchair, and before we left, we told her we were taking the walker to fix the tires. We fibbed and told her they were getting loose. At the time, she was okay with it.

We also brought her some incontinence panties. Again - I struggle with how much to share for her dignity, but I have learned that many folks learn from these "Mom Chronicle" posts, and I hope that this will help someone else. The nurse had told me about underwear that had built-in absorbency liners that are washable. There are various levels of absorbency, and they make them for both men and women. The cloth is soft, so they won't hurt her skin as disposable ones do. She has really sensitive skin. I had never heard about these, so I bought several pairs for her to try. I showed them to her, and I tried to sell them as the next best thing as sliced bread. At the time, she was okay with it.

Well... I got a call from my dear friend Cathy this afternoon. She had brought her mom up there to visit, and Mom was having a melt-down and being uncooperative. She was upset the walker was gone, and she was upset that they were forcing her to put on the new underclothes. These were two major changes in one day for her, so I totally get it. The nurse/aide told Cathy that this wasn't a good time to visit (Cathy-thank you for trying!!) We had the nurse call me and put Mom on the phone so that I could talk to her. She was crying and yelling. At one point, she said, "who am I talking to?" I said, "this is Lori." She started crying harder. I tried several different tactics with her. The one that finally got her to calm a little bit was that I told her that the new underwear would save me a lot of money (which is the truth!) and asked her if she would try them for one week. If she doesn't like them at the end of the week, we can go back to the old way. I realize that she isn't going to remember this conversation, so I will probably have to tell her several times. I'm praying that she will adjust to these and the wheelchair very fast and that this is just another blip in our journey.

I hate it when she's upset and crying. I don't want her unhappy at all. I'm just praying she is having a better evening now and has calmed down some. For those of you who are caregivers, the website I found for the incontinence underwear is **www.wearevérincontinence.com.** Pray she adjusts to these two changes asap!

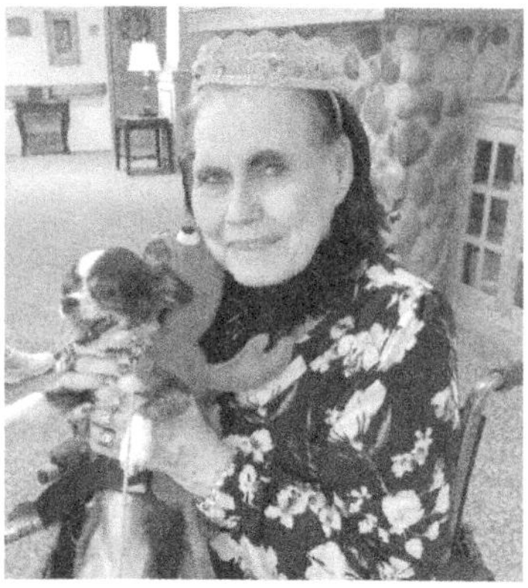

Mom Chronicles October 31, 2017
Sheila's Post: I'm substituting for Lori tonight. We had a great visit today. They had a Halloween party for the residents, and Mom "dressed up" like a princess with her crown. They also had a dog costume parade to entertain everyone. Simi went as a lobster and was super cute (if I do say so myself). It turns out they were judging the dogs, and Simi won 'best costume.' Woo-hoo! She won a cup filled with candy for her family and doggie treats for herself, and a certificate.

Mom was in a good mood and enjoyed the party and her visit with Simi. We called Ted, and she got to talk with him for a bit. Simi and I left shortly after the party began to break up because I didn't want to give Mom a chance to get worked up like she did the day before about the issues Lori talked about earlier this week. Overall, we had a great Halloween with Mom.

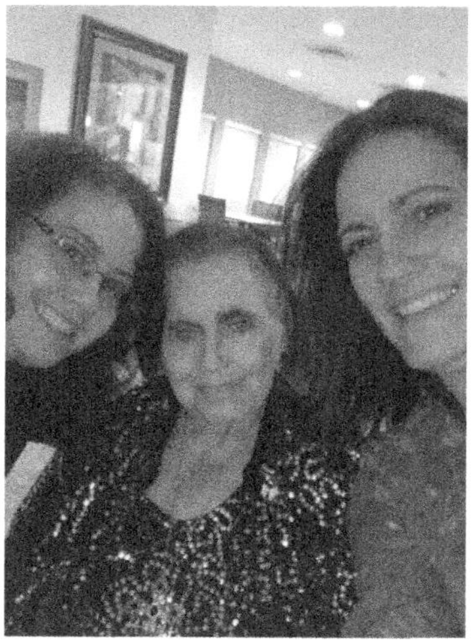

Mom Chronicles November 6, 2017
Sheila and I have been gone for five days, so this is the longest we have been away from Mom since we moved her to the memory care center. (I tried not to worry about her while we were in New Orleans, but it was hard not to since she had a rough week last week.)

We also went over there after 5:00 pm, and with daylight savings time over, it was already getting dark. That's a recipe for disaster with Alzheimer's, but we didn't want to wait another day because Sheila is about to drive home tonight.

When I arrived, one of the sweet little ladies was at the door trying to leave so she could get into her "car to go home." She was sundowning bad. I had to wait a few minutes for the aide to help her walk back into the main room so that I could come inside.

Here is the difference between her and my mom. This sweet little lady came over to the table where I was sitting with Mom. She was just so upset and called the aide a "blankety-blank" for not allowing her to leave. Literally a "blankety-blank." My mom would have used ALL the four-letter words!!

Mom was doing very well. She was happy to see us, and she didn't have any meltdowns. The 5-day absence helped with overcoming the issues she was struggling with last week. It was a great visit!! Whew!!

♥

Memory care centers use doors with codes for staff and family members to enter/exit the center. If a patient tries to leave, an alarm will sound for the aides to go redirect the loved one away from the door. Remember - at this stage, patients may be experiencing delusions and wandering. They will want to get out of the building as much as possible. Many will think their cars are in the parking lot so that they can drive away.

Mom Chronicles November 11, 2017
Mom and Simi are happy to see each other!!

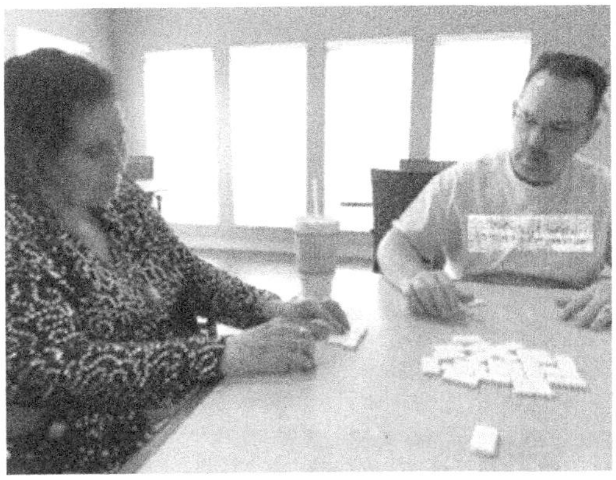

Mom Chronicles November 21, 2017
This was the first time in a week that I have visited Mom. When I got there, she immediately said she was so glad to see me and that things aren't good. So I said, "okay, let's go to the kitchen and talk about it." As soon as I rolled her to the kitchen, I redirected her. In 10 seconds, she went from "things aren't good" to "this place is great, and everyone is so nice to her." (Who remembers 10-second Tom from the movie "Fifty First Dates"?)

Bruce and I then played dominoes with her (well... it's more of a matching game than true dominoes). We would say something like "play the double 2," and she would play the double 4. So we just went with it. Or she would play a domino off a double that wasn't the spinner. She had a blast, and we had some quality time with her, so that's all that matters.

The nurse said she is doing really well, and an aide stopped by our table and said that Mom is one of her favorite residents even though they aren't supposed to have favorites. She was building Mom up about her sparkly gold shirt and teased her that she would take Mom shopping with her to help pick out shiny clothes.

Mom talked about a party that was held in the central area of the center. She said that was the first time she had ever been there. She's been in the main area multiple times since that is where they hold the center-wide activities. It's just crazy how the diseased brain works!! Or "doesn't work," I guess is a better way of putting this. We will visit her again in a few days for Thanksgiving.

Mom Chronicles November 28, 2017
I received a call from the center - I'm always nervous when I see their number - and the nurse said Mom fell a little while ago. She was trying to use her roommate's walker and fell. So far, it seems like Mom isn't hurt other than a carpet burn on her arm near her elbow. She says she's not hurting, so hopefully, that remains the case.

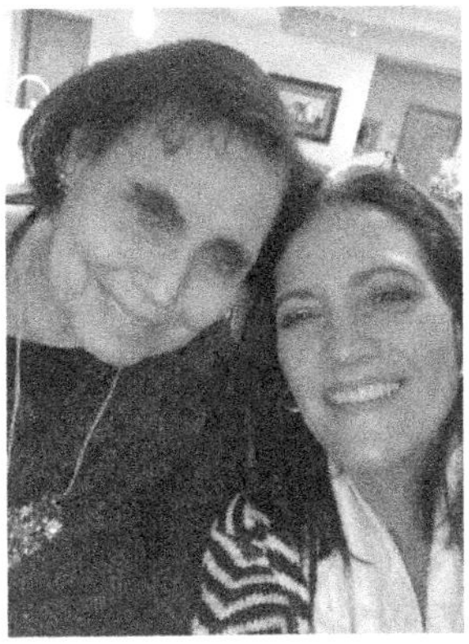

Mom Chronicles November 29, 2017
I stopped by to see Mom after work. It looks like the hairdresser has colored her hair recently, so she looked great! She didn't remember falling last night, and she wasn't hurting, so that is great! Unfortunately, her words were failing her today. I had to ask yes/no questions. I was there at dinner time, so I had conversations (well - as much as you can have with several Alzheimer's patients) with two other ladies. It felt good to help them laugh and smile some. We even were able to witness the vibrant colors of the sunset through the door window. All is well with Mom today!!

Mom Chronicles December 3, 2017

Bruce and I visited Mom today and played dominoes (the number matching type of dominoes). I had her practice counting today. The first time, she did fine. The second time she forgot the # 2. She went from 1 to 3. I held up two fingers, and she said "3". She was a little confused during the third attempt and struggled to find the right words. She was forgetting numbers 8 and 9 but finally remembered. She did okay with the next few attempts at counting. It's just crazy how the disease can have someone remember things one minute and then, not even 5 minutes later, forget something simple like the number 2.

When we were leaving, the aide started to take her into the main area where they were singing Christmas carols. She pouted and wanted me to stay and sing with her. I reassured her I would be back in a few days. That one made me tear up on the way out to the truck. Bruce always can tell when something is getting to me because of her illness, and he immediately started cracking jokes to get me to laugh. He is getting good at redirecting ME!

Mom Chronicles December 7, 2017

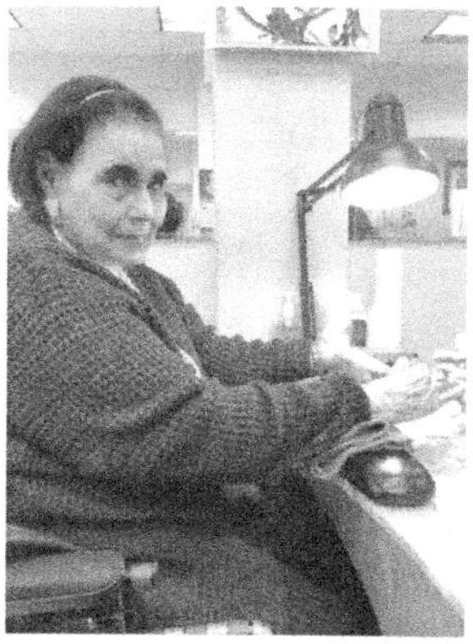

Sometimes taking a half-day of vacation is mandatory for a caregiver. Mom broke a nail this past weekend, and she has been fixating on it (I would be too, to be honest!) So, I picked her up from the center and took her to the nail salon. We are going with a lovely fuchsia sparkly blend today.

Oh, I also learned that her roommate (the other Marilyn) was moved to a different room last weekend. I asked the nurse if it was because of my mom. I wanted to make sure she was playing nice with the kids on the playground. She said it wasn't because of my mom. Whew... I was afraid I was going to have to ground her. The other Marilyn is further along in her journey with this disease, so I am guessing she needed a different level of care in the other wing.

Mom Chronicles December 7, 2017

She's still in a good mood, but while getting her nails done, she is saying over and over that she would like to get moved closer to me. So, I am telling her I will work on cleaning her room, and then I change the subject immediately. The best topic changer so far is about Christmas and what she wants for a present. I have her choosing between a sparkly blouse or jewelry. That is working so far.

Mom Chronicles December 7, 2017

Pretty nails, French fries, and soda make everything better!!

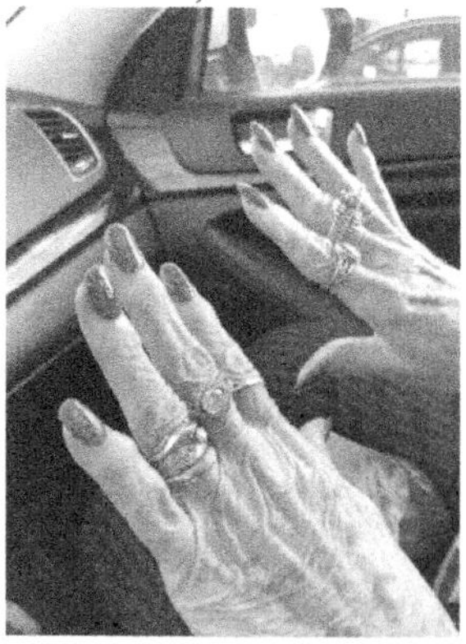

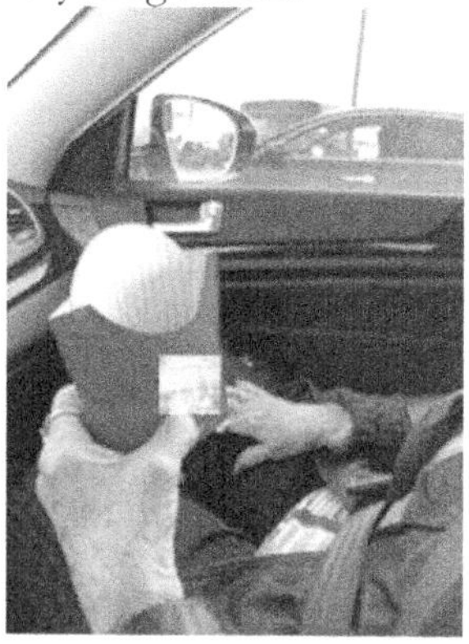

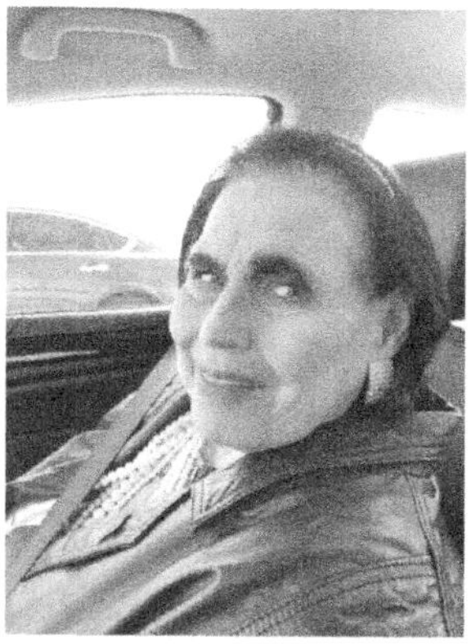

Mom Chronicles December 12, 2017

I visited Mom this evening and stayed a little longer because I knew I would hit a lot of traffic on I-80 going to our new RV Park, where we have temporarily set up the RV. She was in a great mood, thankfully. Names escaped her tonight. She didn't know my name or the names of people in any photos we looked through. She recognized faces but no names. Egypt is a trip that has always stayed on the top of her memory, but she couldn't remember the name of the country or her friends' name who she visited over there.

She wanted to show me her room - she loves to do that with everyone who visits her - and the candy canes she has accumulated. (I'm hoping she's not going into her housemates' rooms and swiping them!!) I'm glad she is happy with it - it eases my mind. We looked through photo albums that my sister had made for her, and it was great to see her eyes light up when she recognized someone. She remembered my dad, which is great because there have been many times she didn't remember him. Aunt Evelyn - she recognized you!! So even though she couldn't remember my name, she was happy tonight. I will take that!!

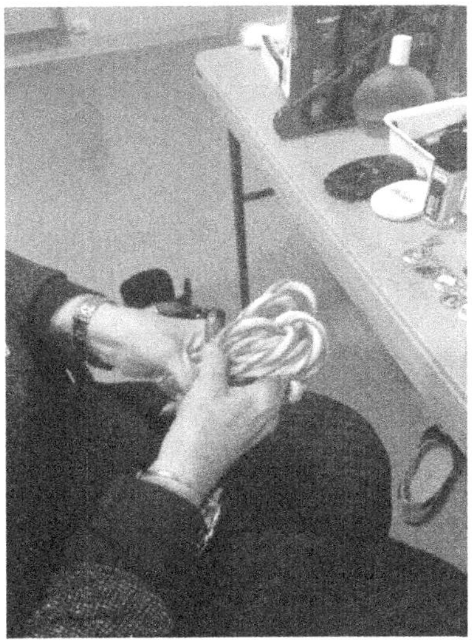
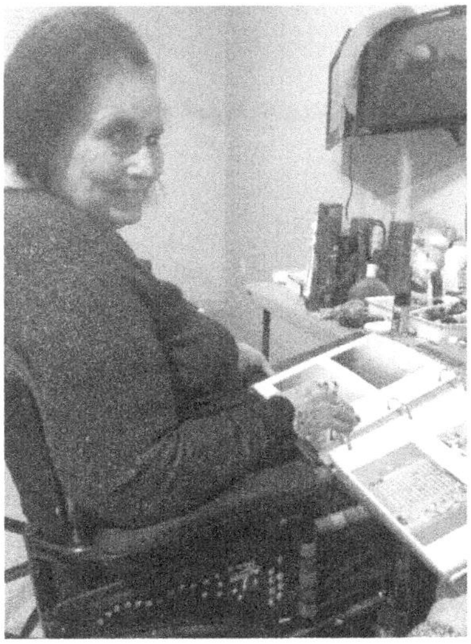
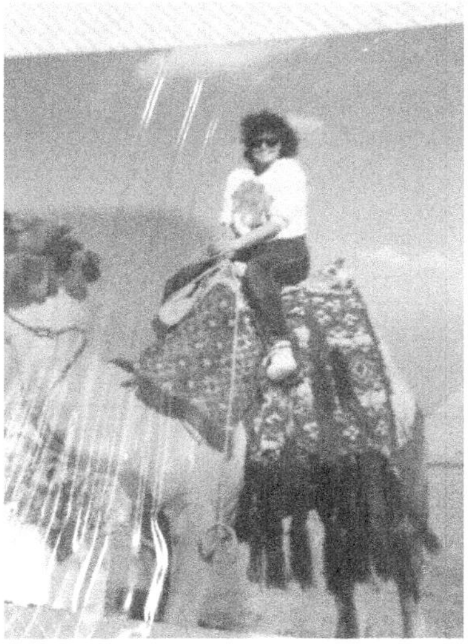

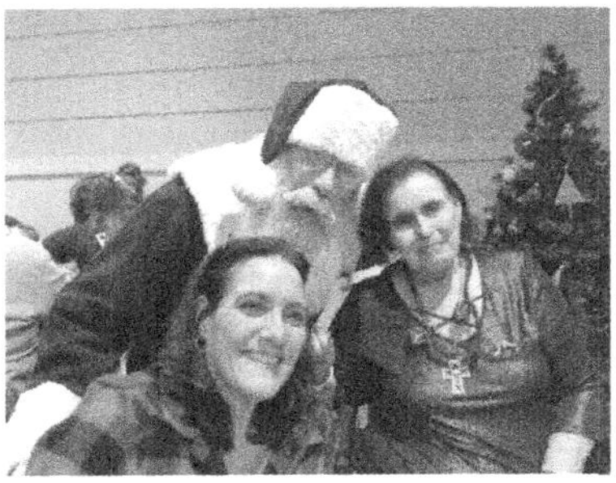

Mom Chronicles December 14, 2017

A Christmas party is not complete without a picture with Santa!

Mom Chronicles December 14, 2017

Here is one more post tonight. She remembered some of the words to the Christmas song, and she knew the tune. It was great having some quality time with her tonight.

Mom Chronicles December 22, 2017

The not-so-fun part of being a caregiver is handling all the bills and correspondence. Today, Bruce and I get the FUN pleasure of getting the address changed for Mom's social security and Medicare benefits. Several people are hacking away here - we need to load up on Vitamin C when we leave. Unfortunately, we couldn't do this online, so we are powering through a lovely few hours at the Social Security office.

Mom Chronicles December 22, 2017

She knows my name today!!

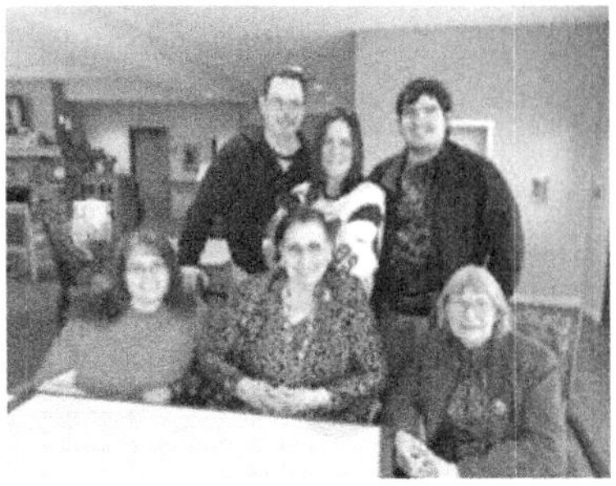

Mom Chronicles December 25, 2017

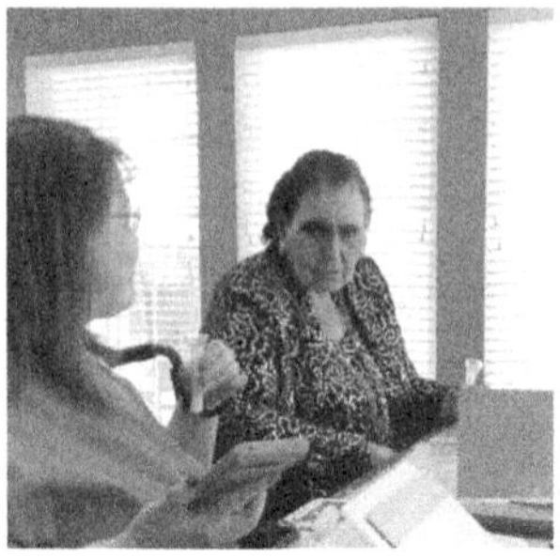

We had a nice visit with Mom today. Cathy and her mom were also there visiting. The very first thing she said to me was, "can I come home?" I just said not today and immediately changed her attention to how pretty she looked. It's like a dagger to my heart whenever she says that, but I know how to deal with it now. Sheila bought her some jewelry and makeup for Christmas. Those are the perfect gifts for her.

We played several rounds of dominoes. Cathy's Mom deals with dementia as well, so Bruce was helping her out while Sheila was helping Mom.

We also bought 4 Ancestry kits, so Sheila, Mom, Bruce, and Josh will send in their samples just to see the results. Sheila and I should be about the same, so we wanted to get Mom's DNA to see what it says. Mom was acting silly today, especially when she was spitting into the tube.

All in all, it was a good visit. We wanted to make it a good one since we aren't sure what next Christmas will be like. So we are packing in memories every chance we get. Merry Christmas, friends!!

Mom Chronicles December 27, 2017

Bruce and I were running errands today, so we stopped by the center to make the January payment. At first, I was going just to make the payment and then leave quietly before seeing Mom, but I just couldn't do it. We almost did that roughly 24 years ago when we were driving by Point Blank with Josh sleeping in his car seat. We were just going to drive by and not stop to see Bruce's folks because we didn't want to wake Josh up. It was getting late, and we still had to buy groceries. But there was something (God's whisper) that said, "Stop and see the folks." So, we did. Margaret had a blast playing with Josh as she always did. We stayed for about an hour or so and then left to shop for groceries and get home in Huntsville. By the time we got home, we had received a call that Margaret had collapsed. They tried everything they could but couldn't revive her. We are thankful every day that God whispered to us to stop and see her. We would have never forgiven ourselves for being selfish and missing out on an opportunity to visit before she passed away.

So, I just couldn't "not see Mom" being so close to her. We never know when we will take our last breath. I was able to have a good visit with her this afternoon. She was holding her picture frame of her and Ted and smiling. She was trying to clean it. Luckily, she didn't ask me about him or ask to call him because I don't have the heart to tell her that he isn't doing well and is in the hospital. Robin (his daughter) said that he would probably be going home on hospice when he is released. Sheila and I decided not to tell her and let the natural progression of Alzheimer's allow her to "forget" him.

I was going through some photo albums with her, and we came across a picture of my dad, sister, and me. I pointed to my dad and asked her if she knew who that was. She smiled and said, "my daddy." I don't know if she truly thought it was her dad or if she just didn't know the term for "husband/ex-husband." It's just hard to know what's going on in her mind. But all-in-all, it was a nice visit. She was smiling and loving looking at the pictures. She didn't ask me to take her home (which made me feel better). We left her with a strawberry shake. She was smiling, and that's all that is important to me.

Mom Chronicles December 29, 2017

Sheila and I stopped by to visit Mom after we had hair appointments today. The store where the salon is housed had some great sales, so we bought Mom a new blouse and necklace. When we got to Mom's center, she greeted us like she hadn't seen us in years and then started crying, saying she wanted to move closer to us. I acknowledged it so that she knew we heard her and understood and then immediately brought out the new blouse and necklace. That brightened her up right away. We then started the puzzle to put her mind on something else.

By the end of the visit, she was fine. She wanted to follow us to the door, which was something new, but the aide followed and took her back to the living area right away. The aides and staff at the center are some of the best!

I think what I'm going to do is start sneaking some of her necklaces out that are hanging towards the back of her closet and just start bringing them in like a present each time just in case I need a diversion away from her being sad.

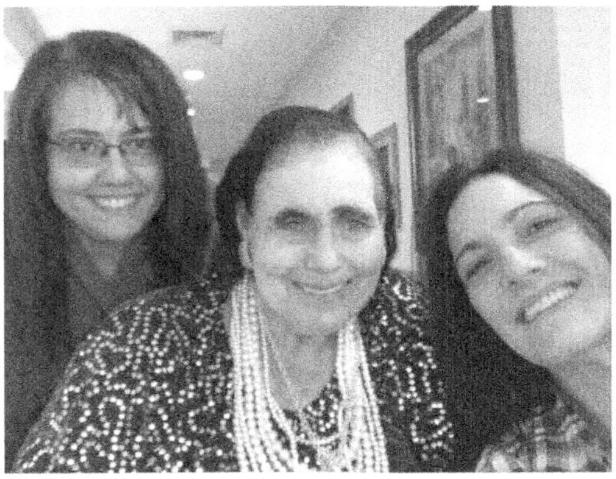

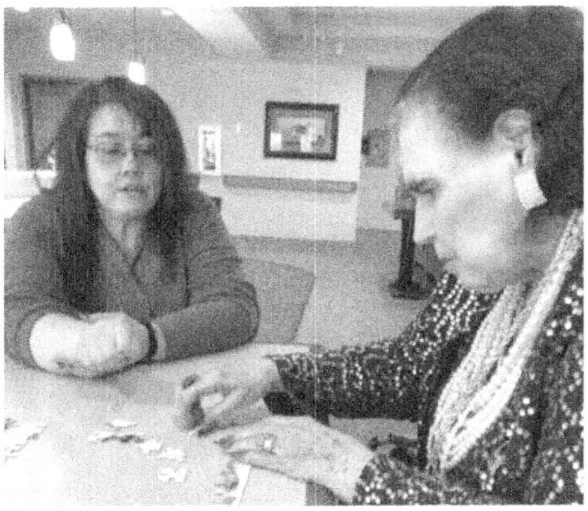

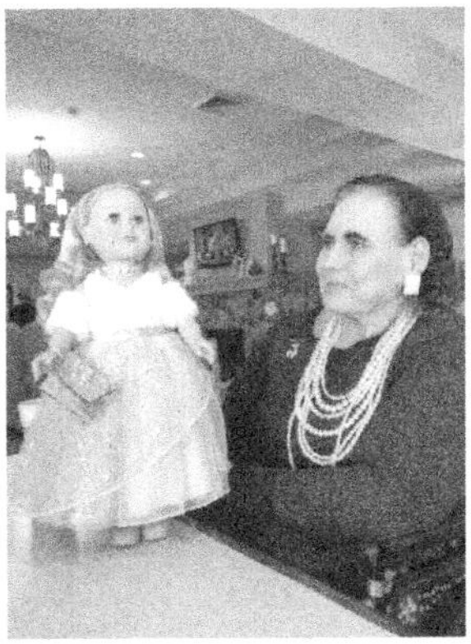

Mom Chronicles January 1, 2018

Happy New Year! Sheila and I are visiting Mom, and we are trying a new thing with her. Many later-stage Alzheimer's patients do well with a baby doll. We saw this one and decided to try it since it is so sparkly. We weren't sure if it would work since it wasn't a "baby," but she loves it so far. She's just staring at it and smiling and trying to show her off to everyone here. We will see if she continues to care for it over the next few days. We love that smile!!

Mom Chronicles January 3, 2018

Hi all, please say a little prayer for my stepdad. He is very close to meeting Jesus face-to-face, and while we rejoice in that fact, we also know that there are family members who will miss him. We have decided not to tell Mom and just let the natural progression of Alzheimer's allow her to forget. I don't want to upset her over and over when she can't remember that he is even ill. He made my mom very, very happy, and for that, I'm thankful he was in our lives.

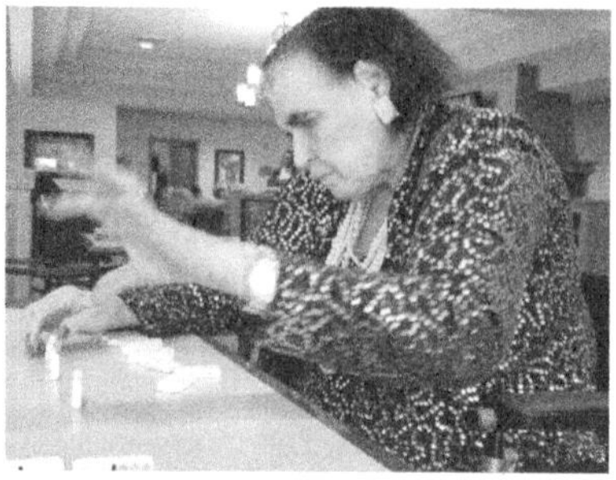

Mom Chronicles January 3, 2018
[Sheila's Post] I had a nice visit with Mom today. She playfully growled at me when I took a picture of her while she was organizing her dominoes. But, she was in a good mood and introduced me as her daughter, so it was a good day.

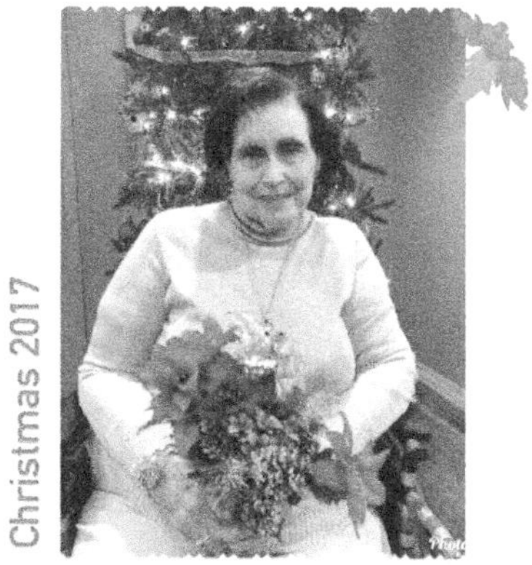

Mom Chronicles January 4, 2018
The activities director just shared Mom's Christmas picture with me. She looks so pretty! I added the date onto it for memory's sake.

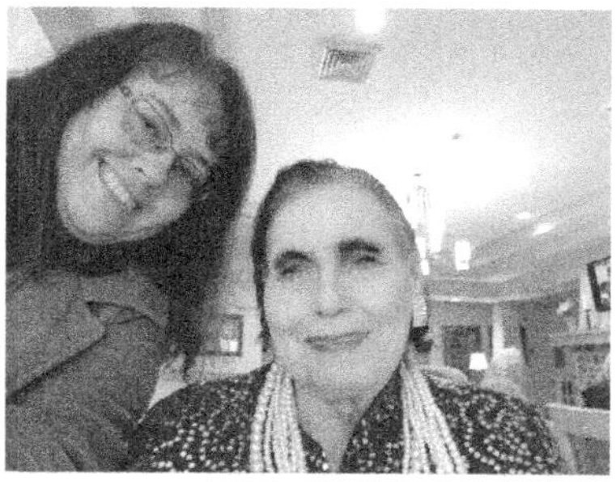

Mom Chronicles January 4, 2018
[Sheila's Post] This was a short but nice visit with Mom today. We tried playing "Go Fish," but it was a little hard for her. The cards had pictures of different fish with their names printed on them, but she couldn't read the words or say what the fish were. Luckily, there were numbers on the cards, so we used those. Lori also told me the center would be making ponchos out of blankets for the residents, so I bought a cute blanket for Mom's poncho.

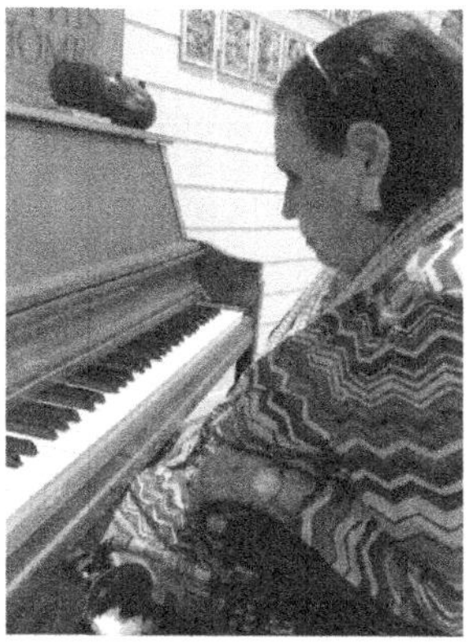

Mom Chronicles January 6, 2018
We stopped to visit for a few minutes, and this time we took her into the middle common room where there is a piano. The last time she played was at the rehab center about a year or so ago.

She only played just a few short minutes, and then the sparkly decorations for the upcoming 50's party grabbed her attention. Piano playing was over for the day!! She was happy today and had no mention of wanting to come home. Yay!!

Mom Chronicles January 7, 2018

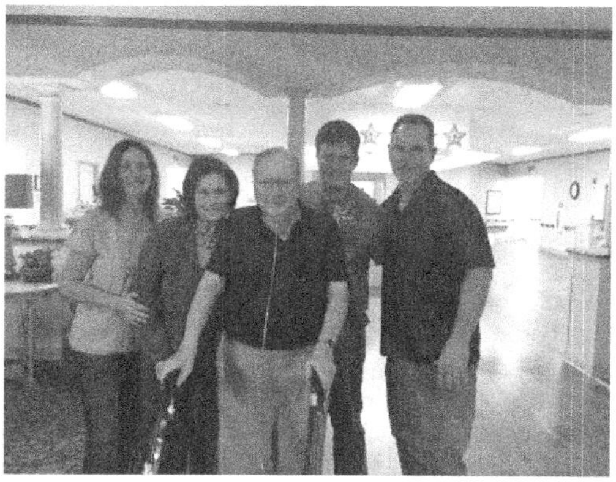

My stepdad passed away this morning just after 3:00 am. I talked to the nurse at the center about him, and she said eventually I would need to tell Mom, but she wouldn't remember. So, I'm going along with the same plan of not bringing his name up, and if she ever asks about him, I will tell her. She hasn't brought his name up in a couple of months, so I don't expect her to now, but you never know.

I'm grateful Mom and Ted were together for as long as they were. Mom did not have successful marriages in her life. Ted was the ONLY one who made her happy. I never heard a cross word about him at all from her. I don't know what his faith life was like before Mom, but she and Ted went to church regularly in California, allowing me to feel at peace that he is playing the guitar with Jesus right now. Robin said he used to sing with his mother as well. Mom and Ted would go dancing every week, and she loved to tell me how Ted would get up on stage and play and sing as well.

Ted was a wonderful "Grandpa" to Josh. Josh would visit them for weeks at a time in the summer when he was younger. He will be missed.

Mom Chronicles January 7, 2018

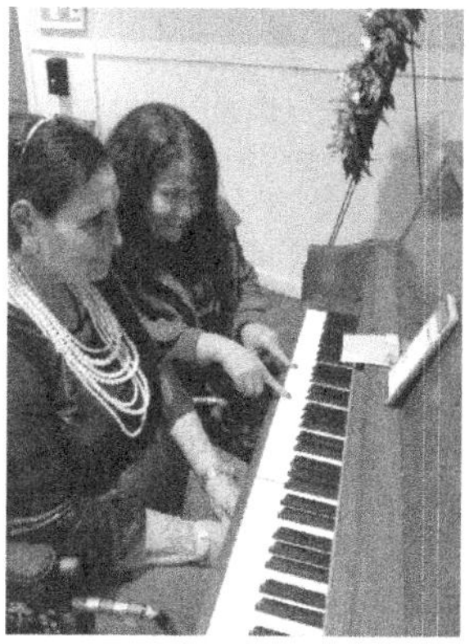

Sheila and Mom are trying to play the piano. Sheila is finding some YouTube videos to watch and listen to while they play. "Chopsticks" and "Mary Had a Little Lamb" were Mom's favorites. She still doesn't quite remember the basics, but she's smiling. She's trying to pull the memories from the deep recesses, but they just aren't coming through. I don't know if those brain cells are diseased now or if it's still possible to come through with some practice. We will keep trying!!

We finished out the visit with dominoes. Thankfully, there is no mention of Ted again, especially today.

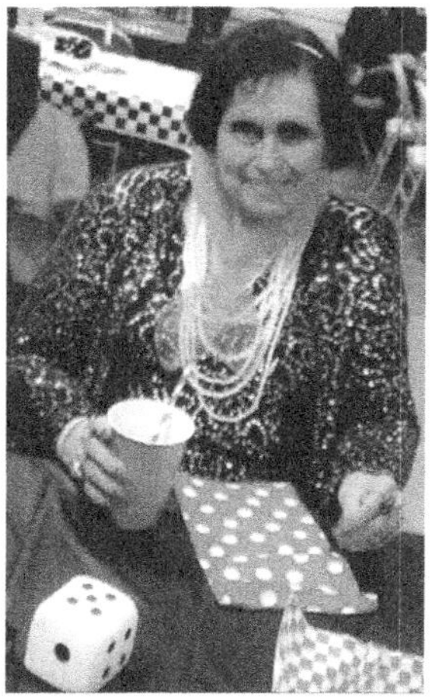

Mom Chronicles January 11, 2018

I wasn't able to attend the 50's Night Party at the center tonight, but Jenni, who is the director, shared this pic with me. Thank you, Jenni!!

Mom Chronicles January 12, 2018
Fridays are usually the best day for me to get Mom to the nail salon, so I went to the center to pick her up after work. As soon as I arrived there, I noticed she wasn't in the common area of her "house." So I went to her room, and she was sitting in her wheelchair in her birthday suit. I don't say this to embarrass her; I say this because it's just part of life with an Alzheimer's patient. I have been at the center before, and one of the residents just started to remove her shirt (no bra on underneath) in the dining room because she was hot. They just don't realize what they are doing.

The nurse aide and I were able to get her dressed so that I could take her to the nail salon. She was a little stressed at first but is better now that her nails are done.

It is getting harder and harder to get her to the salon. I will need to try to transition her away from the fake nails and just have her natural nails polished. I imagine this will be a struggle at first. Her natural nails haven't seen the light of day in over ten years or more!

Mom Chronicles January 12, 2018
We almost had a meltdown when I was leaving. I dropped her off in the dining area to eat her hamburger and then went to sign her back in at the center's front desk. When I got back to the dining area, I gave her a kiss and said I was about to go home. She got a panicked look in her eyes and said no, and then jumbled some words that meant she wanted to go too. I told her she was already home, and she said no, she wasn't. I asked if she knew where she was, and she said no. I then said I would take her to her room. She calmed down almost instantaneously and said, "ok. I know where I'm at." She was fine after that. I think taking her out of her routine just messes with her. (Which is probably another reason I need to keep from taking her to the nail salon again as she progresses further in this disease.) I probably should have stayed just a little longer, too, until she had her bearings straight. I will remember that next time if I take her out again.

It's moments like that which have me fighting back the tears in front of her. I just need to remember how she would calm my fears down when I was a little girl. To end this on a good note, she's eating a hamburger and drinking a soda. She's fine now!!

Mom Chronicles January 14, 2018
Momma was in a mischievous mood today. (Which is so "Marylin"!! When we had a CB radio back when Sheila and I were little, her handle was "Mischief Maker." I have always remembered that!! She would cut up and carry on with all the truckers and CB owners when we would drive back and forth to Ennis from Houston.)

So today, we put a 24-piece puzzle together first (puzzles are getting smaller now), and then I brought the dominoes out. I started turning them over, and she was going right behind me and turning them right side up-just a giggling the whole time. She said she needed to see them! We played one round together, and then she decided she needed to match them all herself instead of playing me. Playing against me just wasn't "in the cards" today. She had her own agenda!!

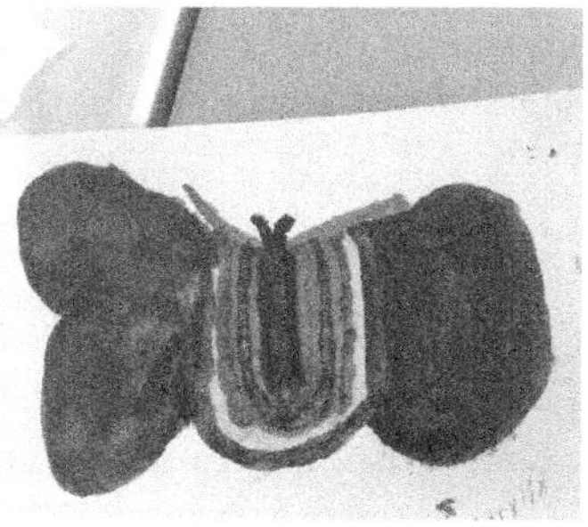

Mom Chronicles January 17, 2018
The lovely staff at the memory care center just shared this with me. Mom was busy this morning! They keep their residents active and engaged. This makes my heart smile!!

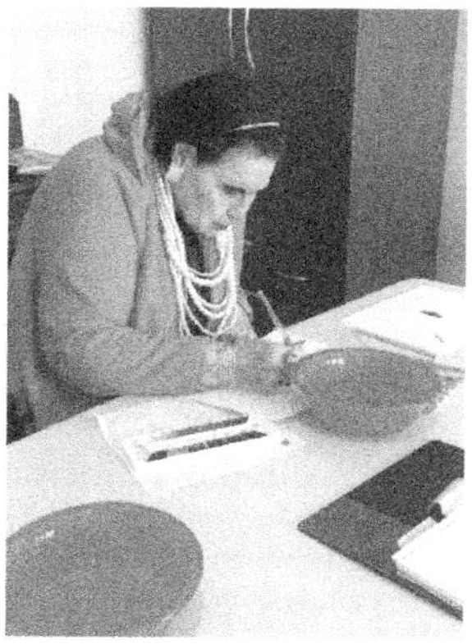

Mom Chronicles January 18, 2018
Bruce and I are at the center tonight at a training/support group type of meeting. I am learning so much! Here is one fantastic tip:

If your loved one is in a story cycle (meaning she is saying the same thing over and over again like a tape recorder rewinding and playing repeatedly), try interjecting a question at different parts of the story to "disrupt" her train of thought.

For example, the director told us how one resident would talk about how she lived in Australia in her past. In one of those "loops," she asked the resident, "is it true that the water in the toilet in Australia swirls the opposite direction?" Think of any question about that story loop that you can ask to redirect and put her on another thought "path."

Mom Chronicles January 19, 2018
Here are a couple more tips I learned last night at the memory care event:

1) some dementias cause hallucinations. If that happens, don't argue with them and tell them it's not there. In their reality, it IS there. Just acknowledge it and then redirect. For example, the director told us of a person who wouldn't go to the dinner table because she saw a bull outside the window. She was afraid the bull was going to attack them. The director said she told her it was okay to eat dinner and that she would stand watch at the window and make sure it didn't attack them or that she would call the authorities to come and get it. Another instance was a lady not wanting to get into bed one night. She was seeing a baby lying on her bed, and she didn't know what to do. The caregiver pretended to pick up the baby and hold it so that the lady could get into bed. The resident was relieved because she didn't know how to get into bed without disturbing the baby.

2) another great tip is that it takes longer for a dementia patient's brain to process a question asked and answer it. We can process a question quickly with a normal brain, and our mouth, vocal cords, etc., can spit the answer out quickly. For a patient with dementia, it could take several minutes for the brain to process the question and deliver an answer. We need to give time for the patient to process the question and try not to move on to the next subject until she can answer. If we repeat the question, it is also essential to NOT rephrase the question. Ask the SAME question with the SAME words to help with the brain process. Also - try to keep the question down to 5-7 words. Keep it short and sweet.

And you all know I try to put humor in these stories as much as possible, so here goes my attempt at a bit of laughter today. If I get Alzheimer's in my future, which is a very real possibility with the family history, and IF I have a hallucination about a big ole potato head staring at me, you can just tell me to rearrange its face and put the eyes in one of the ear slots so that it is gazing in the other room instead of straight ahead at me. So, Josh/Bruce/Sheila – are you getting all of this???? (And oh, my goodness, when I was looking for the perfect potato head image, I found several new potato heads that I DON'T have! I want them!!!) Have a fantastic day, peeps!!

♥

To interject here… I have a vast collection of potato heads (almost 100 different ones) currently in storage, waiting until we have a home again where I can display them. I just LOVE all the different potato head characters they have created over the years!

Mom Chronicles January 19, 2018
As I mentioned yesterday, Bruce and I went to the center last night to go through a simulation of what it is like to be a dementia patient. I found a video clip that is very similar to what we experienced: the soundtrack, the goggles, the gloves, the shoe inserts, everything. The tasks were similar too. It was very eye-opening.

Bruce was the last to go through it, and I can tell you it was tough on him. He almost had a PTSD attack from it that we weren't expecting him to experience. His time in Iraq a few years ago came to the surface. He tried to calm himself down, but we ended up having to leave a little early.

This simulation was eye-opening because if it did this to a "normal" person, what are our loved ones experiencing every day? It's no wonder they have panic attacks so often!!

Here is a news clip by ABC News Nightline, shared by Second Wind Dreams, that I found that shows what we experienced in the simulation. Different room, different people obviously but the "experience" was the same. And when we debriefed afterward, no two people had the same experience. (Second Wind Dreams, n.d.)

https://youtu.be/QEmBmokHU3Q

Mom Chronicles January 20, 2018
Cat Zultner... thank you!!! Mom loved her new jewelry!

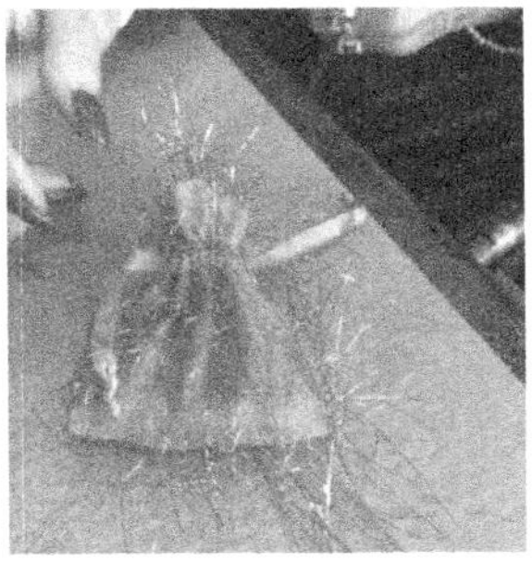

Mom Chronicles January 22, 2018
I'm home sick today, so I'm indulging in the soap operas I don't get to watch anymore. On "Young and the Restless," they have an Alzheimer's storyline. The scene they just did hits soooo close to home. I just want to cry because it's so true. Jack, the son, told his mom that he was going to miss her. The mother (who has Alzheimer's in this story) told her son they would meet again in this universe. Ugh, another dagger to my heart, even though it is so true. I know that I will meet my Mom again in full, picture-perfect health: mind, body, and soul someday. I have that personal faith and belief. I will not visit her this week because I don't want to get her sick. I know she doesn't remember when I visit, but it makes me feel better when I do. She usually greets me like she hasn't seen me in years, and I love bringing that instant joy to her, even if it is only for a few minutes.

Mom Chronicles January 23, 2018
So apparently, Mom is acting persnickety when being rolled into the restroom. Last night, I received a message from the director asking if I could pick up a flashy shower curtain and maybe some wall hangings for the bathroom. Mom holds her arms out and grabs the door frame to keep from being rolled into the bathroom. We hope that having something flashy in the bathroom will draw her attention in there so that she won't fight it so much.

I'm still home sick today, so I just spent some time online trying to find the perfect things for her bathroom. They should be delivered in a couple of days. By then, I'm hoping I won't be contagious so that I can get everything placed. I hope this does the trick! There were matching floor rugs, but those are major trip hazards, so I didn't get those.

Mom Chronicles January 23, 2018
https://www.dementia-directive.org/
I'm sharing this from the director of Mom's facility. It's a difficult thing to think about, but it is absolutely necessary! This is an advanced directive where you can share your wishes if you experience dementia.
(A Simple Way to Document the Medical Care, n.d.)

Mom Chronicles January 28, 2018
We put the new shower curtain up and gold butterflies on the wall of the bathroom. Mom loved them! Only time will tell if this solves the problem. Fingers crossed that it works!

Sheila and I tried the game "Trouble" with her today. She struggled with it. We thought the counting would make it easy, but it wasn't. So we switched back to dominoes, and she was much happier. We even had one of the other ladies sit in with us to play for a bit. She was in a great mood, and we had a really good visit.

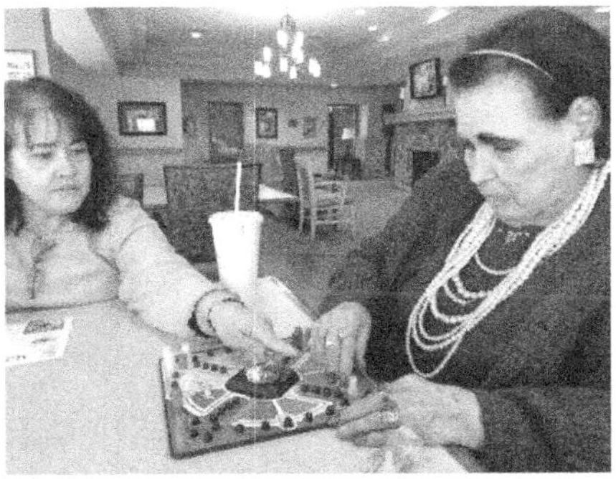

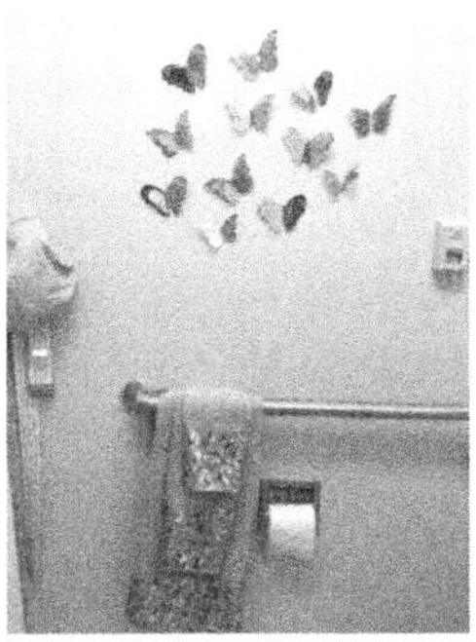

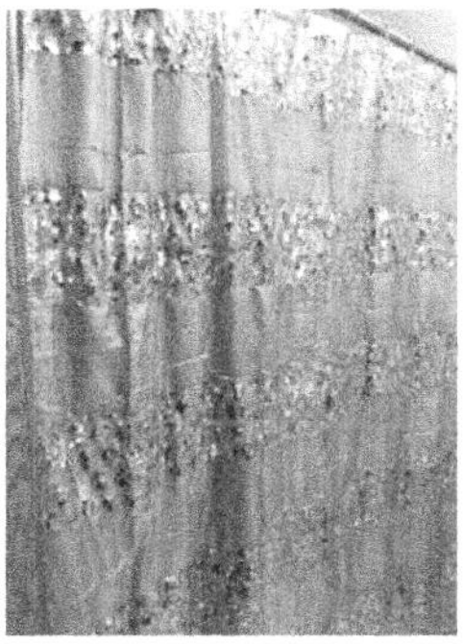

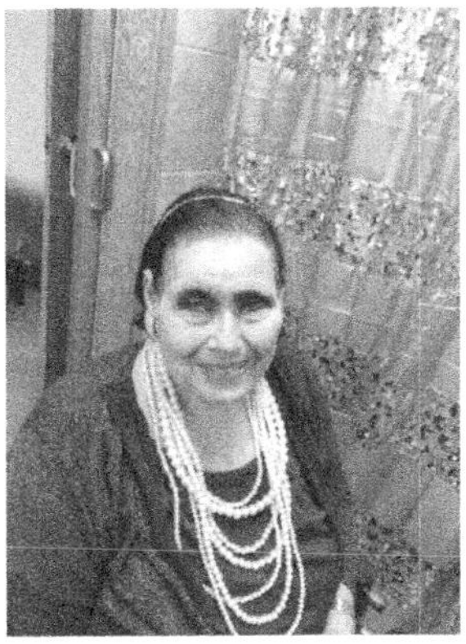

Mom Chronicles January 31, 2018
Mom was in an unusual mood tonight. She ran from one end of the spectrum to the other. When I first got there, she hugged me tight and said she missed me so much. Then she got giddy and said to come and look at something new in her room. She wanted to show me her new shower curtain and butterflies in the bathroom. She had forgotten that we are the ones who brought it to her. I started recording her, and then she kind of remembered that we had fixed up her room. She saw a gold scarf (that I think Miss Janet had given her) on her lampshade and wanted to know if we could put it in

the bathroom too. We convinced her it would be better if she wore it instead, so that's exactly what she did. She pretended to model it and say, "woohoo."

The activities' director came in and asked if she was feeling better. Apparently, her legs were hurting pretty bad earlier today, so she didn't want to get her hair done.

We went back to the dining area to visit before they served dinner. She kept repositioning her wheelchair so that she could get as close to me as possible. She kept telling me over and over how much she loved me. She almost started crying. I redirected her real quick to get her laughing.

I stayed while she ate dinner. I was about to leave when they served her food, but she begged me to stay - so I did. I noticed she had a few issues with managing bite-size pieces of her food. I may need to start coming up at dinner time more often to help her. We will see - I'll take this a day at a time. The staff there must help quite a few with their dinner, so having an extra set of hands there may help. She was feeling better by the time I left. I think she just wasn't feeling good, which may be why she was a little more emotional tonight.

Mom Chronicles February 4, 2018
They had music time for the residents today. Mom knew the tunes but struggled with the words. She did her best on the "Let me call you sweetheart" song. It's so cute to watch the residents recognize a song and try to sing it.

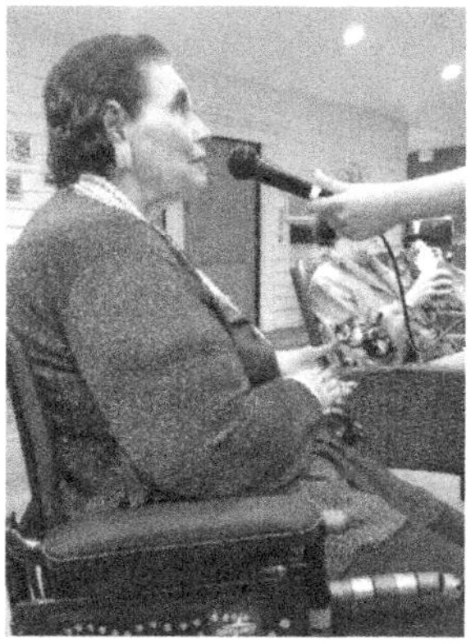

Mom Chronicles February 10, 2018
There will be another post later, but right now, I'm struggling. I mentioned to Mom that we talked to Kathy (my brother's first wife) yesterday. She asked who Tommy was. She doesn't remember my brother. They didn't have a good relationship, but she remembered him a few months ago. It's only a matter of time before she forgets who Sheila and I are. I'm fighting the tears right now. I'm not looking for sympathy - just sharing the raw emotions that come with Alzheimer's. It sucks. (I know that's not a nice word.)

Mom Chronicles February 10, 2018
If you remember about a month ago, I took Mom to get her nails done at a local salon. When I brought her back to the center, she had a brief panic attack of not knowing where she was and not wanting me to leave her. At that point, I decided not to take her out of the home again because it is too disruptive to her routine. I still needed to figure out what to do about her nails, though.

My friend, Monica Munoz, introduced me to her friend, who is a Color Street Consultant. The consultant met me up at Mom's today to walk me through how to place the color strips on Mom's nails. So far, Mom is happy. She is a little disconcerted about two of the fingernails that we covered. The original NextGen nails had popped off this past week, so the nails were shorter. We think once we have all the NextGen nails off and they are the same length, she may feel better. But all in all, she was happy. She loved the purple sparkly color that we picked. They are supposed to last about two weeks, so we will see how it goes for her. Fingers crossed!

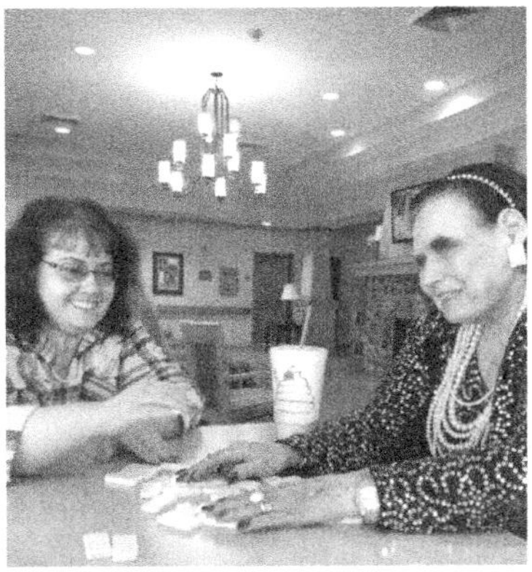

Mom Chronicles February 11, 2018
We are having a good visit so far. Sheila is here, and we are playing dominoes. I also brought Simi for a visit. Simi kept licking Mom's nose, making her giggle.

Mom Chronicles February 11, 2018
[Sheila's Post] I visited with Mom for a while today. We munched on a hamburger and played dominoes. Mom kept blocking me (unintentionally) on one of the rounds and had a good laugh about it.

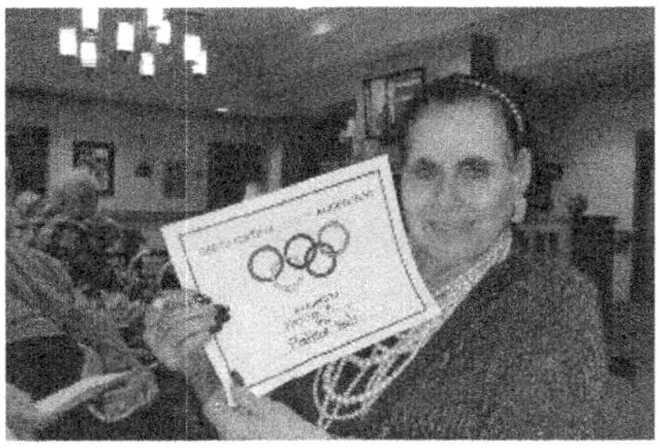

Later one of the workers came by and gave her a certificate that said she had the prettiest nails. Of course, she just beamed when she got that and showed it off to her fellow housemates.

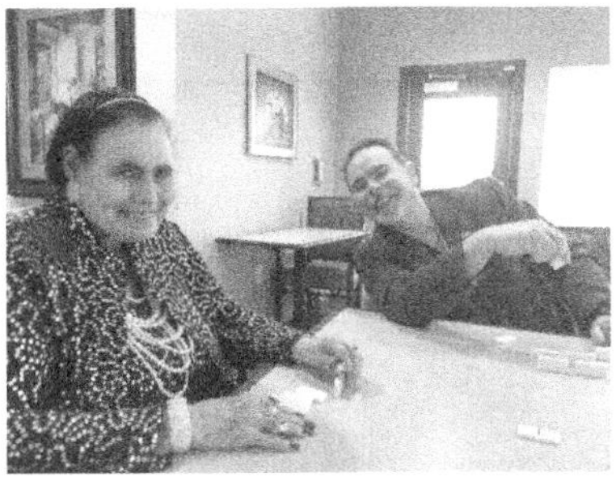

Mom Chronicles February 18, 2018
After church, Bruce and I visited Mom. She was happy to see us as usual. While playing dominoes, we noticed she has a cough that sounds like it is in her chest. I sent a message to the director to have them watch her. Also, one of the aides said she would make a note for the doctor to order a chest x-ray on her tomorrow. I just know how quickly this could turn into something serious at her age.

Mom Chronicles February 19, 2018
I stopped by Mom's after work to check on her cough. The director had messaged me earlier to say they hadn't heard her cough today, and her chest sounded fine, but I'm a worrier, so I had to see for myself. Sure enough, she only coughed one time, so hopefully, she is not getting sick. However, she did promise me they would keep an eye on her. I need to "let it go" and know they are taking the absolute best care of her. The director has been fantastic with answering all my questions lately. I'm so grateful we found this home.

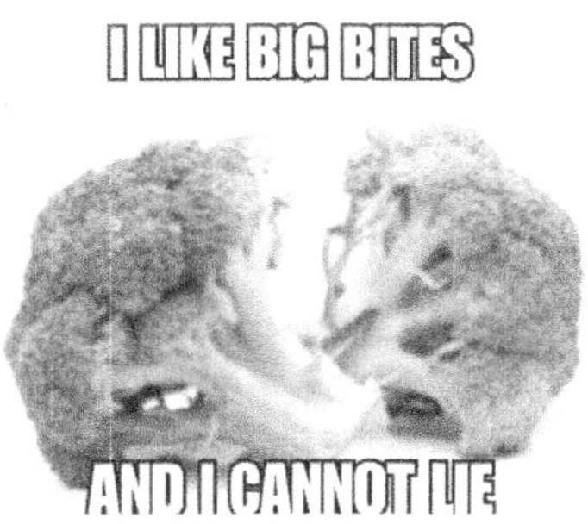

I stayed with Mom while she was eating dinner. I wanted to see how she was doing with feeding herself. She does not understand how to cut her food into bite-size pieces. She picked up a large stalk of broccoli and put the whole thing in her mouth. I'm okay with picking items up with her fingers. I'm just more concerned about the large amount of food she's putting in her mouth. With the lasagna, she didn't understand how to portion a bite-size piece out with her fork. She treated it like layers and pulled the entire piece of pasta off the top, and then put the whole piece in her mouth. I asked if I could cut her food up for her. She said sure. Once I did, she was able to eat much easier. Then when she decided to drink her juice and water, she treated it like soup. She was taking sips with a spoon. I remember her doing this several times when she lived with us.

I sent a message to the director (thank goodness she has a lot of patience with me!) and asked if she could use a cup with a lid or straw and if the staff could help cut up her food. She's not at the stage where she needs to be fed by someone else, but I think these steps would help her.

*Update- the director is fantastic and has already replied. She will ask the doctor to put in an order to have the kitchen staff chop her food up before it comes out to Mom. I can also bring in a couple of dishwasher-safe cups with lids/straws, but I must sign a document saying it's okay for Mom to use different dinnerware. Apparently, the state is very picky about that. So, you guessed it - I'm going to look for a sparkly cup!!

To end with a good note, she asked me how Sheila was when I got there. This is a big deal because she can't remember our names most of the time even though she still knows who we are. So the fact that she just pulled her name out of the air was fantastic!!!

So... enjoy the graphic! As I was commiserating today with a co-worker (Myra Scrabeck) going through something similar with her mother, we have both agreed that "life is an adventure!" Live it the best way you can!!! Keep your sense of humor, peeps. It helps!!

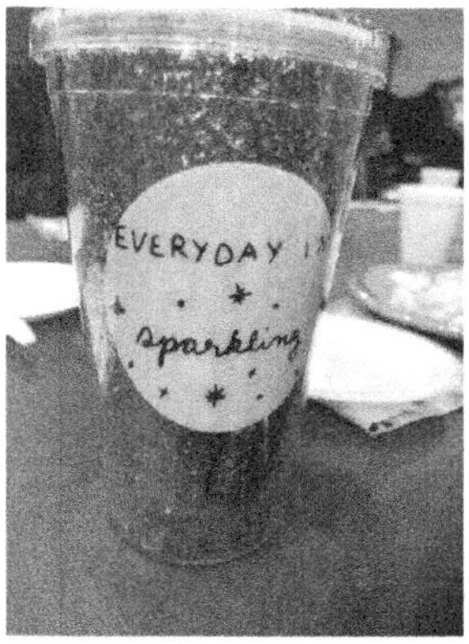

Mom Chronicles February 22, 2018
This post will be a long one. Divine intervention allowed me to see Mom tonight, and I was glad I was there. First of all, I had bought some new cups for her that had a straw or a lid with a slot to drink from because of the experience a few days ago where she tried to drink her juice like soup. I got permission to get these cups for her, and they came in today, so I wanted to drop them off at the center. Divine intervention.

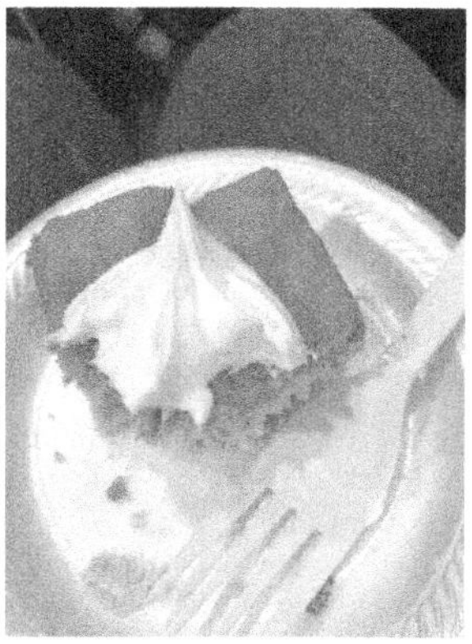

As soon as I got there, she looked like she was unhappy or not feeling well. She was not smiling and bubbly to see me. She was eating dinner and did not like the chicken with barbecue sauce. The kitchen staff kindly went back to get chicken without the BBQ sauce. While waiting for the chicken, the aide gave her a piece of cake. She gobbled that up. The chicken arrived, and the aide was sweet enough to give me a piece of cake too. Mom saw that and gave me the serious stink eye. I asked her if she wanted it, and she said yes. I told her to eat her chicken, and then I would give it to her. (Role reversal here!! Ha!)

She finished her chicken, and then I handed the cake to her. Unfortunately, she started having one of her mucus attacks. She hasn't had one since she first moved in there. When she has one of these, she immediately goes into a full-blown panic attack. That's precisely what happened tonight.

We took her into another room and worked with her to calm her down. The nurse brought her the over-the-counter mucus medicine, and then we just kept reassuring her that she could breathe. When she finally got to a point where she could breathe a little more between coughing fits, I turned on her music playlist. That started to get her attention. As she calmed down more, I did a Google search for Elvis and pulled up images of him. With the music playing, she started tapping her fingernail on each picture. She started with trying to count (1,2, 1, 2, 1, 2, 3, gibberish, 1, 2, 1, 2). Then she started saying the word "him" on each picture as she tapped it. It was almost in a frenzied way. It's hard to explain. Then she saw a picture of Elvis and

Marilyn Monroe and asked if they were still together. I told her I didn't think so. Then she saw an image that said he had died. She asked me if he died, and I said yes. Then I just kept scrolling down the pictures. Finally, after 30 more minutes, I was able to get her completely calmed down and singing and dancing (in her wheelchair) to Elvis. Her lyrics were gibberish, but she knew the tunes.

When I left, I gave her that piece of cake that she originally gave me the stink eye over. She was happily eating while I left the center.

Divine intervention.

Mom Chronicles February 23, 2018

Tonight was another emotional roller coaster. So, some of you know that I have an older brother. He is seven years older than me and is from my mom's first marriage. For the last 12 years, we all have had an estranged relationship. I venture to guess many families have had issues before. I won't go into the details of ours.

Until a few months ago, Mom's memories of him have been on the last negative experience she had with him, so I decided not to find him to let him know about her Alzheimer's. I always felt bad about it, but I needed to protect her and keep her from getting upset.

A couple of weeks ago, she didn't remember she had a son, so the Christian part of me started praying about what I should do. I wondered if I should find him. I wasn't sure if he even wanted to see her at all. I often prayed over it because my mom's health, mental and physical, is the most important thing to me. I just wasn't sure what the right thing to do was. And to be honest, I wasn't sure I was ready to see him either. I know, I know… that was very selfish of me.

God answered my prayer in the way only He knows how to do. My brother's wife found my Facebook profile and Mom Chronicles. They found where Mom lived, and she encouraged him to visit Mom. So I got a message from the director saying that he was there visiting her tonight.

As you can imagine, I panicked. I wasn't sure how Mom was going to handle it. I got up there as fast as I could, and the sight I beheld was beautiful. He had her in the common area and was playing the piano for her. (My brother has a gift with music and can play many instruments.) The aides said that they both cried when they saw each other for the first time. He held her hands several times. She recognized his face, but his hair was throwing her off. At first, I had to tell her he was her son a couple of times, and then I think she finally got it. Since she was crying, according to the aide, I think she knew deep down he was her son.

We visited for a while. He said he is going to start visiting her as much as he can. He is a truck driver now and comes through Dallas every week. His challenge will be finding a place to park the truck and trailer without being towed. Apparently, lots of places will tow the rigs if they are parked illegally.

Yes, there are still some healings that need to be done on all sides. My sister has yet to see him. But it's a start. If anything, Mom and my brother have closure now. God decided to allow reconciliation to happen once Mom forgot about the negative feelings she had for him. Alzheimer's can be a blessing in some instances.

♥

Unfortunately, my brother never visited Mom again. I don't know his reasons, and that's okay. Closure for my mom happened on that night, and any further reconciliation can happen in Heaven.

Mom Chronicles February 25, 2018

Sheila and I are visiting her this afternoon. She's in a great mood today. First, we played a few rounds of dominoes, and then it was time for dinner. The staff served spaghetti today, and she actually remembered how to cut her food using her fork today. A few days ago, she couldn't remember how to cut her food into bite-size pieces. This disease is just so crazy. She can remember things one moment and then forget the next. And then it comes back in glimpses. Just crazy.

She was acting silly too. I caught a picture just in time when she had the breadstick sticking out of her mouth. She was giggling and giggling.

The picture of the apples is artwork she has done here. They had an art show here yesterday showcasing the residents' art. If I could have found a couple of her paintings in the storage unit, I could have brought those up here.

***I added one last photo. She wanted every single drop of that pudding!! Great visit today!

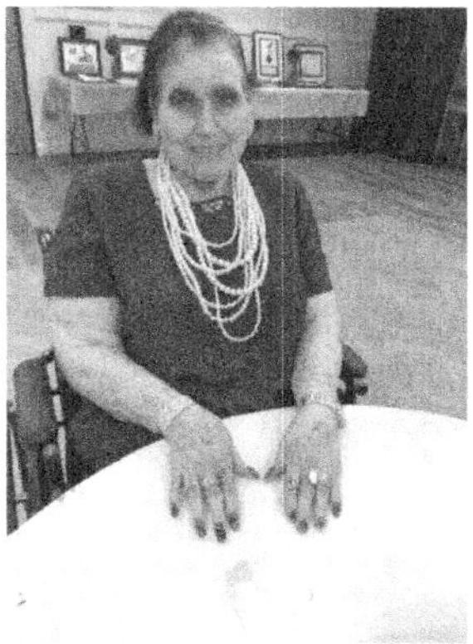

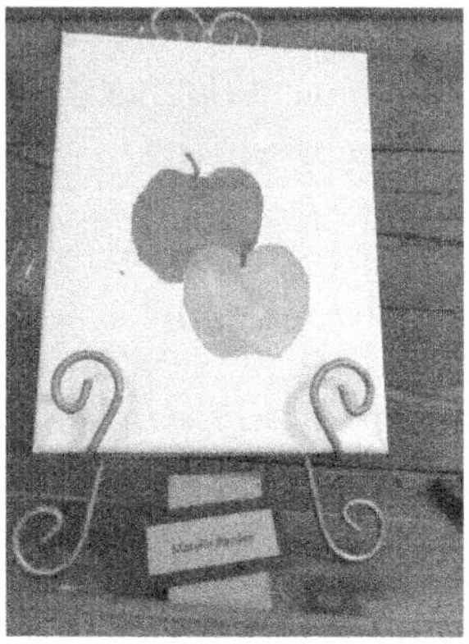

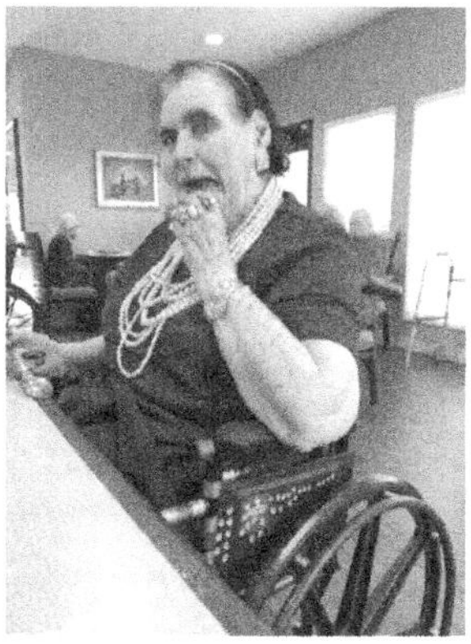

Mom Chronicles February 26, 2018

I had bought Mom some more incontinence products but in 2 different sizes because I just wasn't sure which size was best. The aides helped me determine the correct size for her, and today at lunch, I went to the UPS store to return the rest. The name of the company is "Wearever Incontinence." The clerk read the company name out really loud (first embarrassment), and then he asked what was inside the box. I guess that is something they must do, but I ALMOST was a sarcastic little turkey by answering "jellybeans." I refrained (but I was screaming it mentally!) and responded by saying, "Ummm... incontinence products". (Second embarrassment). What else would be in there with that name of a company?????

Why oh, why did I pick a time to do this when the store was full??

So, how is YOUR day going????

Mom Chronicles March 4, 2018

Bruce is helping Mom to laugh today by being a crazy wheelchair driver!

Mom Chronicles March 8, 2018
Where do I start? Warning: long post.
Now that I live further away, I decided to visit Mom after work today (on a Thursday) because, you know, Survivor night is Wednesday night, and I just can't miss Survivor. I knew I would be staying until 6:30 or 7:00 because I didn't want to fight rush hour traffic.

I had received a call this afternoon from the Life Engagement Director saying that Mom needed some socks. I had forgotten to buy her some more when she told me that she didn't have any socks a few weeks ago. Apparently, her socks sprouted feet and walked away. More than likely, she threw them away. Also, her gel nails have finally all fallen off, and it was upsetting her. The director painted her nails to try and calm her a little bit, which I am extremely grateful to her for doing this. After work, I stopped at a store to buy more socks, and I bought a pretty, pink sparkly nail polish, just in case I needed to do an intervention with Mom.

Once I arrived, she was sitting in front of the TV, and you could tell she was emotional and not happy. I took her into her room and showed her the new socks and nail polish. I also pulled out a gold sequin pillow that I had purchased back in January. I had kept it in the trunk of the car, waiting for an emotional day when I knew I would need something to help redirect her. Today was that day. It helped.

I then proceeded to work on her fingers and toes with the new nail polish. There is nothing like giving your mother a pedicure! Gnarly!!! We had the Elvis playlist going, so the music combined with getting pretty, pink sparkly nail polish on both toes and fingers got her back into a good mood.

Then… it happened. I was about to leave, and the aide came in saying it was time for her shower. She asked me if I would stay because Mom still fights them and tries to hit them when it's time for a shower. She said Mom might be a little calmer if I'm there. Well, I stayed. Mom fought it, crying and screaming the whole time. She didn't hit us, though. The aide asked me if I could come for every shower to help try to keep Mom a little calmer. I think they give her two showers a week. I know one is Thursdays, but I'm not exactly sure what other day she is showered. I will go ahead and just plan on being at the center every Thursday night to help. I'll just pack a change of clothes and shoes so that I don't get my good clothes from work wet from the shower. Hopefully, I can get them to shower her a little earlier than seven so that I don't have to stay as late. It was 8:00 pm before I was able to leave.

After we showered Mom, I brought the sequin pillow out again and played another Elvis song to put her back in a good mood again. She was exhausted, so I put her in bed and tucked her in for the night, promising I would be back on Saturday. Hopefully, she gets a good night's sleep.

On the way home, I allowed myself to tear up for just a minute and then wiped them away. It's just another day in this crazy world of Alzheimer's.

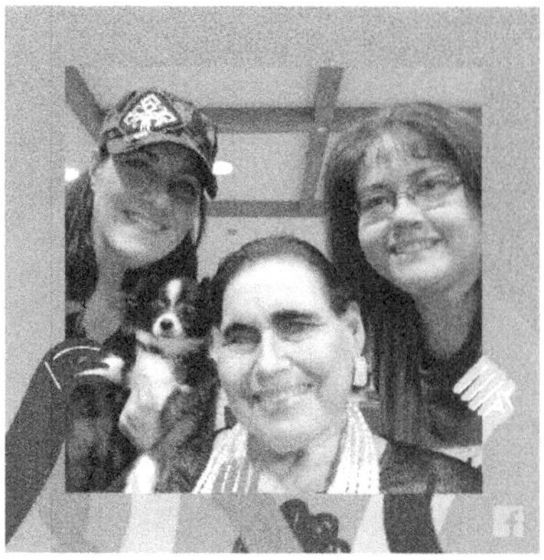

Mom Chronicles March 8, 2018
[Sheila's post.] The two most important people in the world to me. Love y'all.

Mom Chronicles March 9, 2018
Let me tell you how amazing the center is! First of all, the director was willing to be friends with me on Facebook, so as a result, she sees my "Mom Chronicles" and can see the family's side of her residents. I try very hard not to abuse the relationship because she needs her personal life away from work, but she has been absolutely wonderful with an open-door policy.

After reading last night's post, she talked to the new nurse on staff, and they came up with some ideas they are going to try with Mom. There is a video training the nurse purchased immediately that shows how to shower dementia patients, so she will train the staff as soon as it comes in. She also had other ideas to try as well. She mentioned that they would do everything they could to let me be the "daughter" and not the caregiver since that is their job. I appreciated that so much. I'm always willing to help make Mom as comfortable as possible, but I love just being her daughter and enjoying the visits. It hurts my soul to see Mom unhappy and scared at times - that's my "mommy." The caregivers know this is the disease and can put aside the personal side of the job and care for their patients in a loving, caring way. I try, but it's just harder for the family.

Mom Chronicles March 10, 2018
Mom was in a great mood today! Sheila added some gemstones to Mom's fingernails, and then we played dominoes for a little while. I brought Simi with us, so she enjoyed seeing her.

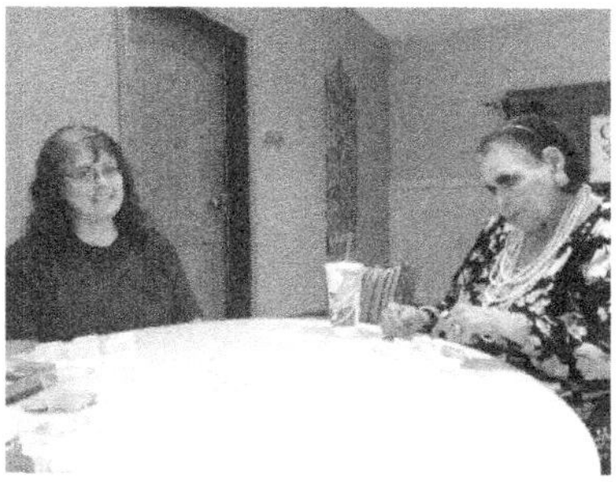

There is another resident there who wanted to hold Simi, so I let her. Mistake!! She almost didn't give her back to me. I was afraid she was going to hurt Simi by not letting me take her back. I know she wouldn't have intentionally hurt her, but she was very strong and didn't want to let her go. So I won't let her hold her again!! The residents always love to see Simi when I bring her. There's just something about animals that they love!

Mom Chronicles March 15, 2018
A friend just shared a study with me called "Spending More Time with Your Mom Will Help Her Live Longer." These were great words of advice! Loneliness can be so hard on people of any age! I'm grateful for the center because Mom has many new friends to help combat loneliness. I have heard more and more that she's refusing to participate in activities, but I imagine they are doing everything they can to encourage her. The article also mentioned laughter. I act like a total goofball with my mom just to get her to laugh. That's usually when she says "I love you" the most. And laughter is great for anyone! Josh deals with depression - I know he won't mind me briefly mentioning this because he wants to help others dealing with it too - but

when I see him "cycling down," I try to act like a total goofball with him too to get him to laugh. It helps for those few moments.

Fill your life with family, friends, and laughter as much as possible!!!

Mom Chronicles March 17, 2018
She's in a great mood today!!

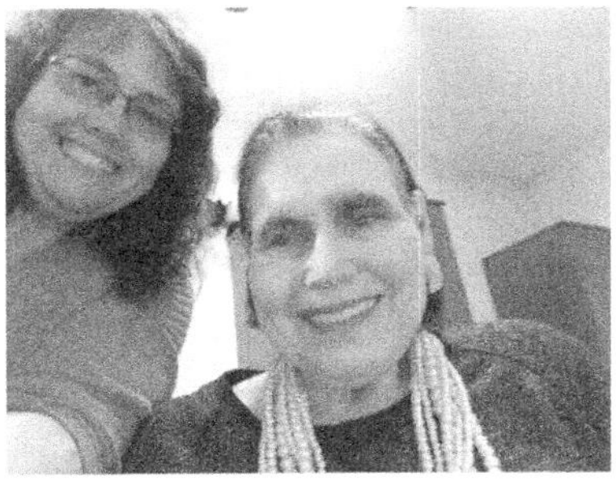

Mom Chronicles March 17, 2018
[Sheila's Post] This was from last Sunday. She wanted to stay in her room that day, so we ate cookies, and she talked about her pictures on the wall. We also looked through her photo albums. I was finally able to talk her into going out in the "living room" and visit with her friends when I had to leave.

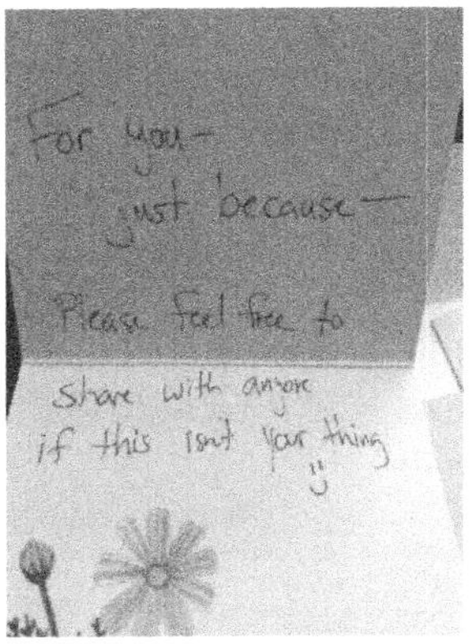

Mom Chronicles March 19, 2018
I work with some of the best people around. I came back from lunch, and this was sitting on my desk. There was no name from the gift giver. I can only assume it is a friend also on FB since this is where I share my family's Alzheimer's journey. So, thank you from the bottom of my heart to the sweet person who brightened my day!

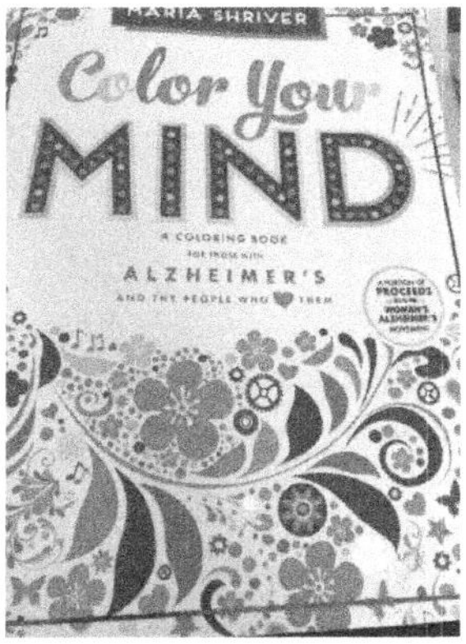

Mom Chronicles March 20, 2018
This one isn't about Mom today. It's about some tips/tricks to help those of you dealing with a Loved One (LO) with Alzheimer's. I spoke with a friend this evening about her mother, and we chatted about some ideas to help her with some changes that have come about in the past few weeks. Her mother has started saying she wants to see or talk to her mother. Her mother has been gone for over 13 years if I remember correctly. The natural thing to do is try to correct them, but in an Alzheimer's mind, it's the truest thing ever, and you can't convince them otherwise. Correcting them only causes agitation. My friend knew this, and she has taught her kids just to redirect whenever possible. (But we are all human and CAN get very tired and want to correct them. It's natural and if it happens, forgive yourself and then find a moment to compose yourself. Your LO has already (or will very soon) forget that you lost your cool!!

This LO also was wanting a phone number to call her mom. So we came up with this idea - Bruce and I have an iPad that has a phone # attached to it for the data plan. The # doesn't take calls but gives a message saying the "person you are trying to reach is not taking calls at this time." So when her LO is adamant about wanting a phone number to call her mother, they can give this number to appease her at the moment. We also chatted about being out in public with a LO. What do you do when the LO is acting strange or saying things that you know just aren't true? Keep some little cards in your purse/wallet that explain your LO has Alzheimer's. I learned that one in one of the blogs I follow. I have used that a few times with Mom over the years. You can buy business card templates at a department store or office supply store and create them with your computer.

I'm keeping my friend's name off the post because I want to respect her privacy, and I didn't ask her if I could share her name, but these are great topics to chat about, and I hope the tips can help someone out there that is going through something similar.

Love and hugs, peeps. As I try to say often - it's not one day at a time - it's one moment at a time!

Mom Chronicles March 22, 2018
She is tickled tonight with that gold pillow. I think that "gift' is a big success. I love hearing her laugh! Oh... and forgive her 4-letter word!!

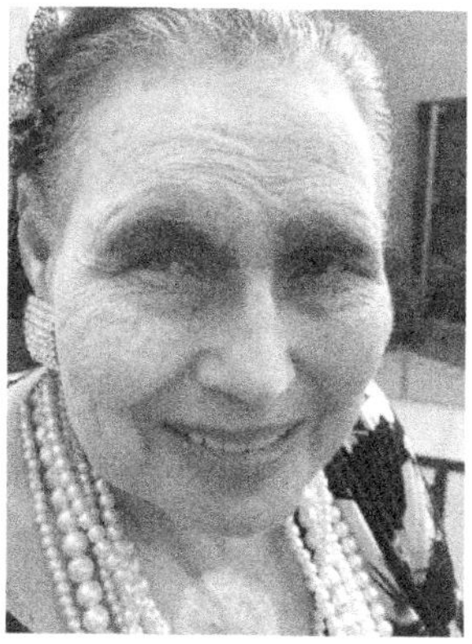

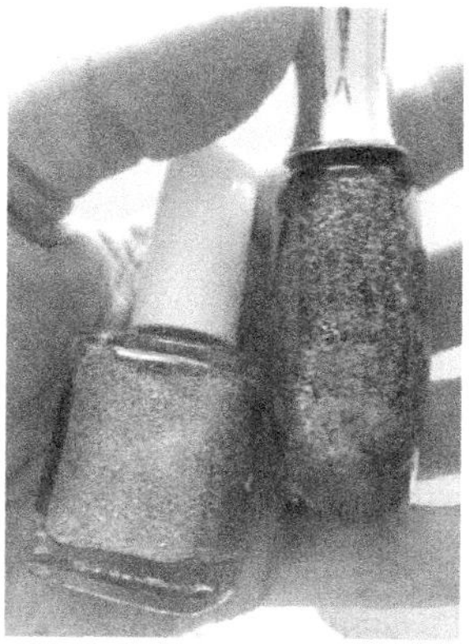

Mom Chronicles March 24, 2018
I'm here for a short visit with Mom, and as soon as I saw her, I notice that her eyelids are more sparkly than usual. I took her to her room to show her some new goodies (sparkly headbands and a hair clip), and she showed me her new "eye shadow." It was the nail polish I had bought a few weeks ago. She decided today that it was eye shadow. Yikes! I'm not quite sure how we are going to get this off her eyelids.

Needless to say, I have already snuck the bottles into my purse to go back home with me. It just goes to show you can't assume Alzheimer's patients know what everyday items are anymore.

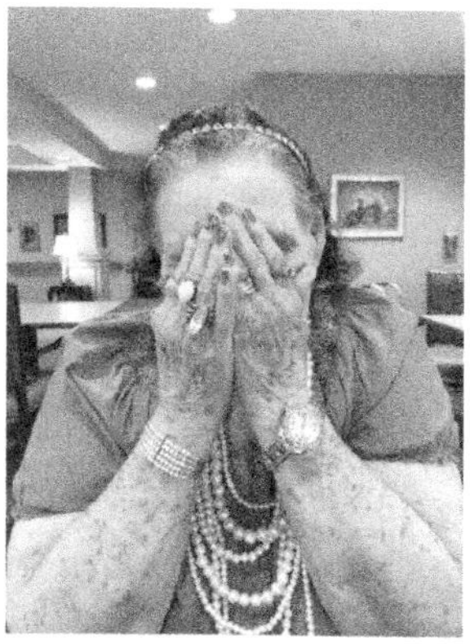

Mom Chronicles Mar 28, 2018
Mom was upset when I arrived at the center because apparently, someone had taken her nail polish off and put stick-on nail wraps today. She had peeled them all off and was not happy at all.

Luckily, I had the new color strips we purchased a few months ago, so I put those on her nails. They should last longer and not be easy to peel off. She was happy afterward.

After that, we played some dominoes. After a few rounds, one of Mom's friends wheeled herself over, and we added her into the game. It was a fun challenge trying to explain how to play to both of them. Mom's friend had a little tougher time because she hasn't played in a long time (if ever) and was having trouble recognizing the color of the dots and the number of dots. She focused more on the colors vs. the number of the dots. Mom gets focused on the larger doubles. I can say "play the double 2," and by golly, if she has the double 5 or 6, she's going to play that instead!! They still wanted to play when it was time for me to go, so I left the dominoes there. There is absolutely no telling how the games went after I left. Oh, to be a fly on the wall with two ladies who can barely communicate and Mom pouting if she doesn't get her way!!

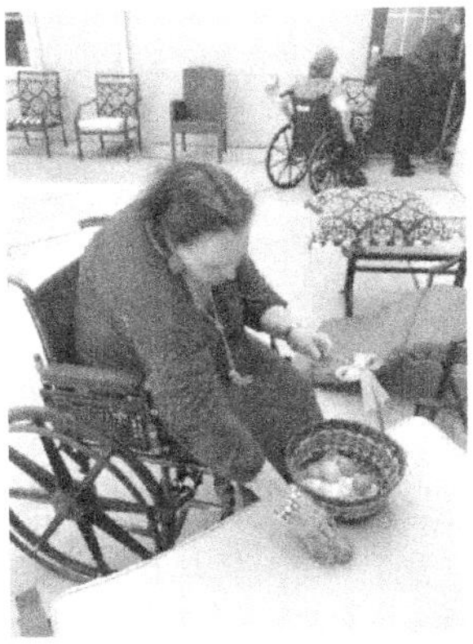

Mom Chronicles March 31, 2018
She is wearing a different necklace today! It's been the pearls for months now (at least on the days I have been here).

The center served Easter egg cookies to them today, and one of the residents here is playing the piano. Sheila is on her way and should be here soon. AND they had a little Easter egg hunt!!

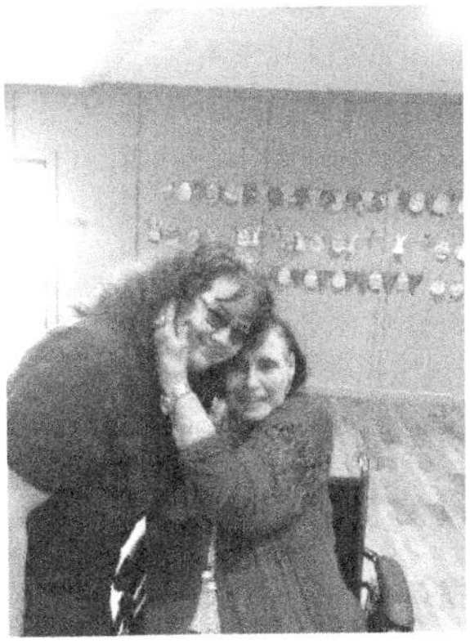

Mom Chronicles March 31, 2018
My momma is a 3-year-old in a 70+-year-old body!! I asked her if she would share some of her eggs with the two people at her table and she frowned and hugged the basket closer to her. Sharing is NOT in the cards today!!

I also bought Mom a new sparkly headband, and she's kind of doing a retro "Cher" look with it.

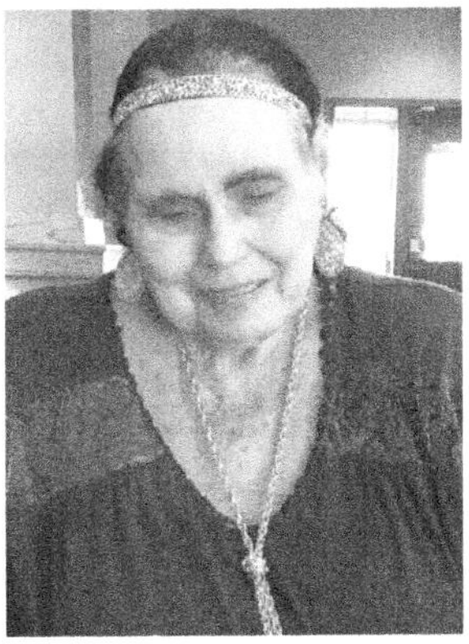

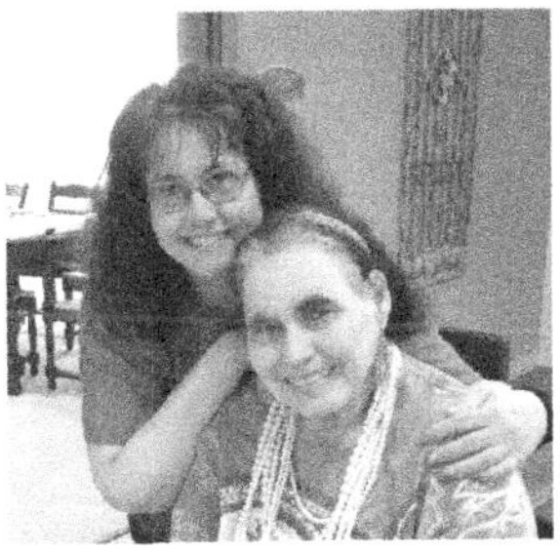

Mom Chronicles April 2, 2018
I had the day off, so Sheila and I went to visit Mom together this afternoon. We played dominoes, and then we played around with a video clip. Sheila and I do our best to make her laugh, and I think we succeeded today. She was really cute. She started singing "You are my Sunshine," and that's about all the words she could remember, but she knew the tune. Sheila and I will treasure these memories forever.

Mom Chronicles April 3, 2018
[Sheila's Post] We played with the filters on my phone today to make her laugh.

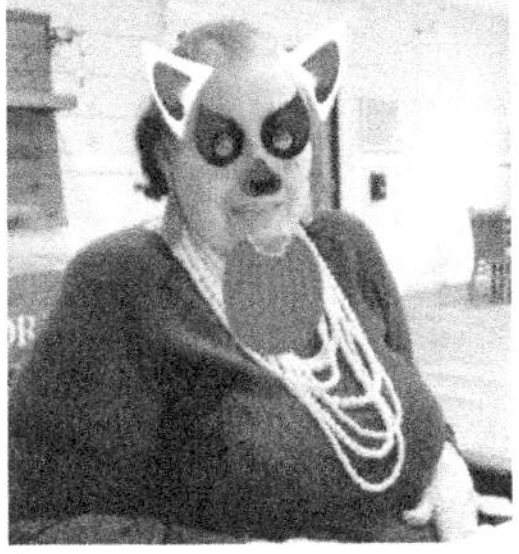

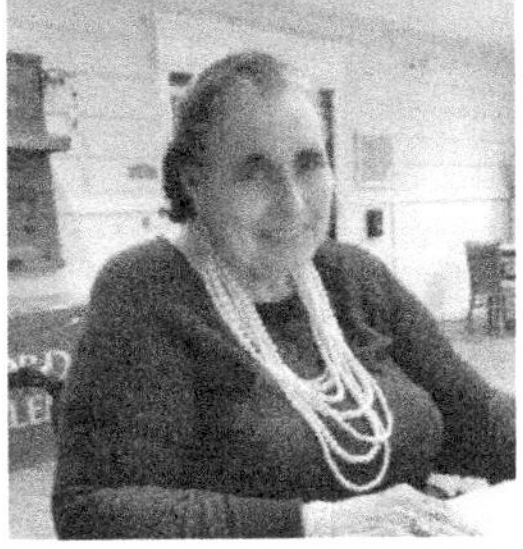

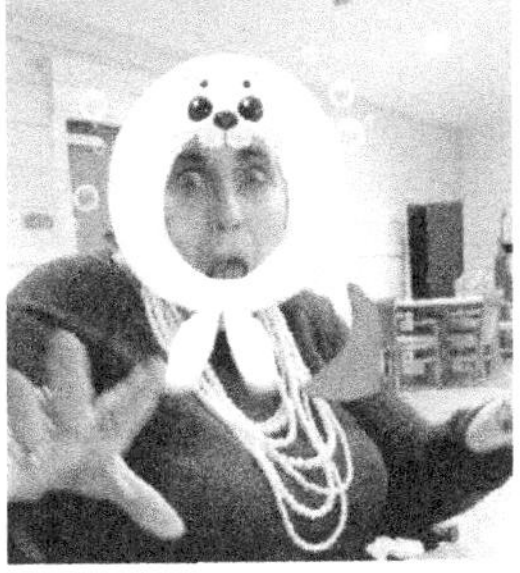

Mom Chronicles April 7, 2018
Mom is helping celebrate a fellow resident's birthday. Besides bling and shiny things, she LOVES flowers. Seeing this picture reminds me that I used to bring flowers home to her when she lived with us. So I am going to start doing that again for her.

And I just noticed Mom holding her friend's hand. She cares for people so much.

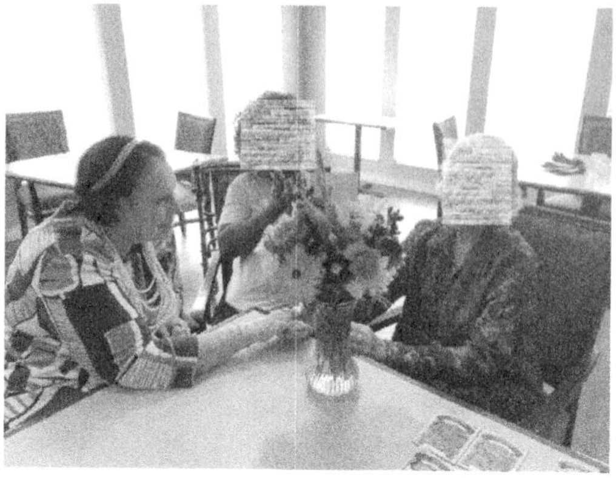

Mom Chronicles April 11, 2018
The home health occupational therapist called me today to update me on her visit with Mom this week. (We had ordered this several weeks ago when I noticed Mom trying to drink her water with a spoon, like soup, and when I saw that she had difficulties understanding how to cut her food to take small bites). Mom doesn't do this behavior all the time, so she hasn't witnessed it, but the center has taken steps to have her food already cut up before being served, which has helped some.

Anyways... back to the update. She talked about Mom's agitation with showering. She told me some steps to use with showering that she shared with the staff at the center. The good thing is that the new nurse purchased a training program for the staff after the incident with my Mom over a month ago. The therapist told me the nurse concurred that the steps she suggested align with the training program the staff has received.

So here it is for those of you who have to shower/bathe a Loved One (LO) with dementia.

1) Move slowly. A dementia patient can't process things fast, so you are scaring her when you zoom through the bathing process.
2) Talk calmly with her. Do idle chit chat - ask her how she is doing.
3) Tell her you are going to start the water. Then, tell her you are just going to listen to the water for a few moments.
4) Tell her you are going to use a washrag to wash her hands. (I remember the nurse mentioning something in the training about starting with the feet, so this is the only thing a little different mentioned between the therapist and the nurse.)
5) She mentioned over and over about moving slowly. Continue to talk to her calmly.

With Mom, they will do one full bath a week and then "bed baths" every other day (with cleanings happening when she has accidents).

♥

Here are some other bathing tips I learned while researching for this book from the National Institute on Aging website. Here are some of the highlights, along with a few other things we learned from doctors and friends: (Alzheimer's Caregiving: Bathing, Dressing, and Grooming: Alzheimer's Caregiving Tips, n.d.)

- Try to shower or bathe your loved one a minimum of twice a week to reduce infections (esp. UTIs in women). Sponge baths are great if you have difficulty adding more showers or baths during the week.
- Make it seem like it's part of a routine. For example, I could get Mom to shower on Saturday nights before church Sunday morning when she lived with us.
- Use positive reinforcement afterward. Use praises and compliments and maybe a special treat that she loves.

- Have all bathing supplies ready. Try to have the room as warm as possible even though it may be uncomfortable for you. Another hint was also to have some soft music playing.
- Use the prescription pad idea mentioned earlier in the book. Have the doctor "prescribe" a bath or shower two times a week for infection control. You can then show this over and over to them and say it's "Doctor's orders."
- Have the bath take place during a time he is normally used to taking a bath. Routine is everything, so if he always takes his bath before breakfast, keep that routine the same. If they prefer showers over baths, use showers. It is safer for showers as their mobility gets worse.
- Dementia can affect how your loved one feels about water. They can become afraid of it. A flexible handheld showerhead can be helpful to ease fears. If they are able, they can use it to control where the water sprays too. Remember - they are also afraid of losing their independence as the disease takes further control. Let them do as much as possible that they are physically able to do. They may need reminders not to forget to wash here or there during the shower.
- When the bath is over, try to have them dry themselves as much as possible. Always praise and compliment as positive reinforcement.
- Some people need to be distracted during the shower. Ideas include singing or giving them something colorful to hold.
- Modesty is a big issue until later in the disease. You can help preserve their dignity as much as possible by allowing them to cover up with a towel while in the shower. You can help wash the skin under the towel to help maintain their modesty.
- Safety is important. Install grab bars and apply non-skid appliques on the tub floor. Shower chairs are good for loved ones who can't stand.
- If you don't have a walk-in shower, your loved one may be afraid of stepping over the tub wall. Try using a transfer board. It's like a stool that has legs on the tub floor and legs on the bathroom floor. Make sure it's long enough that they can scoot from one side to the other.
- Use a calendar and have them mark off the day. This strategy will help with arguments you may get if they say they took their shower already. In addition, the calendar gives them visual confirmation of their shower routine.

Mom Chronicles April 14, 2018
Today I visited Mom for a few minutes while Bruce was at a doctor's appt. The enrichment director had the residents doing some drumming/musical fun. Mom was really enjoying it. Just look at the concentration while she was trying to get the right rhythm.

At one point, I asked if she remembered when she used to belly dance when she was holding the castanets. Nope... she didn't remember. (But let me tell ya... she used to LOVE to belly dance!!) I've got pictures somewhere in an album in storage!! ;)

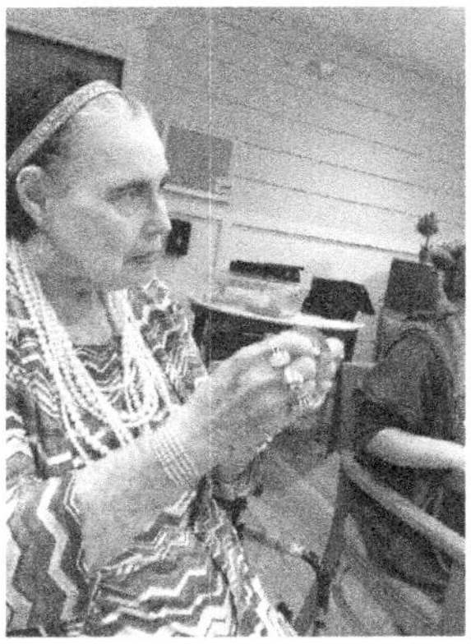

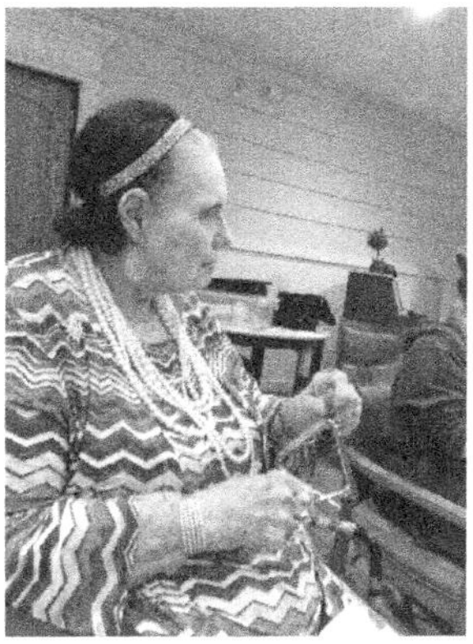

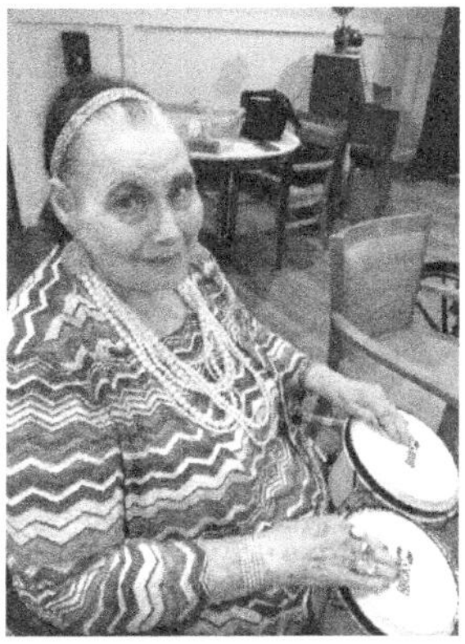

Mom Chronicles April 21, 2018

Sheila and I visited Mom today. Sheila has a cool nail kit and worked on her nails today. It's her way of connecting with Mom in a fun way. I have the nail strips for days when Sheila isn't here, and Mom has a "nail emergency."

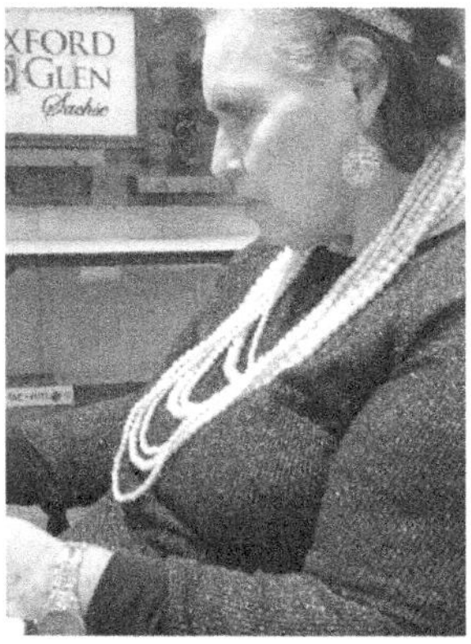

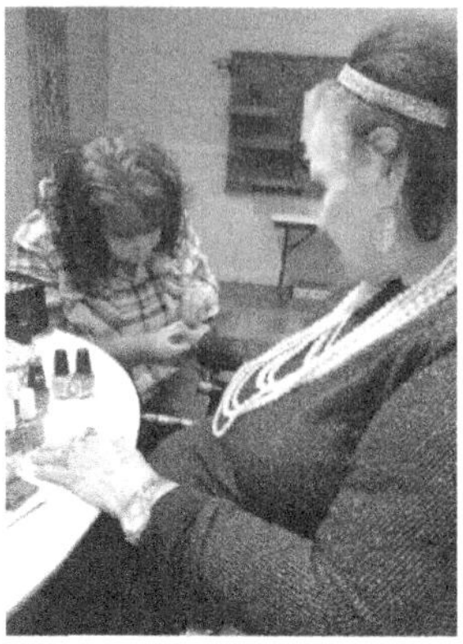

Sheila used some stuff that she put around the nails so that if she accidentally gets the polish around the nails, it will go on this pink stuff. Then all she needs to do is peel it off. We explained this over and over to Mom, but she couldn't understand it. The one pic where she looks mad or in shock is just one of the pics taken where she made this look at the pink stuff.

All in all, it was a good visit. Mom was in great spirits and happy to have sparkly fingernails again.

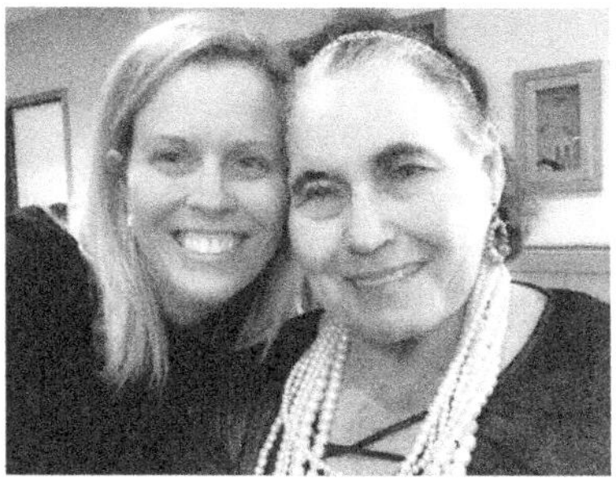

Mom Chronicles April 23, 2018

Jenni just shared this pic with me. She said Mom is laughing and sharing stories with the entire group. It looks like she's having a great day! (But goodness knows what kind of stories she's telling!!!)

The only sad part about this is that they were gathered for a small memorial service for one of their housemates. I hadn't seen this resident in a while, so now I know why.

Mom Chronicles April 26, 2018

Tonight was Family Night at the center. They had a lady playing the cello, and it was wonderful! I never realized just how beautiful that instrument sounds! Mom loved the music. She also had a nail emergency, so I'm glad I had another set of nail wraps to save the day.

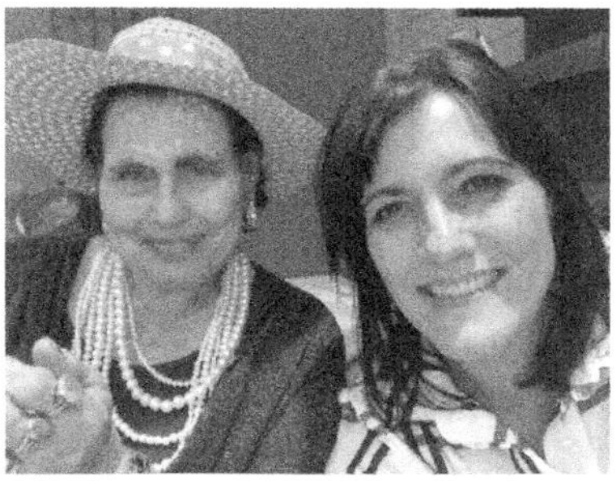

However, even with this wonderful evening, we learned this morning that my uncle (Mom's brother) is in the hospital and could use some prayers. We came close to losing him. The good news is that he did improve some during the day today, so we are hopeful.

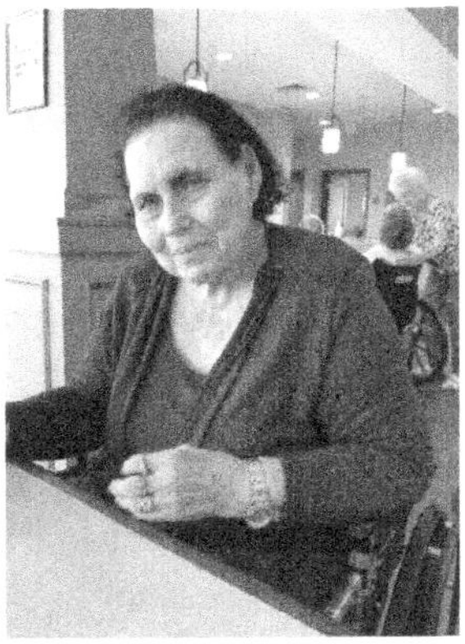

Mom Chronicles May 2, 2018
First of all, for those who follow our Chronicles, what is wrong with this picture?

She must have been having an "off" day. I didn't have a chance to ask the aides if they knew anything about her day. I hadn't seen her without jewelry (necklace and earrings) since her last hospitalization a year ago.

When I first walked in, she was sitting at the kitchen table sound asleep. My heart always stops for a second when I see her with her head folded to her chest. I always look to see if she is breathing. It took me a little bit to wake her, and when I did, she was a little confused at first.

The other big stories of the night are about three other precious ladies in the "house." The first one came up to me and acted like I was her daughter or something. She hugged me and told me she was glad to see me and that she loved me. Of course, I went right along with it. She is one of the newer patients. A few minutes later, she walked over to the dining room window and took her pants off. The bad thing about dementia is that they have no clue about social norms anymore. The aides were with other patients, so I went to find one to assist her.

The second lady is also a newer patient. She is still transitioning to living there. She goes back and forth from crying because she's afraid and angry because she can't get out. She came over to me and started yelling at me to let her out. I kept playing dominoes with Mom because I knew she would lose her train of thought and move on to her next emotion. I feel so sorry for her.

Then the last story is about one of Mom's closest friends there at the center. She was there before Mom moved in, so I make it a point always to say hi. She likes to play dominoes with us but needs more help than Mom. She has fun, though, so that's what is important. When I was leaving, I hugged Mom and told her I loved her. Mom's friend asked quietly if she could have a small hug too. I gave her a big hug, and she just smiled. I hope Mom perks up by this weekend. This version of my mom is unsettling.

Mom Chronicles May 5, 2018
Sheila, Simi, and I visited Mom today and had a nice visit. Whatever was ailing Mom this week is over because she seemed okay and had all her jewelry on. We noticed that it looked like she had put gold nail polish on her eyelids again, which confuses us because we had removed all of it from her room. We found another gold nail polish bottle in her room when we looked again, so we removed it.

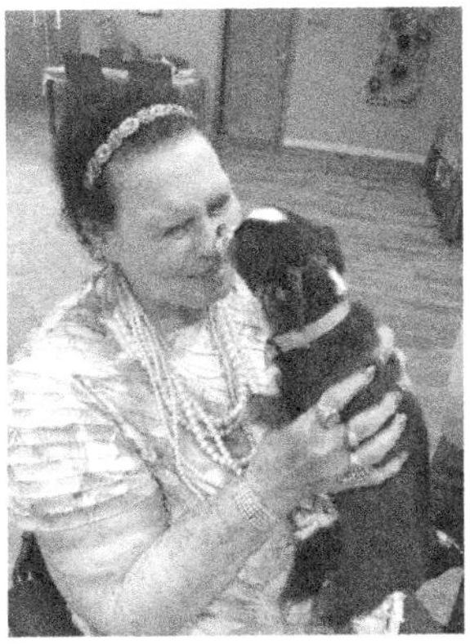

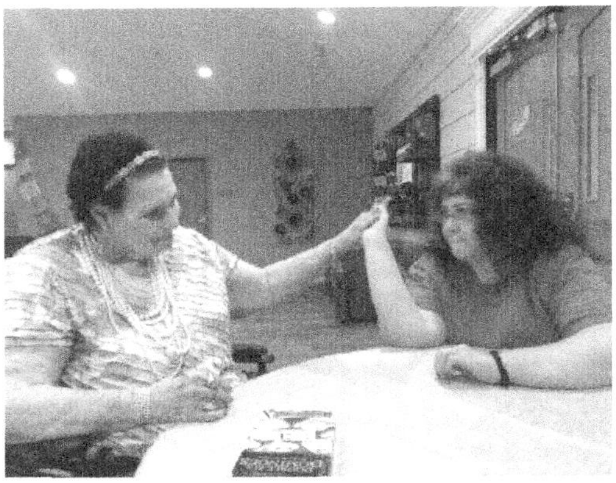

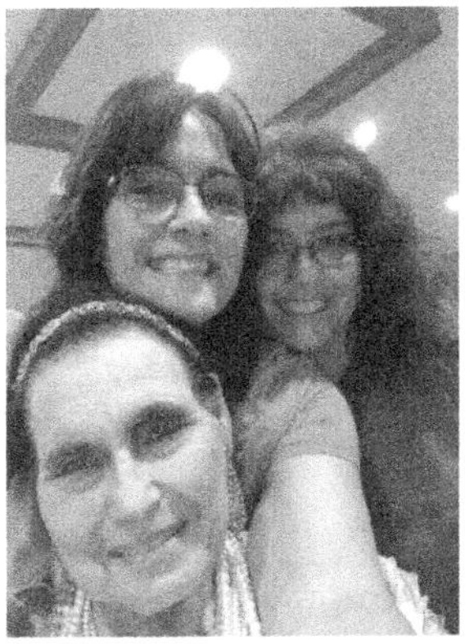

Mom Chronicles May 6, 2018

[Sheila's post] This is just a short one tonight. I need to get on the road. We had a good visit. She was in a good mood, and the stinker did her usual blocking while playing dominoes. And, of course, I had to play with the stickers to make her laugh. It's hard to leave, but I think to myself it's just two weeks.

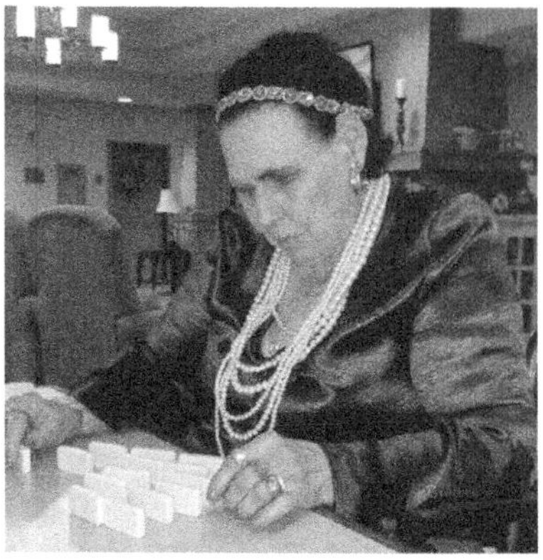
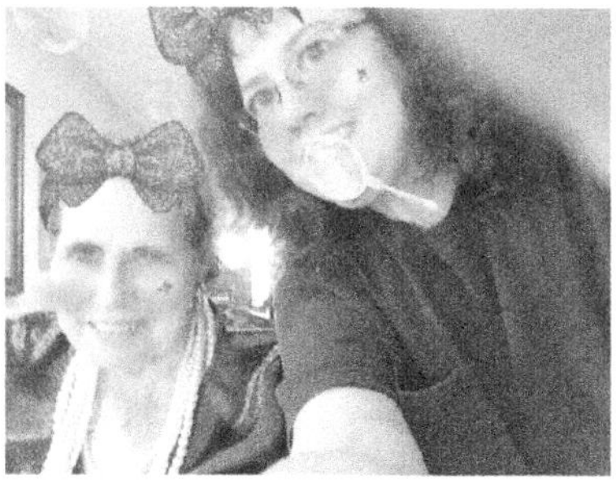
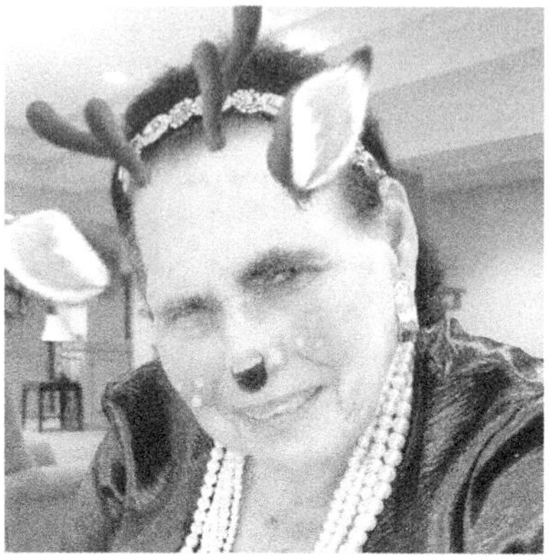

Mom Chronicles May 10, 2018

I'm currently with Mom. She is more out of it tonight. When I first arrived, she was trying to get the last drop out of her dessert. She was so hunched over she didn't even realize who I was when I arrived. She finally looked up at me and said hi, then went promptly back to trying to get the last drop. I don't think she knew who I was at first.

I have her in the middle room now playing dominoes. She just seems so out of it today. The nurse called me earlier and said her legs are very swollen (and they are!!!), so the doctor is changing some meds to try and help. She is also "shaky" tonight. She also complained of her back hurting, so they gave her some pain medication.

The nurse also told me that she removed her jewelry several times today, but they helped her put it back on. So that's another sign that she just isn't herself today.

We Skyped with Sheila, and she perked up a little, so that was good to see. Hopefully, she will start feeling better tomorrow when she begins taking the new medication.

Mom Chronicles May 11, 2018

They are having a little afternoon tea at the center in honor of mothers. Mom is feeling a little better today but still doesn't quite seem 100% yet. But doesn't she look cute?!

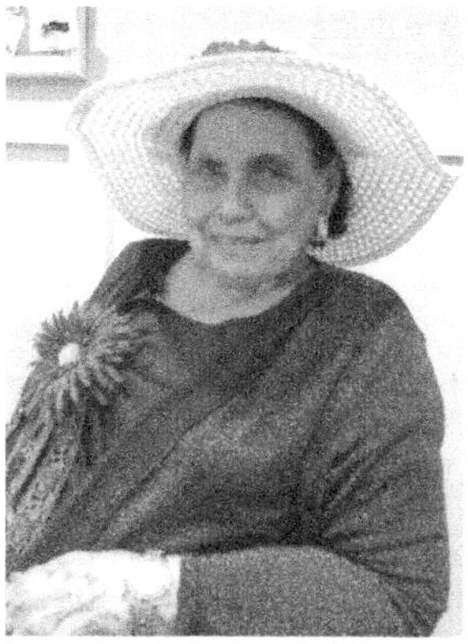

Mom Chronicles May 13, 2018

Today was rough. When Bruce and I arrived at the center after church, Mom was very upset, and the aides were doing their best to calm her down. Her main complaint is she doesn't want to wear incontinence pads. She also physically is having a hard time standing anymore to get moved to the wheelchair.

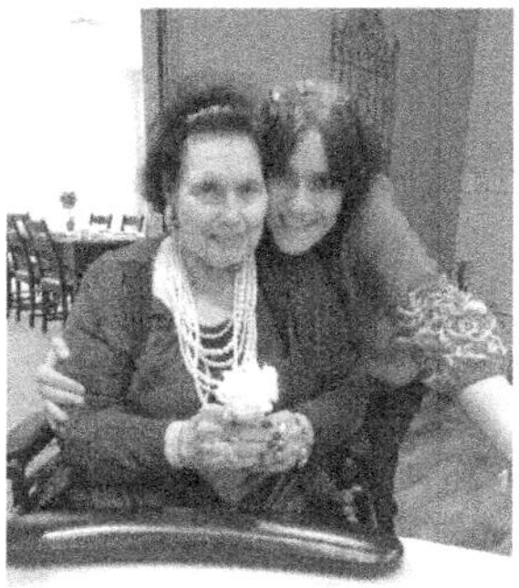

I just had a talk with the director via phone (thanks, Jenni, for always being there to calm me down!), and she is going to talk to home health tomorrow to see about some options to help her since she is declining so much. I was scared I would need to move her to a nursing home, but Jenni assured me she could get things done to help Mom.

But to end this on a good note, after we got Mom to the wheelchair, Bruce and I wheeled her into the other room and put some Elvis music on. Then I fixed her fingernails. By the end of the visit, she was no longer upset. I think Bruce even has some blackmail video of me singing with Mom. (Remember - I can't carry a tune in a bucket, so it wasn't pretty. But Mom smiled, so that's what is important.)

Happy Mother's Day to my momma. I don't know if this will be my last one with her or not, but she was smiling at the end of the visit, so that will be my good memory from the day.

Mom Chronicles May 13, 2018

The director at the center is fantastic! She is up there at the center this afternoon, and she let Mom video message me so that I could see she is having a better afternoon. Thank you, Jenni!

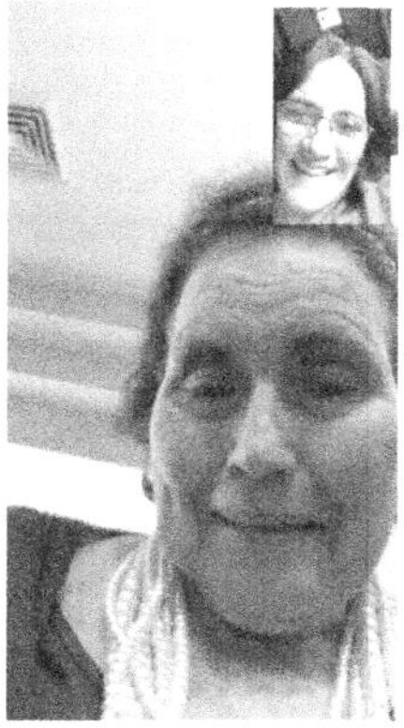

Mom Chronicles May 14, 2018

The beauty of Mom Chronicles is that someone viewing these "moments" has either gone through one of these issues, knows someone who has, OR some of the suggestions shared here will help someone else. A fantastic friend from work, Richard James, just shared with me that they used this "Stand Aid" device with his loved one. I sent this video over to the director where Mom lives to see if this is something we can get for her. I know she is contacting home health care to get Mom evaluated, so they may have another suggestion to help transfer Mom from the bed to her wheelchair and vice versa.

Hopefully, this will help someone else out there needing assistance with helping a loved one to stand up and transition to another chair/bed/toilet.

https://www.youtube.com/watch?v=j6p6IUNvHJI&feature=youtu.be

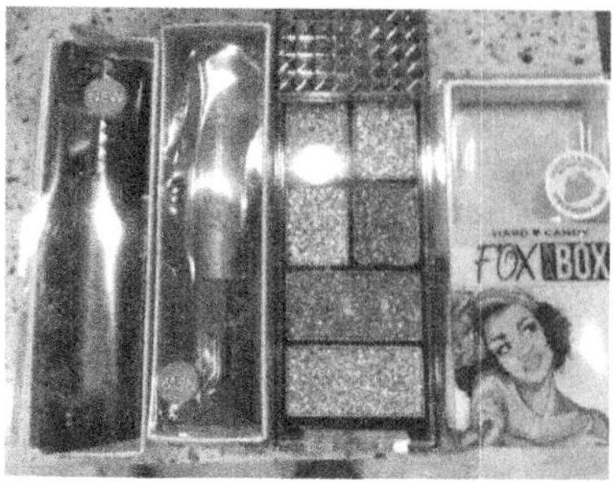

Mom Chronicles May 14, 2018

I know someone who is going to be very happy when she sees me tomorrow. Glitter eyeshadow is much better than glitter nail polish on her eyelids. Yes, we have the potential of looking like "Mimi" on The Drew Carey Show, but it makes her happy so bring on the glitter!!

Mom Chronicles May 15, 2018

She is feeling much better tonight. So enjoy watching her sing Jingle Bells and giggling!!

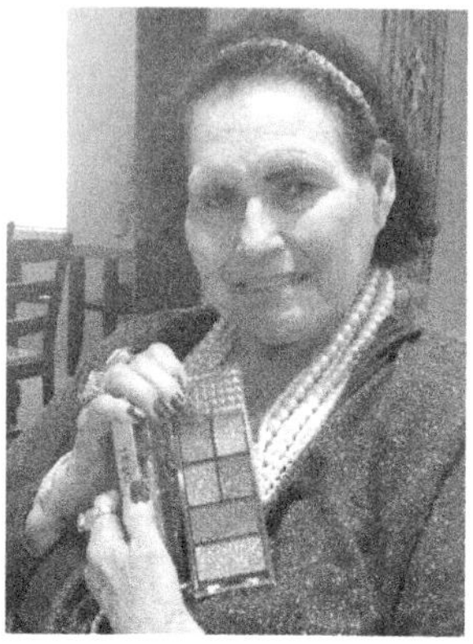

Mom Chronicles May 17, 2018

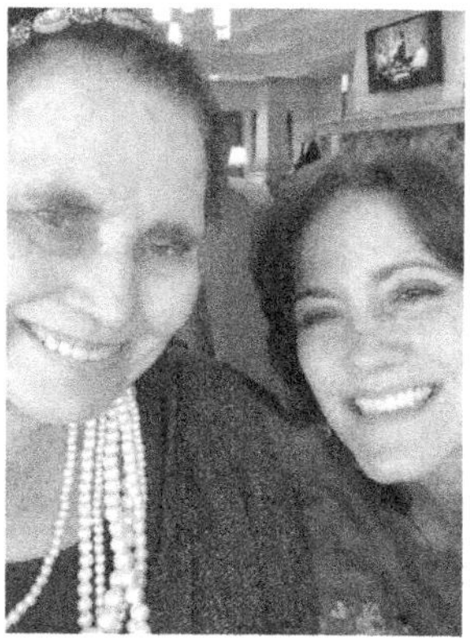

I'm with Mom right now while she is eating dinner. The support group starts at six o'clock, so I have an hour to spend with her. The main meal is always cut up for her now, but I wasn't paying attention to her fruit cup for dessert. The grapefruit was cut up into bite-size pieces, so I assumed all the rest was too—silly me. I shouldn't assume! Before I knew it, she put a huge slice of peach in her mouth. I couldn't get her to put it down fast enough so that I could cut it for her. She was able to chew it enough and not choke, so all is well. It's just so weird to me how Alzheimer's patients can forget the basic skills we learn first in life.

Also, when I got here, I noticed that she had red splotches all along her hairline. At first, I thought they were scratches, but I saw that it was red lipstick after closer inspection. I also noticed that it was all in her hair. I'm not quite sure why she decided to put lipstick on her hairline and in her hair. I guess she just loves color and is going to put it in every place she can!! Maybe she wants to become a redhead??? I took a selfie of both of us and showed her. She said it looks like she isn't wearing lipstick. Wellllll... it's because she put it on her hairline instead of her lips. I didn't have the heart to tell her that. But on the positive side, I have my very own, life-size Mrs. Potato Head!! She can rearrange her lips any way she wants!!

If I learn some new things in the support group tonight, I will share them. Have a wonderful night, peeps!!

[Update - I learned later that the reason she put lipstick on her hairline was that her gray roots were starting to show, so she was trying to cover them in the only way she knew how.]

Mom Chronicles May 17, 2018
In the support group tonight, we mainly helped a man whose wife of 60+ years has recently been diagnosed with Alzheimer's. He was at a total loss. The rest of us offered as much advice as we could give without overwhelming him. You must chew this elephant one bite at a time!!

I did learn something new, though! When your loved one is anxious, try a weighted blanket!! I'm going to shop online tonight for one to see if this helps Mom. We also talked about fidget blankets to keep their hands busy.

I'm glad I went to the support group. I have to admit in the 3+ years of this adventure, I have never gone to one. I should have been doing this all along. I think we are going to start one at church this fall. A few of us are meeting with Pastor Ken on Tuesday to begin planning an Alzheimer's series after summer. This stupid disease affects so many of us!

Mom Chronicles May 19, 2018
Here are a couple more resources that I learned about in Thursday night's support group:

A weekly journal: www.alzheimersweekly.com

And a book called Chicken Soup for the Soul: Living with Alzheimer's and other Dementias. (I'm picking this up today!)

Mom Chronicles May 19, 2018
Sheila Parsley is saving the day by fixing her nails. Josh joined in on the visit today too.

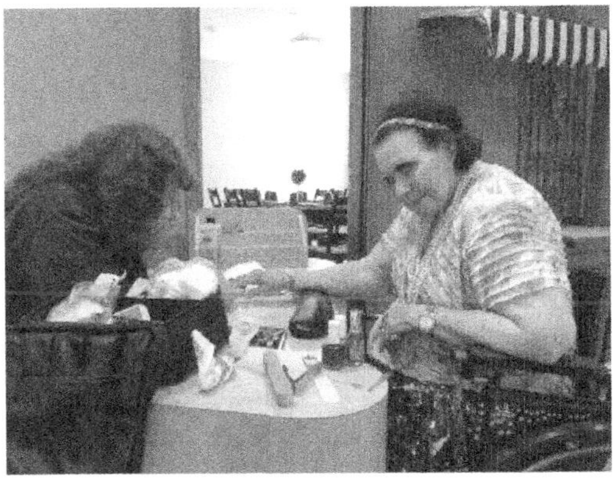

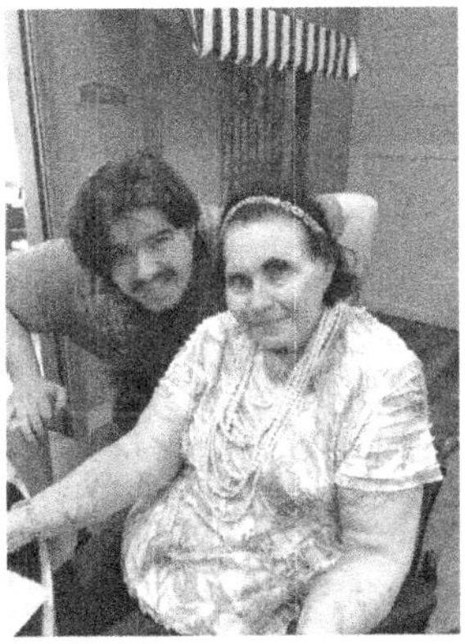

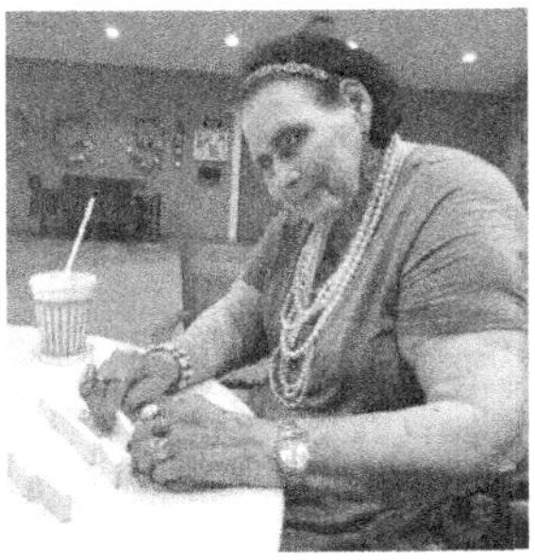

Mom Chronicles May 24, 2018
I stopped by to visit Mom for about an hour tonight. When I got there, she was in her room with an aide, trying to get her composure. Apparently, something went down the wrong pipe, and she had a coughing fit.

I have to admit that my first thought was, "Is this the beginning of the end?" I looked back at my Mom Chronicles post from the last neurologist appt. It was August 2017. He told me that at the rate she was deteriorating on the MMSE test, he expected her to be at the severe stage of not being able to swallow in about a year. That's coming up soon. Too soon. More than likely, it was just a simple wrong pipe episode that we all have. But I can't help wondering when she will make that turn to stage 7? I keep telling myself that I'm prepared, but I know deep down that I'm not.

I also bought her a weighted blanket. Her first use of it will be tonight. I told the aide about it so that she could monitor if it is helping or if it makes her too uncomfortable. I wasn't sure what weight to buy. The online site said to get one that is 20% of the person's body weight. We will see. I learned about weighted blankets in the support group with Shauna at the center recently. After reading up on this, it is supposedly helpful for autism and other issues where people need comfort and to feel safe. So I bought one for myself too. It's like being wrapped up in a big, huge hug. I think mine is a little too heavy, but it does feel comforting. I just need to be sure the AC is turned down really cold.

Mom Chronicles June 7, 2018

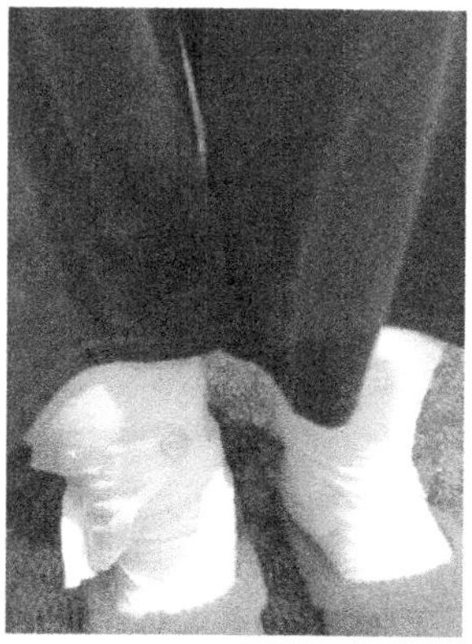

It's been a week since I've visited Mom. We had to move our RV last weekend to a different site, and then I sprained my foot and had to stay off it for several days. I didn't think that I would miss her that much, but I realized I did miss visiting with her as I was driving over there after work. Let me tell ya, that revelation surprised the heck out of me.

Anyways... as soon as I got there, she had finished her dinner and was sitting in her wheelchair in front of the TV, sound asleep. I eased up to her and gently woke her up. It took a few seconds to get her bearings, and then she just started stroking my face and saying over and over how much she loves me. Finally, she asked if she could come live with me. I immediately diverted her to other things to get her mind off that topic. It's been a while since she has asked me that. It's always hard to hear.

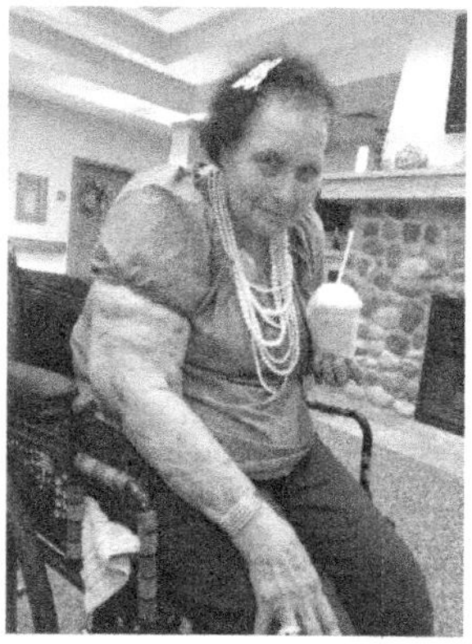

She is still dealing with swollen legs, and her leg wounds are still wrapped in bandages. She thinks something is terribly wrong with her when she points to the bandages. I just tried to explain it is just a few sores that are trying to heal and that she will be better soon.

Playing dominoes was a little more challenging for her tonight too. She had a hard time matching the numbers tonight. I also Skyped Sheila in for a few minutes. She just kept telling Sheila over and over how much she loves her. She tried to stoke Sheila's face on the screen too.

I think she was just sundowning more tonight. The sky was darker because of some rain about to blow in, and it was after 5:30 pm. I will be visiting her on Saturday midday, so I expect her to be better then.

Mom Chronicles June 9, 2018

Bruce and I visited Mom for a few hours. When I got there, they were changing her. She is down to wearing diapers instead of washable padded underwear. I also saw that she has quite a few sores, one a little bloody, from sitting all the time (understandable) and because she is refusing to get changed when she gets wet. The nurse asked if I could talk to Mom and encourage her to allow them to change her more often. Well, I know she won't remember me talking to her, but I told the nurse they could call me when she refuses to see if I can convince her over the phone. I have also sent a message to the director to find out if there are any other strategies we all can try as well. Dominoes makes her the happiest, so we played the entire time. She was very loving towards Bruce today. She reached out several times to hold his hand and leaned over to kiss him on the cheek. We also Skyped Sheila in for a few minutes. All in all, it was a good visit. After we left Mom, we went to a builder's supply store. We had just left the plumbing aisle, ironically, when I got a call from the aide. Mom was refusing to get changed. I was able to convince her to let the nurses change her, thank goodness. I can only imagine how the conversations will sound when they need to call me at work to talk to Mom. But at least I work with the most understanding folks!

Mom Chronicles June 10, 2018
I just want to shout out again about the center. The director called this morning, on her day off, and explained what they would do to help Mom. She doesn't mess around. She gets things done because she genuinely cares about her patients and her staff. I know beyond a shadow of a doubt that Mom would not have this same level of care at a nursing home. Thank you, Jenni and Shauna, for loving and caring for my mom!

Mom Chronicles June 19, 2018
Lots to share today... I was kind of emotional on part of it.

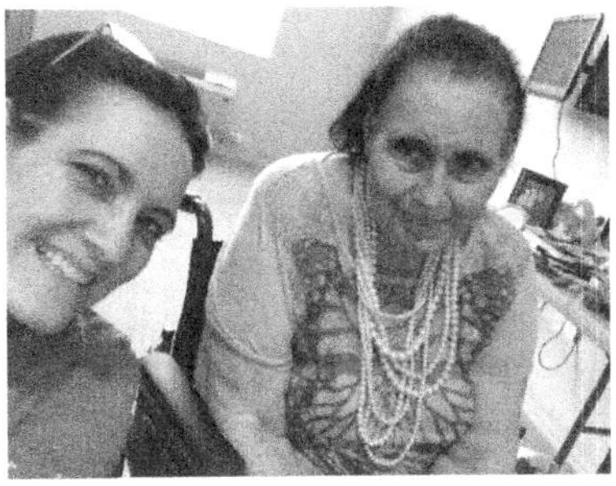

First... I received the quote from the traveling dentist who visits the center. They reported that Mom has four cavities and needs a deep cleaning. She doesn't have dental insurance, and this amount is way more than I can float right now. Which credit card do I max out for that??? I am struggling with the right thing to do. One - I don't think she's having pain in her mouth, but I think the staff would let me know if she does. Two - I honestly don't think she would sit there and let them work on her. I remember the fiasco of trying to get the shot in her hip last year. You would have thought she was being murdered. Three - I've always heard that infections in the mouth can lead to complications elsewhere, so is it wrong for me to not get them fixed??? As I said - this one is a struggle, and I will pray hard on this one.

Next... during our visit, we looked through photo albums. I videoed a lot of short clips so that I could grab reactions. I won't post them all here, but I am going to post one. She came across a picture of Ted. She said that was her "baby." I knew what she meant and prompted, "Ted - your husband"? She said yes. Then she quietly asked me if he was still alive. I took a few seconds because I had decided several months ago when he passed that I would not tell her. For some reason, I couldn't this time. I told her he had passed away. She then picked the picture up and kissed him. She quietly said, "I love you." I nearly lost it when she did that. My eyes are tearing up now as I type this in. She kept on looking through pictures and laughed and smiled about him. We then moved on to other albums. She didn't bring it up anymore, and honestly, she probably has already forgotten it.

My mom didn't have much luck in the marriage category (8 marriages), but I can tell you she and Ted had the best relationship out of them all. She was with him for more than 15 years, and I never heard one cross word about him. And believe me, I was always the first to hear when a relationship went south. They adored each other.

So yeah... today was a little emotional. But she was smiling and laughing when I left, so she's okay. And don't judge me on her fingernails when you watch the video, peeps!! I'll paint them in a couple of days!!!

Mom Chronicles June 21, 2018
I visited Mom today for about 30 minutes before the support group meeting at the center. Her eyes were very bedazzled with glitter eyeshadow - on her eyelids and under her eyes. She would never do this before Alzheimer's hit. But hey, it makes her happy, so I will always provide her with glittery makeup until... well... just until. When I first got there, she had finished eating dinner and was sitting in her room facing the bedroom corner, looking down towards the floor. I walked around to stand in front of her, and she looked

up and started crying (not a hard cry - just a "tears in her eyes and her voice" cry - telling me she's glad to see me. She looked so down and dejected, so I was not sure what was going through her mind at that moment.

After several hugs and letting her hold my face for a few moments, she pointed to the air conditioner and said it was "hurting her." I asked if she was cold, and she said yes. It was 78 degrees in there, but I remember Mamaw Annie Mae (Bruce's grandmother) sitting in her hot house in the dead of summer in Texas wearing a sweater, so I understood. I looked for her sweater but couldn't find it, so I will try and dig up another one.

To get her smiling again, I brought out the goodies. I had bought a $5 purple bracelet from a friend who sells costume jewelry. I bought a new pink watch even though she doesn't know how to tell time anymore. Her last pink watch broke, so she needed a new one. I also brought her more makeup and some scented body lotion. I also Skyped Sheila in for a couple of minutes. Sheila just saw her last weekend, but Mom said it had been a long time since seeing her. Time has no meaning in her world now. She was smiling when I left to attend the support group. It made my day.

After work, the dentist called me to try and talk me into getting Mom's teeth deep cleaned and filled. After carefully considering a friend's advice (who had been in my shoes as a caregiver), I decided not to go through with having Mom's cavities filled. The dentist even told me he had a hard time just doing a simple cleaning on her. He said they could give her anxiety meds, but she's already on that, so what good would that do? No... she simply can't handle anything remotely painful or stressful. She cries out when we push her cuticles in, for Pete's sake. She just can't handle anything anymore. I realize I'm taking a big chance in her getting bacterial infections. My sister and I talked it through, and she is backing my decision.

My friend who had given me advice about Mom's cavities was the caregiver for her father, who had Alzheimer's. Her father had been a doctor himself and had written out all he wanted to be done medically when he progressed to the later stages. He wanted to be off all medications except for pain control so that he wouldn't extend his life through the rough parts of this disease. I've thought about this for my mom, but I just can't do this right now. I, however, am going to write out my wishes for Bruce and Josh so that they don't have to agonize over any decisions regarding this disease. With family history, I will probably get it. I'm praying I won't, but I'm going to be practical. I want Josh to have the easiest time possible if and when the time comes.

At the support group tonight, there were four new people there. It was nice getting to visit and trying to help each other. Shauna from the center does a great job of facilitating the discussion.

So, all in all, it was a good day. I strolled down to the lake with Simi and took in God's beautiful creation to end the day almost perfectly.

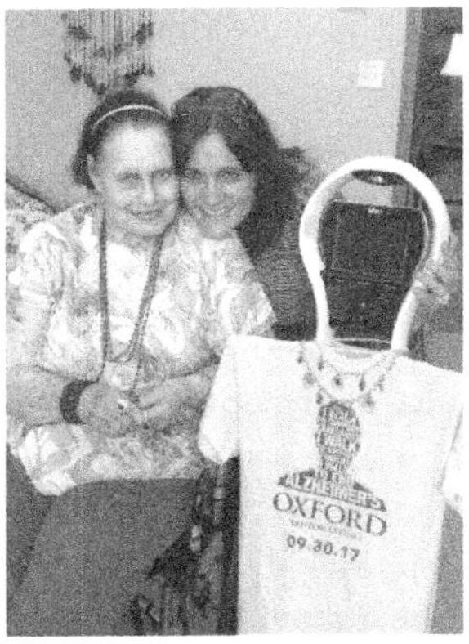

Mom Chronicles June 22, 2018

With permission from my director, I was able to bring a robot from our Reggie's Robots program over to the center to do two things: 1) they have a robot activity in a little over a week, and they asked if I could bring one of the robots out to showcase and 2) do a trial to see if families would log in to visit with their family members and to see how their loved ones would react to this. If it works out, they may consider procuring one to help enrich the lives of their patients.

Since the robots are not in use during the summer for their original intent with homebound kids, we are trying this out at Mom's facility.

I took one robot out to the center to test the WiFi this afternoon. It worked okay in the front office and in one of the houses. Mom was with me the whole time I tested it. (And I made sure to do this on my own time so that I wasn't using my work time for this. I want to be careful not to cross any lines to jeopardize our fantastic program.) Mom was pretty confused seeing me in person and on the robot simultaneously, but I think she will process it better when I try logging in during lunch or from home.

We put a shirt with the center's name/logo on it, and we let Mom pick out a necklace on it. The only thing I worry about that is that she is extremely possessive now with this disease, so she may see the necklace later and want it back. She's like a child who hasn't learned to share.

We temporarily named the robot "Roxie." However, that may change since it was a spur-of-the-moment name.

Wish us luck as we try it out with families there at the center. I can see this being a great way for families to help redirect or help encourage a loved one to get cleaned up or even to see their loved one say hi.

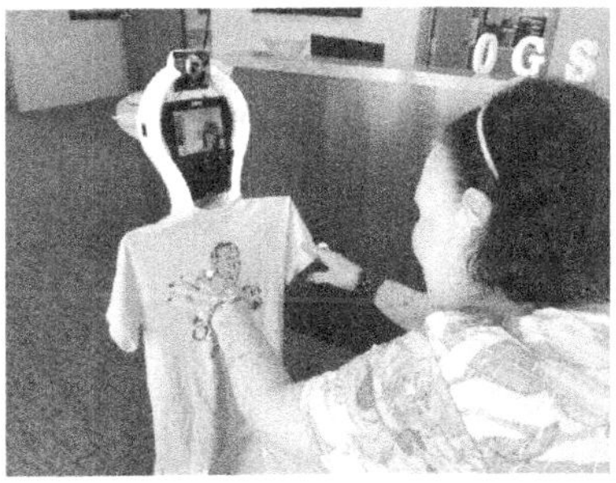

Mom Chronicles June 22, 2018

Jenni just shared this photo with me. It's my favorite one from today. I was in Jenni's office, logged in to the robot, and Mom was in the reception area with the robot. When she saw my face on the robot, she reached out to hug the robot. So darn cute!

Mom Chronicles June 25, 2018

I don't like to wait too many days between visits, so since Friday was my last visit, I decided to stop by there today. I got there at dinner time, and the first thing I noticed is that she was not wearing a bra. That is the first time I have ever seen her in public without a bra unless it was one of her sexy low cut evening gowns she would wear going to a party or out on a date. I'm not sure what to think of that. I know that dressing is more of a challenge as the disease progresses. I know she also has a hard time matching colors quite a bit now. I just wasn't expecting the braless look that I've seen some of the other ladies who are further along in this journey. All these little changes just hit me in the gut, and then I'm okay after I sleep on it.

As for dinner, they had lima beans, spaghetti, and a roll. Because we have Mom's food cut up before it arrives at the table, the roll was already cut up. She wasn't eating it. I told her to eat her chicken. She said, "that's not chicken." I swear it looked like chicken!! So, I took a bite and said, yep... that's not chicken!! I have no idea why I would think they would serve chicken with spaghetti!! But she didn't eat it - she didn't like it. Her tastes have changed over the last several years.

Towards the end of her meal, her left-hand knuckles started hurting badly. I think it was arthritis. Since she quit eating, I took her to the middle common area and played dominoes to get her mind off the pain. It worked for a while, and then the pain started up again. I turned on one of her favorite songs to divert her attention. They couldn't give her anything for pain since she had already had some pain meds at 4:00 pm. I'm hoping it eases up so that she can rest. Also, the nurse/aide said that she had one of her coughing panic attacks earlier in the day. She said she sat with her for a long time to help calm her down. I'm so thankful the staff genuinely care about their patients.

I did also learn that Mom still fights them on showering. One of the nurses showed me a scratch on her arm that Mom did to her a few weeks ago that is just now healing. I hate to hear that Mom is hurting them. God bless anyone that does this job.

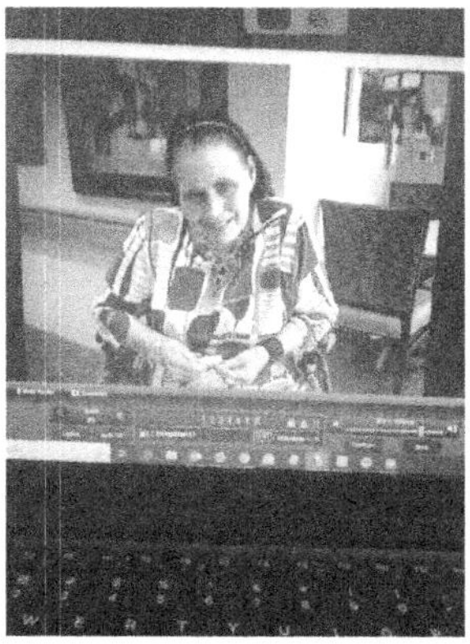

Mom Chronicles June 26, 2018

I visited Mom briefly through the robot this afternoon. We wanted to test the WiFi in one of the houses from someone logging in from outside the center before going public to the rest of the families. We finally found one "sweet" spot near the kitchen in House 1 where the WiFi signal was strong. Mom seemed to do very well with the call. Josh even popped in for a minute to say hi, which thrilled my Mom. She loves him so much!

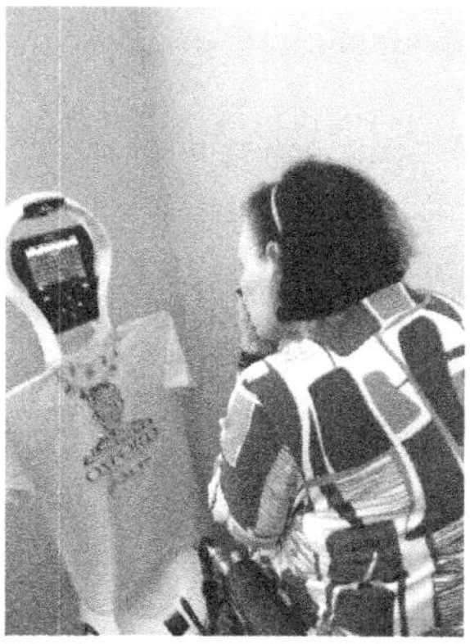

Anyways, the call went well. It's a little more complicated since verbal communication isn't the best. Playing dominoes or listening to music takes the pressure off of having meaningful conversations. So, talking through the robot will require some new skills on my part to figure out questions to ask her that she will be able to answer. Most of her words are jumbled now, so it's a challenge. I still think this is a fabulous opportunity for families, though, even if it's only for a few minutes.

The funny part is that when I logged off, she was bound and determined to have the robot placed in her room. She had one of the staff members take it there while Jenni had stepped out to the office. When Jenni walked in, Mom was looking at the robot and pressing buttons (I can only assume to try and bring me back on the screen.) Jenni had to convince her that she needed to take the robot back to the office to be charged up.

I'm excited to hear how other families work with the robot. Fingers crossed that this is a successful program over the summer!!

CHAPTER 4: ALZHEIMER'S STAGE 6 ♥ THE MIDDLE/LATE STAGE... CONTINUED

Because I started chronicling our journey a little more once she moved into a memory care unit, I'm splitting up Stage 6 into two chapters. Continue following our journey as we learn more about Alzheimer's and inch closer to Mom's final stage of the disease.

Mom Chronicles July 3, 2018
Mom and her best friend at the center are looking at the pictures on the wall and talking about how they recognize the people in the photos but can't remember their names. Mom has no clue I'm here. I'm just watching her from behind and listening to them laugh and try to talk to each other.

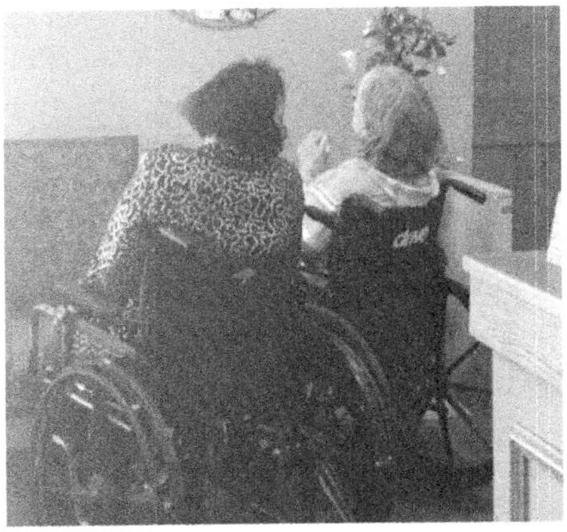

Mom Chronicles July 4, 2018
In one of the blogs I follow, I saw a video by Teepa Snow. It was fantastic! I then looked on YouTube and found a whole bunch more, plus I found her website. I think I just found another very valuable resource. It looks like she uses a different set of words for the stages, like Emerald, Diamond, and Pearl. I need to read more about that. She's funny but full of great tips and info.

Several things struck me in this video. First, Ms. Snow said 4 out of 5 families fall apart because of caregiving stress and this awful disease. All I can say is that I am completely and utterly blessed to be in the 1 out of 5 families that stay together. My hubby, son, and sister have all been 100% behind all the decisions we have made to care for Mom. My sister drives 3 hours every other weekend to come up and visit. When Mom lived with us, she gave Bruce and me the time we so desperately needed to be away for a few hours. My hubby has been supportive and willing to uproot our lives for several years. Josh would come over and sit with Mom when we needed him.

Another thing that stood out was being empathetic. Sometimes (well, truth be told - ALL the time), it gets frustrating hearing the same thing over and over again or when the loved one acts a certain way that you know is not her norm. She said to never get in their face and say "calm down" or tell them you have already heard this 15 times. Just come from an empathetic point of view and say, "it sounds like you are upset or sounds like you....". Remember, they no longer have a filter and will say things that they usually would never say. Growing thick skin is very important for us as caregivers!

The final thing I got out of it was "breathing." By breathing in and out deeply, you are not only calming yourself down, but you are also calming your loved one down. Try to get them to look at you and give visual cues to breathe in and out. If they aren't looking at you, give them a light touch to get their attention, and then do these deep breathing techniques. They will start mimicking you. Do three deep cleansing breaths five times a day. A study shows it brings the cortisol levels down for both of you! Here is her website: **www.teepasnow.com.**

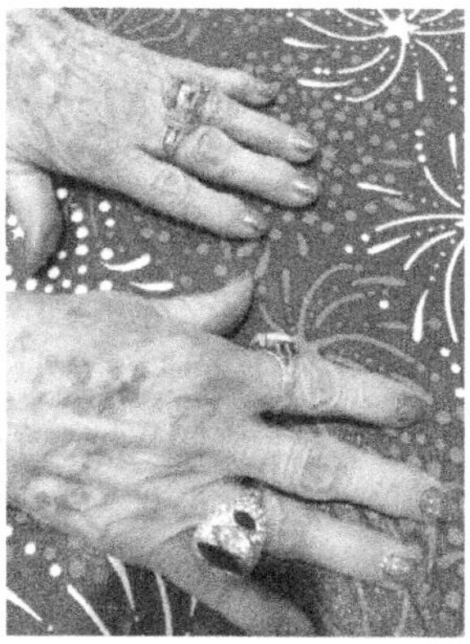

Mom Chronicles July 8, 2018

After church, Bruce and I went to visit Mom. She had just finished her lunch, so we took her into the common area. I worked on her nails. She wanted purple, but I was out of those nail strips, so I used the sparkly light blue. She liked them, but just not as much as the purple, so I will be ordering more this week.

I also worked on her toenails, and I noticed she had some sores that weren't bandaged on both of her heels. They were oozing onto her socks (sorry to those of you who are squeamish). I was lying on the floor looking at them and scared the part-time nurse half to death. She thought something was wrong with me! I explained to her what I was looking at, so she looked too. She then looked at Mom's chart and called the home health nurse right then. That nurse will be coming out this afternoon to bandage them both. They weren't bad, but they did need bandages. Bruce was a wound care technician many moons ago, so I trusted him on this.

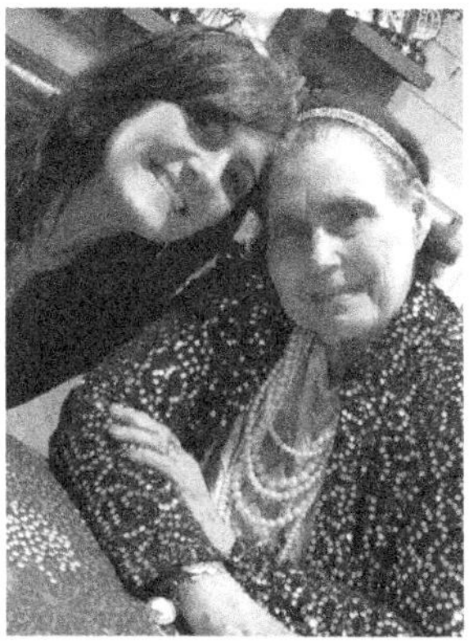

We played dominoes for a little bit, and then it was time for all the residents to come into the common area for a sing-a-long. I started to put Mom's socks and sandals back on. That's when I noticed her pants were soaking wet. That's probably my fault because I think their routine is to take her to the restroom after a meal, but I interrupted that routine. The thing that bothers me is that she didn't even realize she was wet. She used to get upset if she had an accident. Now she doesn't even realize it.

We got her cleaned up and changed, and then I took her back into the common area so that she could participate in the singing. I told her I was about to leave, but she held on for dear life and begged me not to go. So, Bruce and I stayed just a few minutes until she was distracted by the sing-a-long. I told her I would see her in a few days, and she was fine then.

Mom Chronicles July 9, 2018

The director knows that she can call me if the staff ever needs help redirecting or calming Mom down. Well, today was one of those days. Unfortunately, I can't afford a private room for Mom, but luckily, she has been by herself for most of the time she's been there. However, today, they needed to move one of her housemates into the same room. It is one of the ladies that she always eats meals with, so they are friends. But they both were upset. Change is tough for anyone, but especially for someone with dementia/Alzheimer's.

Mom was crying and saying no; she can't do it. She was very worked up. Jenni video called me so that Mom could see my face and hear my voice. It took me a little bit, but I was able to get her calmed down. Josh even stopped by my office at the perfect time, and he helped too. He usually doesn't stop in my office during the afternoons, but I think that was divine intervention so that she could see another face she loves dearly.

At one point, my boss was calling on my office phone. So I had to answer and tell him I would call him right back. Thank goodness I work for a director who understands what's going on with my mom.

Mom Chronicles July 12, 2018
The visit today was... epic!!

Mom and I started our visit off in her room. It looks like she and her roommate are getting along, so things seem to be well on that front.

Mom was in her wheelchair and showing me all her sparkly party hats. And then I Skyped Sheila in to chat for a few minutes.

One of the residents was roaming the house and was near Mom's door when it was time for her medicine. The nurse brought the meds and a cup of juice to her. Well... here is the epic part. I made the mistake of smiling at her and making small talk by saying it was time for her medicine. I always try to talk for a few moments to the residents in the house. Mistake. Big mistake. She took her meds, and then with the juice she had remaining, she walked over to me and proceeded to pour the juice all over my hair, shirt, and pants. She was just laughing away! She didn't do it out of malice. It's just that folks with dementia don't know boundaries anymore. How in the world could I get mad? Mom was laughing. I was laughing. #stickyhairdontcare.

After that, Mom and I played dominoes for a bit while my hair and clothes dried out.

Yep... epic. Lesson learned: don't make eye contact with this sweet lady at medicine time!!!

Mom Chronicles July 14, 2018
Mom is in the midst of one of her panic attacks. Please pray she gets over it soon. It's been going on for an hour, and that's usually how long they last. I'm hoping the meds kick in soon so that she can calm her fears.

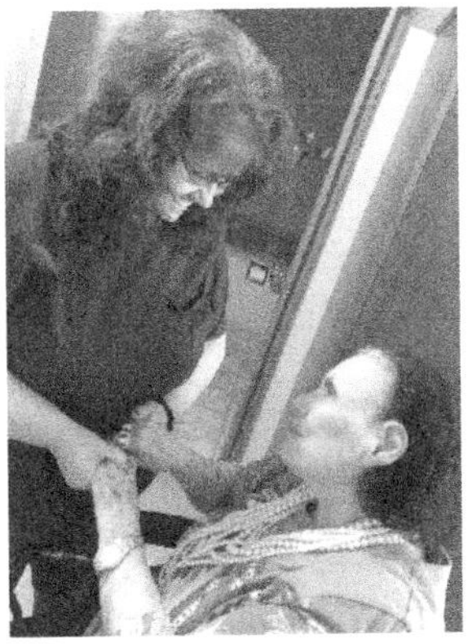

Mom Chronicles July 14, 2018
She's better. It took music and finally a photo album to calm her down. We will be a little late for our painting class tonight, but we couldn't leave her until she was calm. The director called and asked how Mom was doing. She was willing to come in on her day off to help calm Mom down. I love this place. Thank you, Jenni! You are a wonderful director!!

The photos are of Sheila getting a hug from Mom afterward.

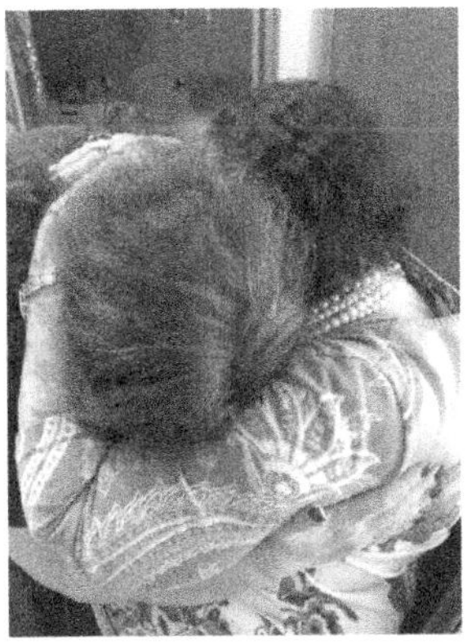

Mom Chronicles July 16, 2018
When I walked into the center this evening, dinner was wrapping up. The first thing I noticed was that she was wearing a glittery, star-spangled banner party hat. No one else was wearing a hat. After that, all I could think of was that commercial on TV where the dad lets his daughter wear her princess outfit all week, and then one day a week, she plays a sheriff so that he could wash her princess costume. It's just so surreal that

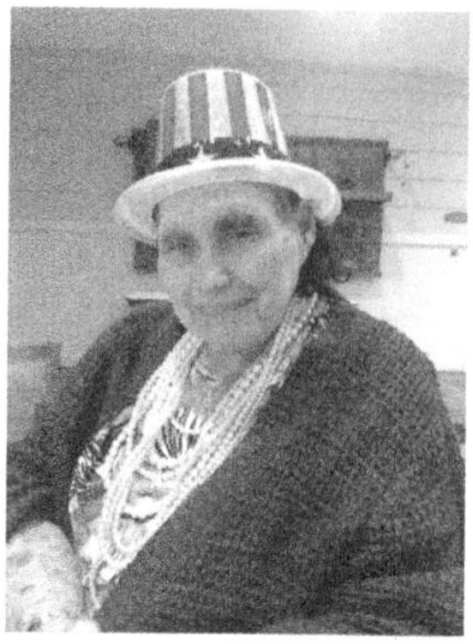

a 76-year old woman is acting like a young girl. There were many times when I was growing up that I felt like I was raising her instead of the other way around, but now it's truly real!! I wonder if I could get away with grounding her when she's acting like a patooty during shower time???

After she finished dinner, I took her into the middle room to change out the blue nail polish to her favorite purple. For some reason, every finger was hurting tonight. I could barely touch any of her fingers. Bruce wondered about neuropathy, but her feet didn't seem to be hurting, so we aren't quite sure what's causing it. She has shown pain in her fingers lately, but those times almost seemed to be like arthritis. Tonight, her fingertips were hurting. I was able to get it done, but it was a struggle! I hated hurting her!!

When I was leaving, one of the sweet, sweet residents slid out of her wheelchair. It wasn't a "fall," it was just a slow slide down to the floor, but the poor sweetie was lying on the floor. She couldn't move by herself. The aides were with other residents at the moment, so I went to get an aide's attention for help. He had to call the nurse on duty because they needed to make sure she wasn't physically hurt. I love this attention to caring for their patients. The only reason I bring this up is that Mom saw me with her, and she immediately started moving her wheelchair closer. She was so concerned and wanted to help. There is nothing that Mom could have done, but it just shows that Mom truly cares about people, and hopefully, that is something she never forgets.

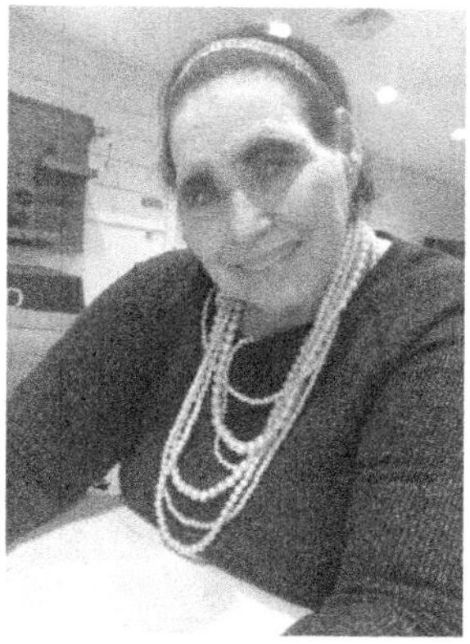

Mom Chronicles July 19, 2018

She wasn't wearing her star-spangled party hat tonight, but she was still dressed to the nines! Her hair was freshly colored, and she was in a great mood! I need to get her a few more pairs of clip-on earrings, though. She has either lost most of her earrings, or they have broken. That's the only thing that was bothering her.

After visiting her, I attended the monthly support group. We had a new lady there whose husband has early-onset Alzheimer's. He started showing signs when he was around 56. That is so scary!!

I also learned tonight that the daughter of one of the residents in my Mom's house (the sweet lady who poured juice on my head) is a mutual friend of my college roommate!! Small world!!

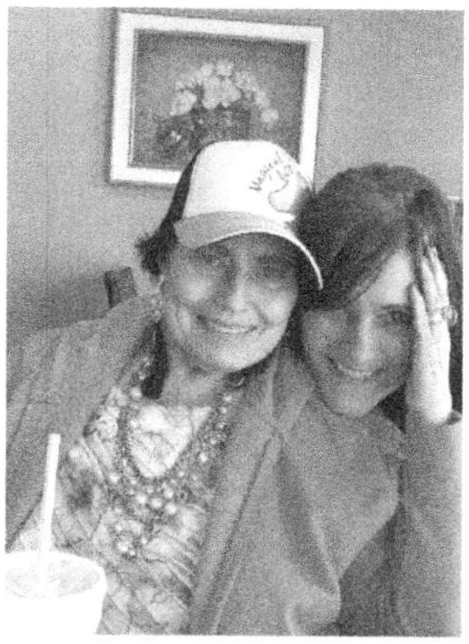

Mom Chronicles July 22, 2018

This was just a simple visit today. We brought her some new earrings and a sparkly unicorn ball cap. I am saving four other sets of earrings for redirection emergencies.

Mom Chronicles July 25, 2018

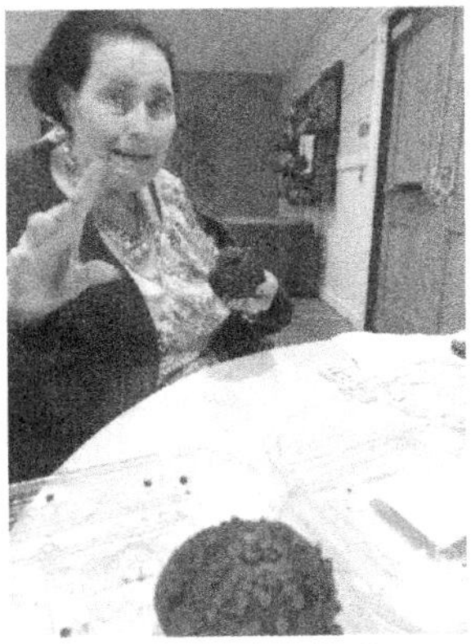

I arrived at the center when Mom was finishing up dinner. She is a very picky eater now and didn't eat the main course. Mom used to eat everything! She was a very adventurous eater and never minded trying new things. Soooo... because she didn't eat her dinner, I shared with her my leftover sandwich from lunch (minus the cheese!!) She loved it! A little bit later, I brought out the chocolate muffins that I had bought at the store this morning. I noticed she was about to bite into the paper lining, so I held out the muffin in front of me and slowly removed the paper from my muffin. She watched me like a hawk and followed my lead. Once she got the paper lining off, she went to town. She had the most intense look of pleasure on her face. I mean, really... it's chocolate. You can't go wrong with chocolate. (I still haven't made the switch to keto yet - I'm just not sure I can give up my chocolate!!).

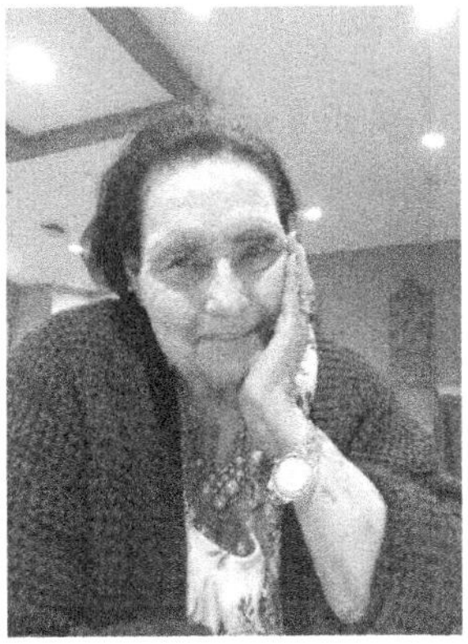

We did our usual routine of playing dominoes and listening to Elvis. I've heard Elvis so much lately that I find myself humming his songs instead of my 80's music.

Oh, and one final note. She didn't have makeup on today. She had the jewelry on but no makeup. I missed my "Mimi"! She looks so different without makeup.

Mom Chronicles July 25, 2018

I'm sharing in case this helps anyone else with a loved one in a memory center or has a caregiver when you are away from home. This morning the director asked me to make a series of short video clips to share with Mom when she is persnickety. (My word - not the director's term!!).

I did one for freshening up ("freshening up" was our way of preserving her dignity and getting her brief changed), for going to the restroom, for showering, and for putting on pajamas. Josh did one too. He felt bad about it because he felt it was lying since he doesn't get over there as much as me, BUT I explained that Mom would still love to see him in the video, and by the time she freshened up, she would have already forgotten that we said we would be coming soon. Besides, "soon" is relative, right??

Mom Chronicles July 28, 2018 - AM

We will be visiting Mom this afternoon, so I'm sure there will be a PM post.

I truly believe that sometimes we are put on a path, not out of punishment but to help others experiencing similar situations.

For example, Bruce and I now help other couples on the brink of divorce because we went through a divorce and found our way back to each other through God's Grace, help, and a lesson in forgiveness. We have personally helped two couples find their way back to each other before divorcing. It was not all our doing - completely God - but we were one small part of sharing His message.

So, what does this have to do with Mom? Well, last night I talked to a friend for quite a while on the phone. Her mom has some type of dementia. The poor lady experiences lots of hallucinations. This friend had lots of questions and just hasn't been able to share her feelings with anyone. She desperately needed to talk to someone who understood. One of the things she said was, "I miss my mom." I totally get that, but one of her relatives didn't. Why would you miss her? She's right there. Well, no. She's not. Her "shell" is but not the Mom we remember, know, and love. Don't get me wrong. We will always love our moms. But it's not the same person!! We must dig deep, pull up our memories, and love our moms using those. Our current moms sometimes have different personalities, which can stretch a person's patience to the extreme. Again, we must dig deep and remember our loved one is afraid but can't express that fear, so they express it in the only way their diseased brain allows them.

I'm glad I was able to be a sounding board for my friend. God put me on this path, so I will hop, skip, and jump all the way down it until the path comes to a dead end. I may just do a u-turn then.

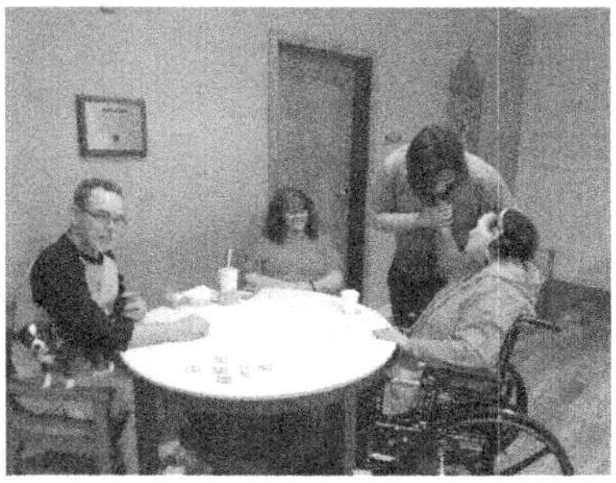

Mom Chronicles July 29, 2018
From yesterday's visit with Mom.... they were having a karaoke activity when Josh got there. It was perfect timing since Josh loves karaoke!! It was more of a sing-along, but it was still fun.

Mom Chronicles August 6, 2018
It's been almost a week since I visited Mom. I admit I decided to be selfish and lazy, and I stayed home over the weekend instead of visiting.

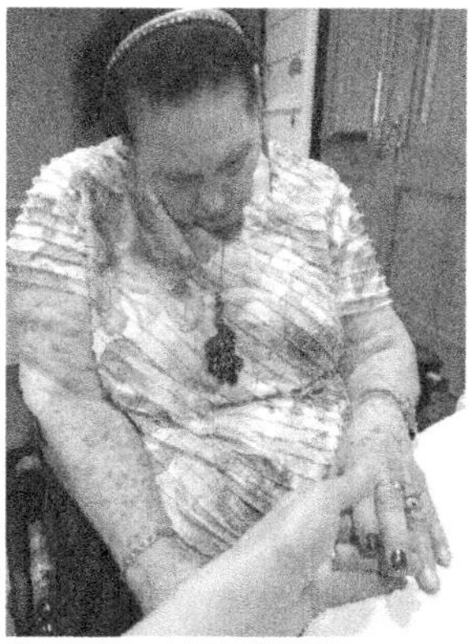

When I got there, the first thing she mentioned is that she didn't have any socks. She didn't word it that way. She just pointed to her feet and said something was wrong. So, for the next 30 minutes, I went through her closet and organized it. I found eight pairs of socks. I want to "thin out" her clothes because I remember hearing that dementia patients don't need a lot of choices to choose from. However, with Mom... if she doesn't have a "lot," she freaks. She was a hoarder for as long as I can remember. At some point, I will be able to thin things down, but for now, I will just reorganize often to make sure she knows what she has.

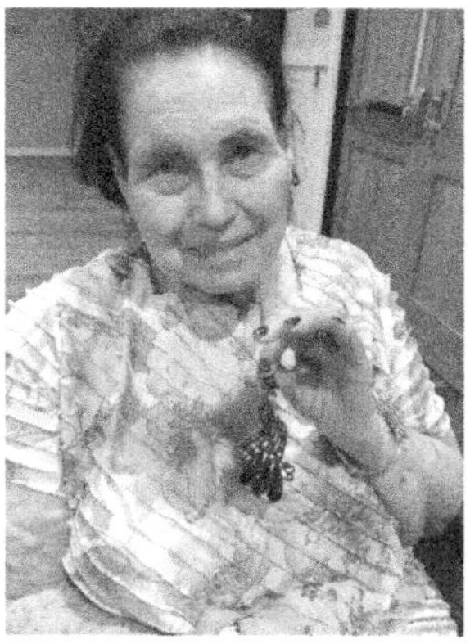

The only other fun thing is that after cleaning her closet, I worked on her nails. I had Elvis playing, and by the time I was on her 3rd nail, she was sound asleep. It was so cute. She kept jerking her hands while sleeping, which is a challenge when trying to work on nails. When she would wake up for a few moments, she would hum the song playing. I told her she was falling asleep, but she would deny it. All I could do was just agree with her.

She woke up to pretty, purple nails that matched her peacock necklace. It was a good visit.

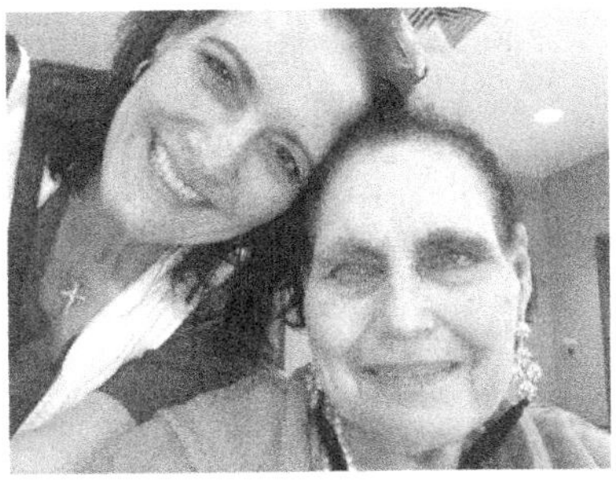

Mom Chronicles August 9, 2018

Mom was rocking a sparkly, purple raccoon look today. It took me by surprise at first, and then I settled into the new norm.

By the way... her 77th birthday is coming up on Aug 20. Do you have any ideas for us to make this as special as I can? She doesn't understand birthdays anymore, but I do, and if by chance this is her last, I want to know I did everything I could to make it special. I'm thinking Mylar balloons so that they will last for a while. And of course, I will get a cake and probably a couple of blingy jewelry pieces wrapped in pretty paper. What else can you think of that might make it special under these circumstances? Her photo albums are way back in our storage unit, or else I would pull old photos out for her. Ideas?

Mom Chronicles August 11, 2018

Sheila and I had fun with Mom today. Sheila has an android phone with stickers, and Mom doesn't like them at all. Her speech was better today too.

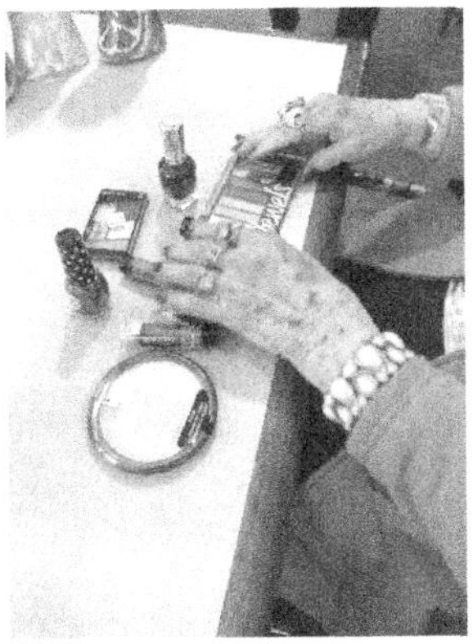

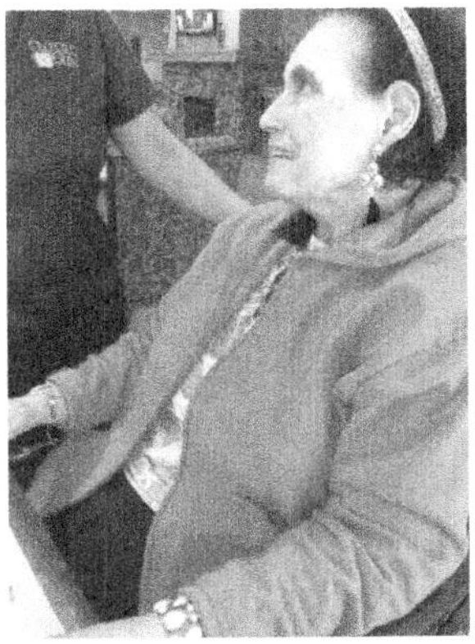

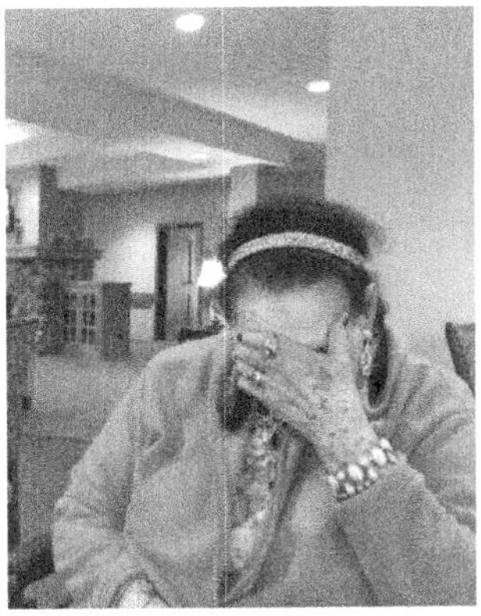

Mom Chronicles August 15, 2018

I visited Mom after work today. It was just a simple, normal visit. The only thing noteworthy is that she struggled a little more with choosing the right dominoes. For the last few months, we have noticed she struggles with the "blank" half of a domino (the 0). She doesn't seem to process mentally that when a blank is played on the table, she can match it with one of her blanks. It was even more noticeable tonight.

I mentioned this to Shauna one day, and she wondered if it's because it is the same color as the table. So I might try bringing a colored tablecloth with me to see if that helps her "see" the dominoes.

Mom Chronicles August 16, 2018

Tonight, I was tired and was planning on skipping the Alzheimer's support group, but I decided to go anyway. I arrived at dinner time, and as it usually happens, it's a good thing I decided to go.

First, Mom was extremely upset. She had just spilled water on her table and plate. It looks like she was almost finished with dinner, so I don't think she was still hungry. The staff members were with others because dinner is a hectic time when they help many residents eat. I helped get her table dried and put the plate up so that it was out of her eyesight. Second, she was freaking about the ice in the juice cup (they give two cups of liquid - one water and one juice). She couldn't tell me the word "ice." She was just freaking that there was something in her cup.

I had brought a "throw-down bling bracelet" and the nail supplies, so I immediately wheeled her into the common area since I still had 45 minutes before the support group meeting. I gave her the new bracelet and then started fixing her nails. I also played the latest songs I had downloaded (thanks to everyone who suggested the other songs besides Elvis from the 50s. They were a hit!) Within the 45 minutes of new nails and new music, I had her calmed down. Whew!

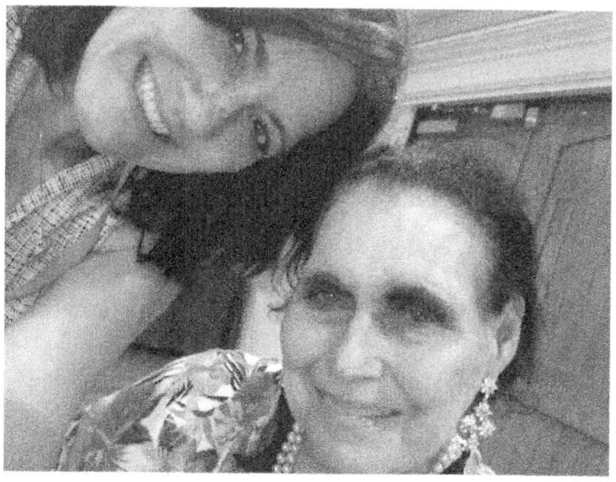

Second, the support group was small tonight. One of the nurses led the group this time and what I immediately loved is that she asked permission if she could lead us in prayer first. I really loved that. Tonight's focus was on caregiver feelings, frustrations, and guilt. All three of us had a chance to share from our hearts. Guys - being a caregiver is HARD! Luckily, the center handles the physical part of this for Bruce and me now, and that is truly a blessing upon blessing on how we were able to arrange this, BUT it's still hard. There is guilt on the feelings of wondering when Mom will pass away so that financial stress will be lifted. Or there is guilt for wondering when I will be able to have my life back. And then the moment I have these thoughts, I immediately feel guilty for even thinking it because I know beyond a shadow of a doubt that I will miss her when she's gone. I'm just being honest here - if you have never been in this type of situation, it may be hard to understand. Make no mistake; I love my Mom tremendously. Sure - there were decisions she made in her past that I wasn't too happy about, but who am I to throw that stone? It just took me a long time to get to that point - and I truly believe God put us in this caregiving situation for me to come to terms with how much I do love her.

So, long story short. I am glad I showed up to the center tonight - 1, because Mom needed me, and 2, because I needed the support group.

Mom Chronicles August 20, 2018

Hi all, two quick things. 1) I got a call this morning at 5:45 from one of the nurse aides that Mom fell last night. She's okay, but they always let us know whenever this happens. And 2), I created a birthday "event" for her since today is her 77th birthday. She probably doesn't even understand the concept of "birthday" right now, but Sheila and I do, so if you will take just 2 seconds to wish her a happy birthday on that event page, Sheila and I would be most appreciative! I'll show her this tonight when I visit. Then I will show her again when Sheila comes up this weekend to celebrate a little more. Thank you!

Mom Chronicles August 20, 2018

Thank you from the bottom of my heart to Terri Tamayo and her son for taking time out of their day and going to visit Mom. Terri gave her several pairs of clip-on earrings and a purple sparkly birthday balloon. I have only met this lady once, but we have become friends virtually on FB through the commonality of our mothers dealing with dementia/Alzheimer's.

I'm trying to figure out how to get the videos off my messenger to post here because they were super special. In the meantime, here are some of the pics. Thank you again, Terri!! You have a heart of gold!

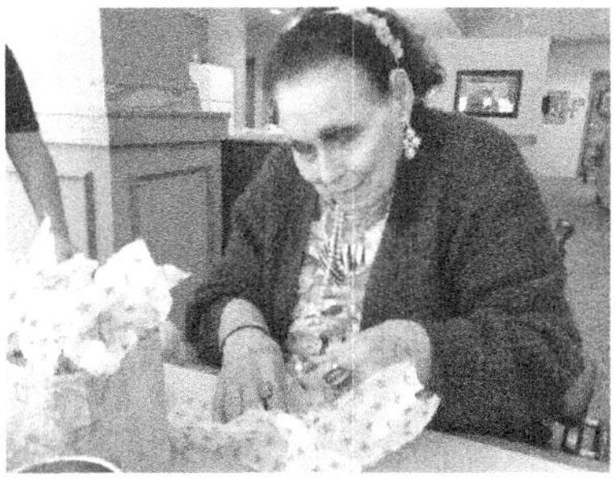

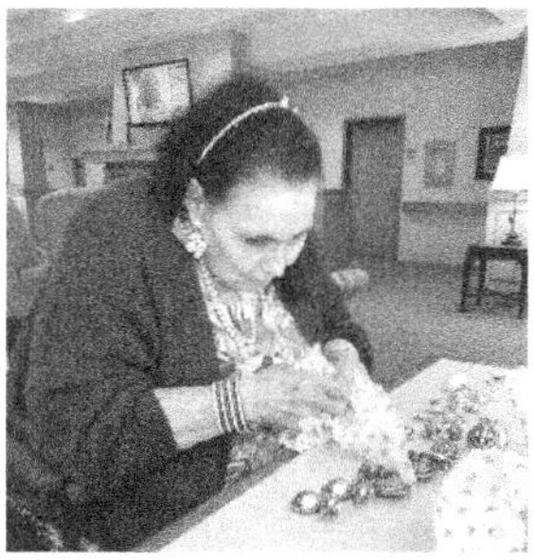

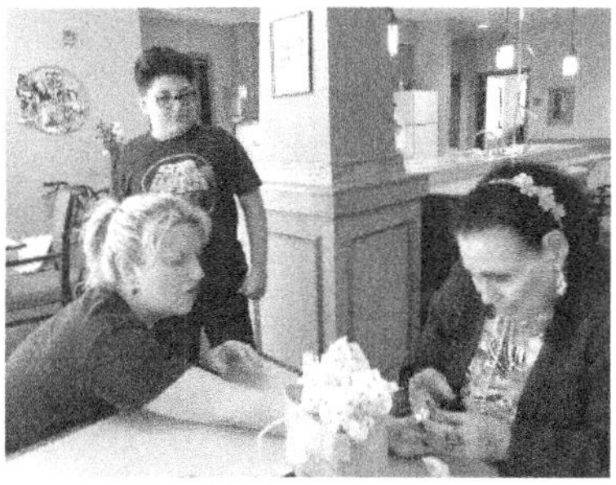

Mom Chronicles August 20, 2018
I spent a few hours with Mom for her birthday this evening. I stopped by the grocery store near the center and picked up a cake, more balloons, and flowers. I freaked a little at the cost of the prettiest flowers that I thought she would like, but I bought them anyway. She can't enjoy flowers at her funeral, so I want her to enjoy them while alive!! They were pink and gorgeous!! (Buy or pick some flowers for your loved ones while they are still alive!! It doesn't have to be expensive!!)

I also picked up some magazines like "Better Homes and Gardens." She ooohed and awwwed over the pictures inside. She loved to garden when she was younger.

She also got one pair of earrings from me since she made out like a bandit from Miss Terri earlier today. So I'm saving the other earrings for the bad days.

Over the years, I always had a hard time picking out birthday cards and Mother's Day cards for my mom. It was hard to find the right sentiment because I honestly couldn't relate to the "perfect Mom" poems. So I usually picked generic cards out. I can honestly say I picked out a card this year that had more heart in it. This journey has changed ME a lot. God is clever that way... sly dog!!

I also read the birthday wishes and showed the video clips from you all. Mom loved them!

I FaceTimed Sheila in, and we both sang happy birthday to her. Mom blew out the candles and had a couple of pieces of cake. She licked her plate entirely so that there were no icing or crumbs left. I was able to give a few residents some cake. They had just finished dinner, so several weren't hungry, and a couple couldn't have sugar because of their diabetes.

One of the residents sat by us for a little while. She is a resident that tends to cry a lot. It breaks my heart every time, but this time when she started crying, I played Mom's playlist. She stopped immediately and started dancing and laughing with Mom. Mom was boogieing with her shoulders, and this resident also shook her shoulders for a few seconds (I think trying to mimic Mom) and then reverted to dancing with her hands. It was fun to watch them. We sang (they garbled phrases and tried to match the tune) and danced for about 30 minutes to Elvis and several new songs that many of you recommended. It felt great helping her to stop crying and then also seeing Mom dance and laugh.

We are going to celebrate again when Sheila gets up here on Saturday. All in all, it was a great birthday!

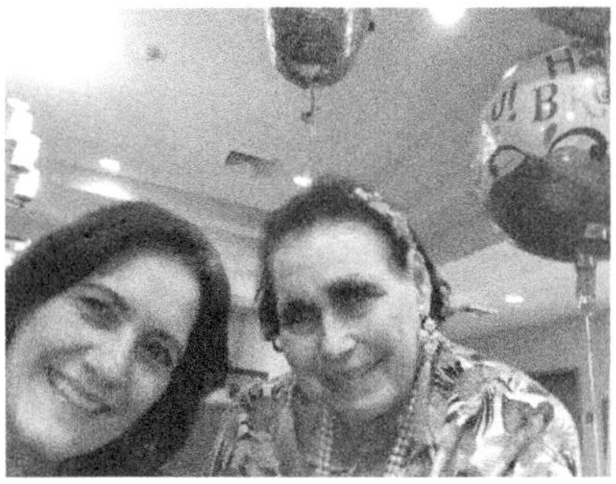

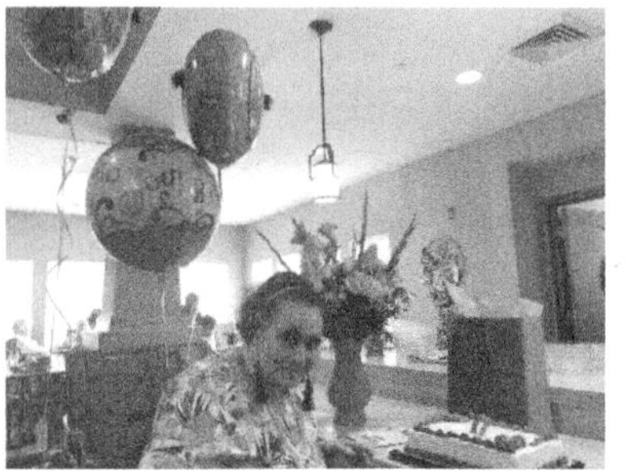

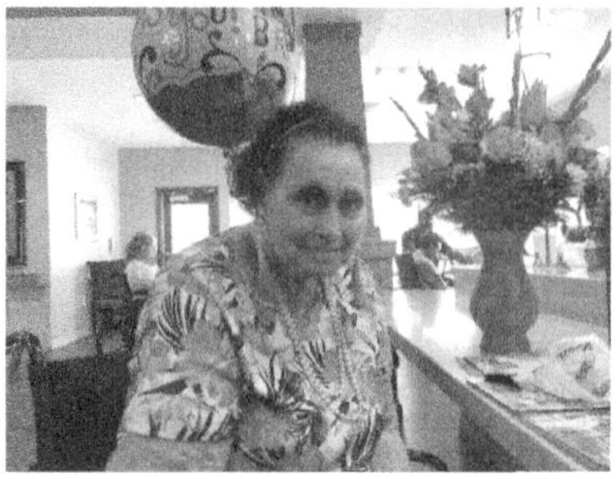

Mom Chronicles August 23, 2018

I did get to visit with Mom today for a couple of hours. They were in the middle room eating dinner as a large group and listening to a trumpet player. I watched her eat, and she did well with her spoon and picking up the vegetables, but she ate the diced chicken with her fingers. She picked them up and ate them like finger foods, which I have heard is a great way to let Alzheimer's patients eat when they get to that point. It's just weird to watch. And she still licks the bowl or plate clean if it tastes good - as she did with her birthday cake on Monday or the ice cream tonight.

Also, I have been talking to a Hospice agency for a few days to see if Mom qualifies yet. The doctor for Mom at the center called me today and said she's close but not there yet. A few well-meaning friends and folks along this journey had told me that if it is a life-ending illness, which Alzheimer's is, one can qualify. Well, not really. According to the doctor and the hospice agency I talked to, they need to be in the last stage to be eligible. Mom has several of the signs that would lead to approval but not enough of them yet.

Even though hospice sounds scary and sad, it comes with some great benefits that will help Mom when the time comes. For example, they provide a nurse to visit regularly, an aide 3-5 times a week to help with bathing or other daily routines, a volunteer to just sit with her and keep her company, and a chaplain. In addition, they provide medical equipment as needed, and they pay for prescriptions and supplies related to her illness, like incontinence supplies.

Here is what I found as signs for eligibility on several hospice sites for dementia patients:

- a life expectancy of six months
- a diagnosis of other conditions as COPD, CHF, cancer, or congenital heart disease
- an increase in hospitalizations, doctor visits, or ER trips
- a diagnosis of pneumonia or sepsis
- weight loss or dehydration due to challenges in eating/drinking
- communication is limited; speech limited to six words or less per day
- difficult swallowing or choking on liquids or food
- urinary and fecal incontinence
- unable to walk without assistance such as a walker or now requiring a wheelchair
- unable to sit up without assistance
- difficulty holding head up
- no longer able to smile

(Hospice Eligibility, n.d.) and (Hospice Eligibility Criteria Dementia, n.d.)

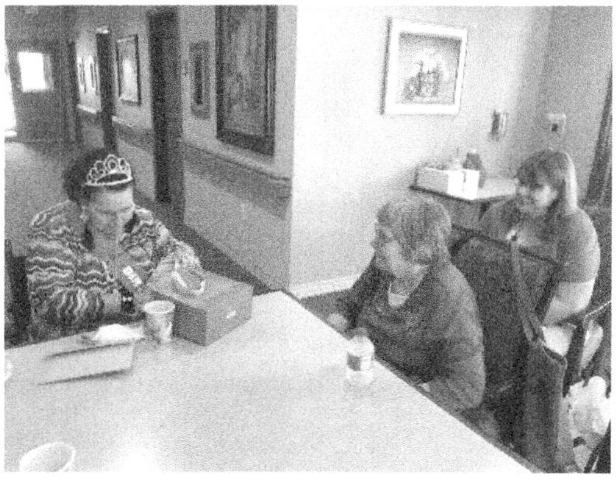

Mom Chronicles August 25, 2018
We are having our 2nd birthday celebration today since Sheila is here this weekend. Ms. Janet and Cathy came over to visit as well. Mom made out like a bandit. She got some scented shampoos, lotions, body washes, a necklace, a crown, an Elvis pillowcase, and a charm bracelet.

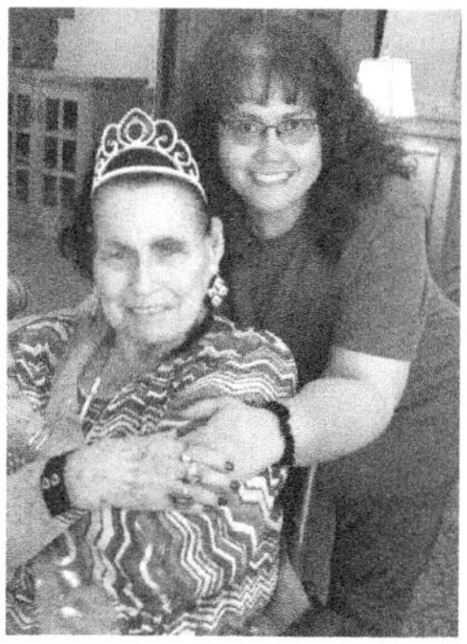

Mom Chronicles August 29, 2018
Janet Nell, this one is for you. These sparkly slippers are what I bought with the birthday money you sent for Mom. Thank you! We love you!

Mom Chronicles August 29, 2018
This video shows how happy she felt after putting the slippers on. She was so cute dancing and singing with her new slippers. Enjoy!

Mom Chronicles September 2, 2018
Today was a simple visit. No issues. She was dressed to the nines, and makeup wasn't all over the place. I knew the flowers we had bought for her birthday would be dead by now, so we bought a fresh set to put in her vase. No scent, but they were pretty with vibrant colors. She didn't want to put them in her room. She wanted them out in the main area for everyone to enjoy.

Bruce doesn't get a chance to visit often, so he played several rounds of dominoes with us.

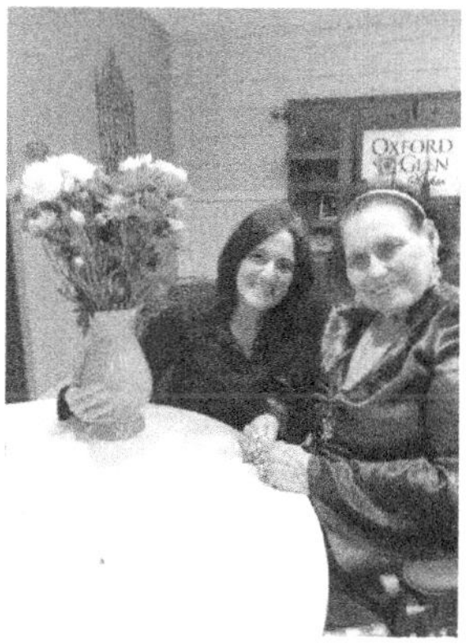

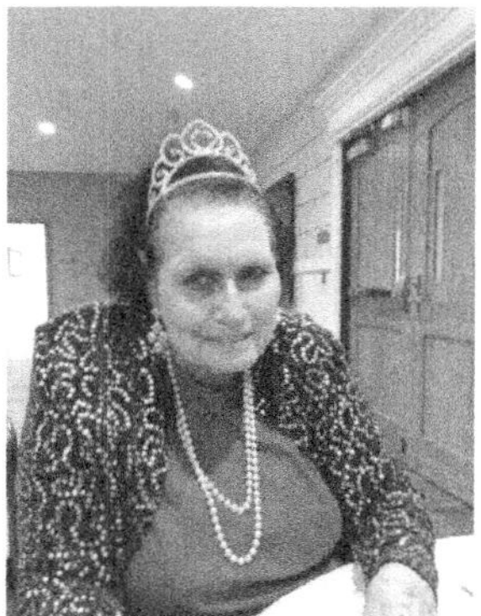

Mom Chronicles September 5, 2018
Kim Gilson, the crown idea for Mom was a hit. I walked in today and found her wearing it at the dinner table.

Mom Chronicles September 5, 2018

I showed Mom the photos I found this weekend. Watch the video to see her reaction. Enjoy!

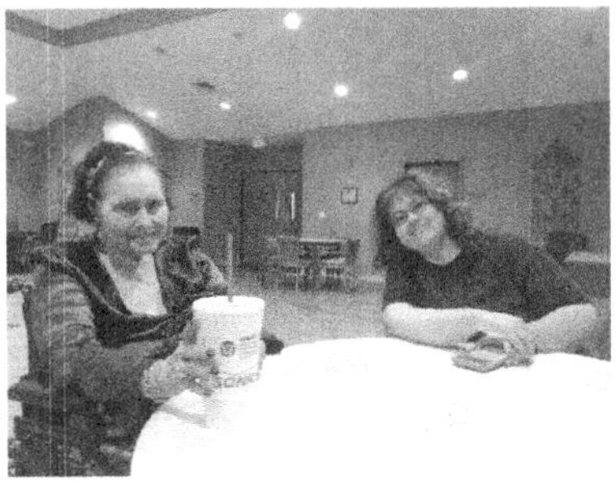

Mom Chronicles September 16, 2018

Sheila and I visited Mom for a short visit this time. She was in a good mood but didn't have any makeup on. She also wasn't wearing a bra again, but she still looked beautiful.

The only sad thing about this visit is that I learned one of her housemates passed away last week. This is the lady who had slid out of her chair a few months ago.

Mom Chronicles September 18, 2018

I was able to get to Mom's by dinner time so that I could observe her eating "skills." She did well through the main course but then choked during dessert. I think it just went down the wrong pipe. She was able to get back under control after a couple of minutes.

After that, I worked on her nails and then played a few rounds of dominoes. Other than the "choking," it was a good visit.

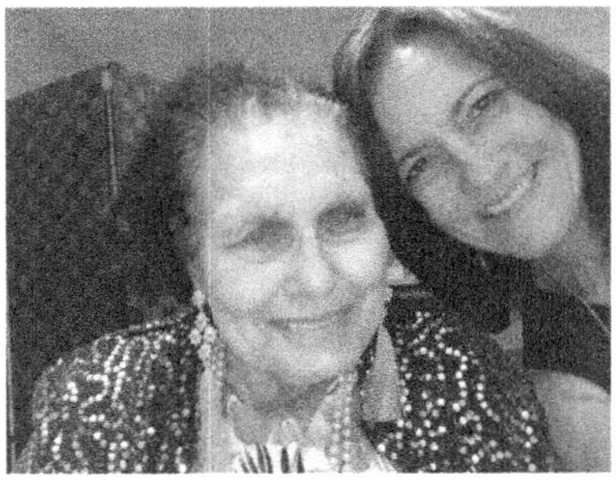

Mom Chronicles September 20, 2018

I arrived right at the end of dinner with a strawberry shake for her. Her friends and tablemates asked where their shakes were, so I promised to bring them drinks on Monday. They were so cute!!

After dinner, and thankfully Mom didn't get choked today, we played dominoes. Unfortunately, I couldn't find her colored dominoes, but I did find another set with the standard black dots in her closet that she pilfered from someone. She struggled with playing tonight since they weren't the colored dots. I think the colored dominoes set helps her with matching.

At 6:00, I took her back to her house and then went to the Alzheimer's Support Group. We had four ladies plus the home's marketing director tonight. We talked about quite a few things, including the stress that this disease puts on family relationships, the stress of the caregivers, and the pain of watching the housemates decline and pass away. They aren't family, but we do get to know them and care for them. One of the attendees mentioned she just put her mom in hospice this week, and it was a difficult subject for her to talk about. We talked about how it seems that many are just going along fine, and then all of a sudden, they start a very steep, fast decline. How in the world do you prepare for this?

The only comic relief for me tonight was that one of the housemates was on a tear tonight. I say "comic," but it's not funny. But, if you don't laugh at some of these situations, you will go crazy! She came out of her room without her clothes on and was yelling at everyone. One of the aides had to get her back in her room ASAP and help her get a nightgown back on. The aides are always so professional and kind and do their best in some very difficult situations. They have been trained very well. I also noticed that one of Mom's friends had a swollen, red eye. Miss "A" told me that the same lady who was streaking had hit her last night, and she had to go to the ER. Knowing how Mom doesn't always get her stories right, I can't say that is what happened, though. Miss "A" may have gotten her story wrong. I'm just hoping my mom didn't do it!!! I imagine I would have gotten a call if she did, though.

When the support group was over, I made the mistake of going back into Mom's house to tell her bye. She had already forgotten that I had been there visiting her and couldn't understand why I would just show up and tell her bye without visiting. Luckily, I still had a cookie in my purse from lunch (don't judge me!), so I redirected her quickly by giving it to her. I told her I would be back in a few days and leaned down to kiss her on her cheek. Mom's best friend was sitting next to her and asked if she would get a kiss too. Well, of course! I leaned down and kissed her forehead. Like I said earlier, we start caring for the housemates!!

One last thing... I was punching the door alarm numbers to leave the house when I looked back. Mom's roommate was trying to walk between Mom and the room support column so that she could sit on the other side of Mom. Unfortunately, there wasn't enough room, so my dear sweet Mom got a little persnickety, raised her voice to her roommate, and said just to go around. Her roommate replied right back with a little bit of a raised voice and said, "well, okay!" I'm not worried about it because I know within 2 minutes, they will both have forgotten they were upset and will be best friends again.

The life of an Alzheimer's patient... it can be comical sometimes!

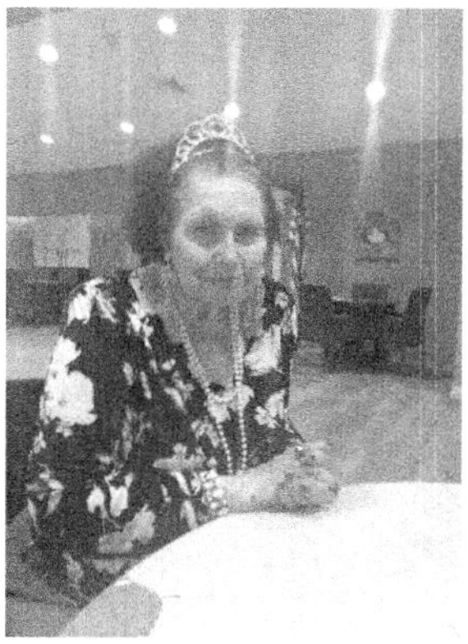

Mom Chronicles September 24, 2018

I arrived at dinner time with four milkshakes for the lovely ladies who all sit with Mom. They always mention how the shakes look good whenever I bring one in for Mom, so I asked them what their favorite flavors were when I was there. Mom's roommate knew hers (chocolate), but Mom's best friend couldn't tell me hers. She just pointed at Mom's strawberry shake and said that one looked good. The 4th lady is always different at the table, so I bought a vanilla shake because I didn't want to leave anyone out at the table. I figured vanilla would be a safe flavor that most people like. (I did confirm with the aides that it was safe to bring them shakes since some residents have diabetes.)

They all looked like a kid in a candy store when I gave them their shakes. It was so cute!

I did notice that Mom was wearing her birthday crown and hardly had any makeup on. She also appeared to be slightly shaky at dinner. Not bad-just a slight shake. By the time she finished dinner, though, the shake was gone. She also swallowed her food just fine tonight. Nothing went down the wrong pipe.

She did make more mistakes in dominoes tonight. We had her colored dominoes, but she missed quite a few matches. It's usually the blanks that she misses, but she was missing other numbers tonight too. Maybe she was just more tired tonight.

She hummed a lot to the music but hardly spoke any. She also was shifting in her wheelchair a lot, so I think her hips were hurting. I imagine weather changes are not helping her arthritis at all. We will see how she feels in a few days.

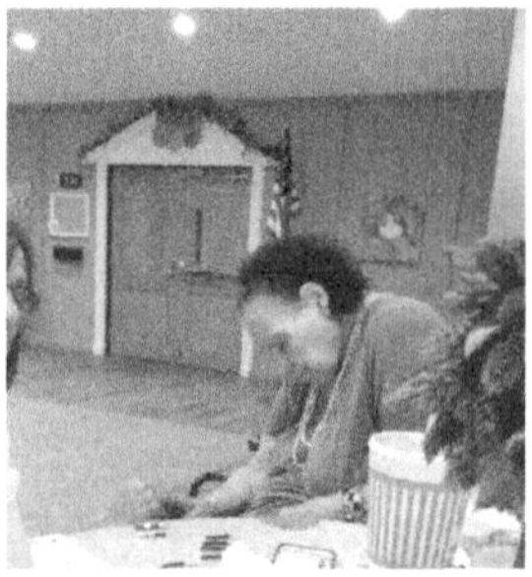

Mom Chronicles September 30, 2018

After church, Bruce and I visited Mom. When we first got there, she was in the restroom panicking a little bit because she saw blood from a sore on her hip. Unfortunately, she has such tender skin (she has had thin, sensitive skin her whole life), and the diapers just don't help. The staff are doing everything they can to protect it - I could see how much cream/medicine they are using to try and protect her as much as possible. But she still freaked when she saw fresh blood. She just kept saying she didn't know what was "wrong with her."

The aides put more medicine on her and freshened her up. Bruce and I then took her into the middle room for our visit. Her fingernails needed to be redone, so I worked on fixing those for her. She's always so happy when her nails look pretty.

As you can see from the pic, she fell asleep again while I was working on them. It's a challenge because her hands jerk when she's sleeping.

I also noticed she didn't have makeup on again. I don't know if she's just not wearing it any more or if I just happen to be visiting when she's not wearing it. She is still wearing her jewelry, thankfully.

It's just weird to see these small changes in her.

Mom Chronicles October 3, 2018

It's a royal crown or crown royal kind of day!! Actually, she's doing pretty good. It is just a short visit today after a long day at work.

Update... Mom was a patooty last night, according to the aides. They said she said, "they are not her friends anymore." She didn't want to shower or change clothes for bedtime. I can just picture her crossing her arms and being stubborn.

Of course, Mom doesn't remember any of this. She just laughed when they told me about it.

Mom Chronicles October 6, 2018

We are celebrating Sheila's birthday with our Mom today with a lemon-flavored "Nothin' Bundt Cake." Mom had to lick all the icing off the candles. We now have another recording for a wonderful memory of Mom singing happy birthday to her.

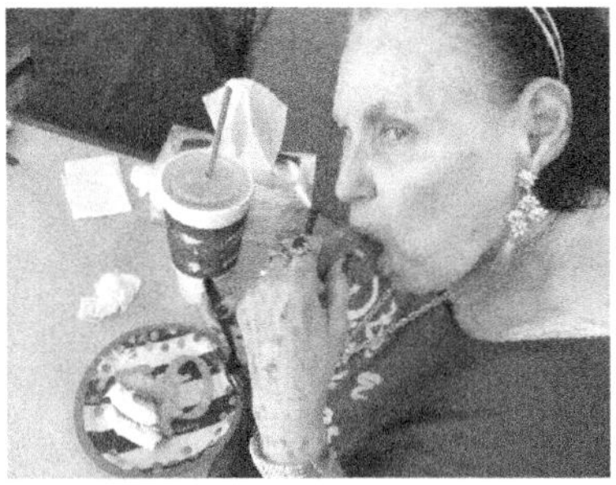

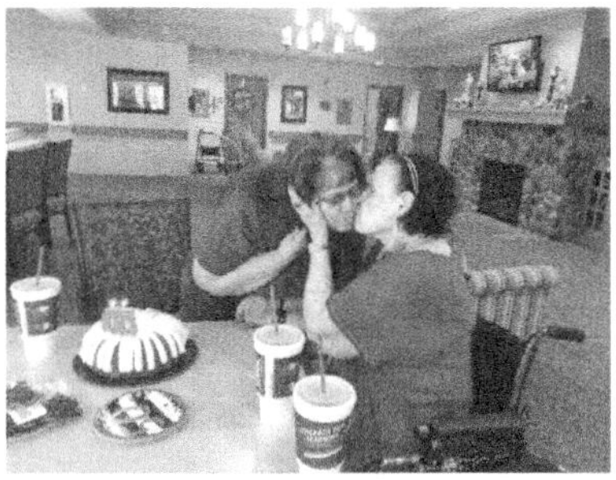

Mom Chronicles October 6, 2018
Mom's best friend at the center is one who talks in phrases that make no sense at all. She's a sweetie, but the phrases she says are humorous. She came over and sat down between Mom and me. Mom reached out and patted her hand and said, "honey, you will be okay." Her friend exclaimed, "your ice cream is COLD!!" All we could do was laugh.

Mom Chronicles October 7, 2018
Mom looks so different without makeup, and my sissy loves the filters on her phone. Mom kept trying to hide behind me when she realized what Sheila was doing to her pictures. It was funny!!

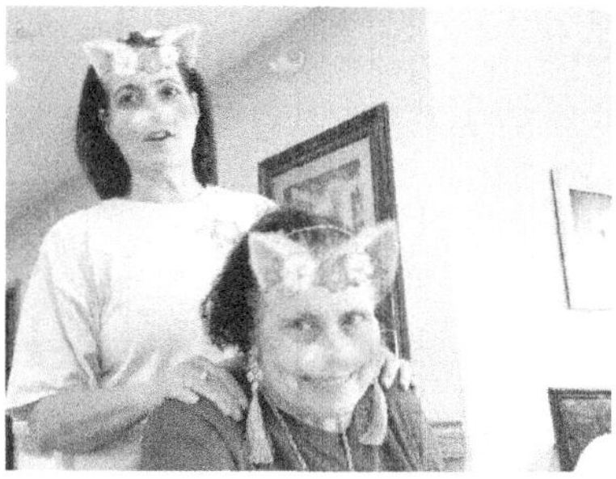

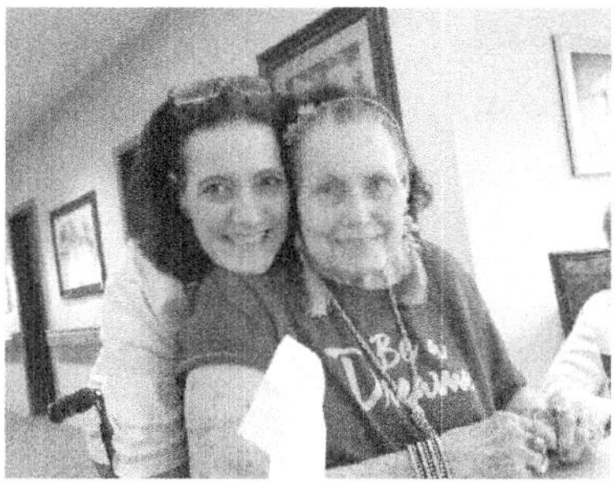

Mom Chronicles October 10, 2018
Mom has her crown on again, and she had eye makeup on.

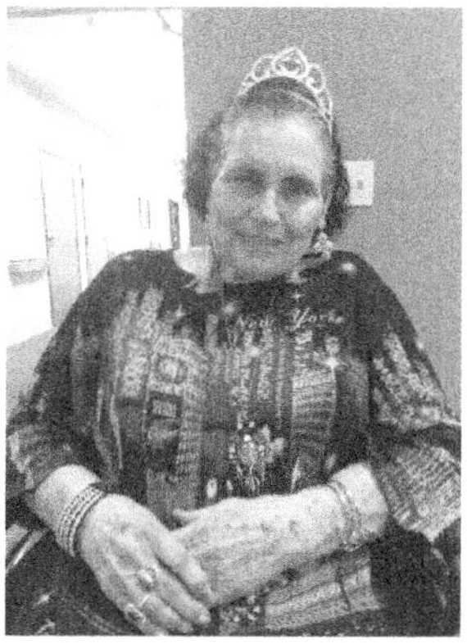

I also put on a different nail wrap color, and I could tell she's not that happy with it, but surprisingly she didn't want me to change them. Usually, she acts like a 2-year-old and wants things her way. So I will probably have to switch back to the sparkly purple next time.

Her vocabulary is getting smaller. I hardly got any coherent phrases out of her tonight. She could only get a few words right in the songs, but she could still hum the tunes, so that was good.

Her go-to phrase that she can still say is "I love you." She also can still introduce me as her daughter to her friends most of the time. So all-in-all, things are good in the grand scheme of things.

Mom Chronicles October 15, 2018
This one is so cute of Mom! I was able to visit with her for about an hour today and took this pic of her.

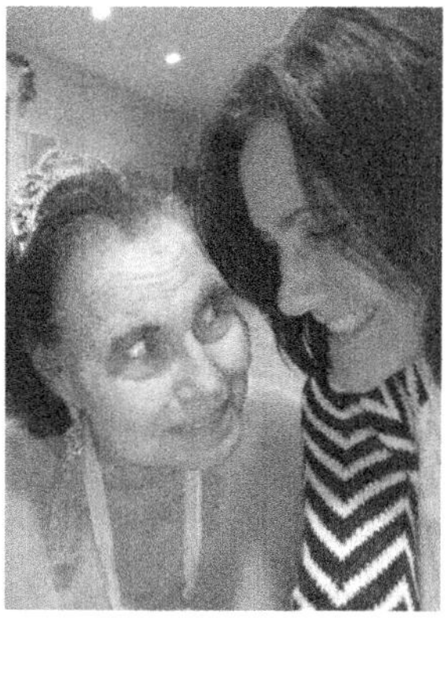

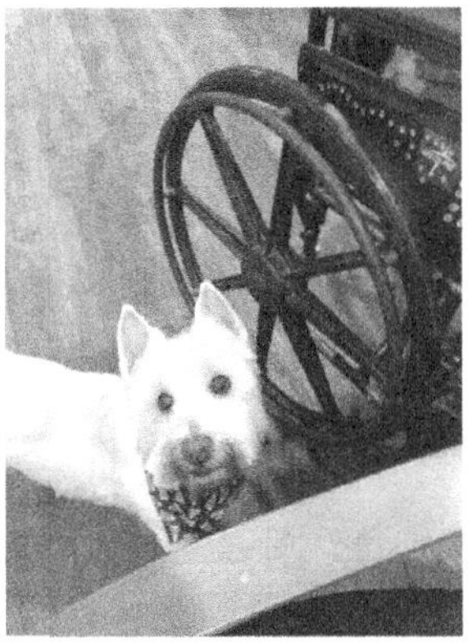

Mom Chronicles October 18, 2018

I decided to treat Mom to a hamburger, fries, and soda. That meal used to be her favorite. She loved it at first, but she was getting more frustrated as the toppings kept falling out. She finally said she was full (in her limited words) when she was about halfway through with the burger. I showed her the chocolate chip cookie, and of course, she had room for that!! Oh, and Shauna's dog, Buddy, tried hard to get a French fry! I had to take a pic of him. He was adorable!

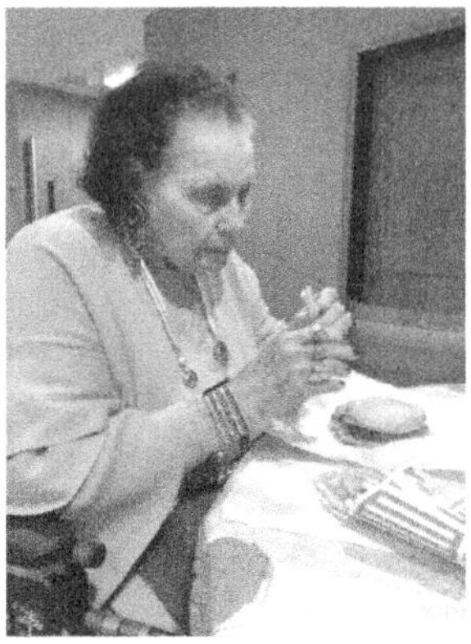

We then played dominoes for a little bit until the support group started at 6:00 pm. At the support group, we had a new family visiting whose husband/father lives at a different facility. We also worked on relaxation techniques which I still fail miserably at. The group leader did say that it takes practice, so there is hope for me yet. My mind just races constantly. It's hard to turn it off. I cringe every time I look at my Fitbit sleeping pattern. It looks more like a heartbeat during a 5K race instead of a flat line. She said that so many of us stay worked up, and we don't realize just how stressed we are because it has become a new normal or baseline for us.

There was also a counselor-in-training at the meeting, and she recommended a book (*Creating Moments of Joy Along the Alzheimer's Journey* by Jolene Brackey). She said it consists of lots of small stories about different Alzheimer's topics.

We ended it with the question of what we wanted to talk about next time. I volunteered a suggestion about ways to communicate with Mom. Her vocabulary is so small now, and I desperately want to hear her talk to me again. I didn't think it affected me that much, but when my eyes teared up suggesting it, I realized it does. I also know that I need to let that go. She will never be able to "really talk" to me again until I see her in heaven.

They did say that she can communicate in different ways. They are going to look up suggestions to talk about next month, but they did mention these things to try:

- Art. Ask her to draw or paint a picture of her house when she was little.
- Sorting objects. She might be able to pull some basic words out about the objects.
- Put together a box full of objects that would mean a lot to her and then just talk about what I think those objects mean.
- And I know I need to bring the photo books out much more. She always loves that.

Mom Chronicles October 24, 2018

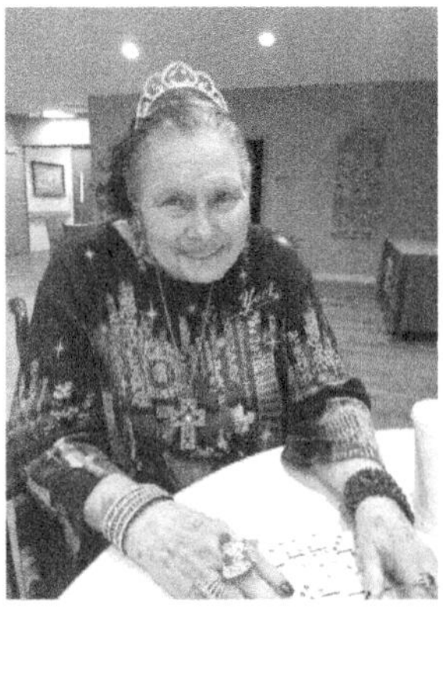

Well, we had a little extra confusion tonight. Maybe because it was raining, so it was darker outside when I got there? Who knows... Anyway, she wanted to scramble the dominoes dot side up this time. She also decided to use two spinners during one game. As you may also notice, she is still sporting her birthday crown (going on two months now), and she is also wearing a birthday ring from one of the other resident's recent birthday party. This woman keeps me on my toes!! I never know what to expect!! And finally, Josh FaceTimed in for a few minutes so that she could see his face. When we were going through the photo album, she saw his picture and said she hadn't seen him in a long time. She knew who he was, though. She just couldn't remember his name. (She doesn't remember my name either, so that is to be expected.) So, I called Josh to see if he was available, and he was.

Mom Chronicles October 26, 2018
We get off work early on Fridays, so I arrived at Mom's center by 3:15. When I got there, she had her hands and arms crossed over her lap. I asked if she was okay. She pointed to her lap and tried to tell me she was wet. Sure enough, she had an accident, and her pants were completely soaked, and so were her blouse sleeves. She was so embarrassed. I quietly told the aide and then quietly took her into her room since she didn't want anyone else to see she was wet. Because she was so wet, they decided to do a bed bath for her and get her completely clean. She didn't fight them at all. She just kept saying she was sorry over and over.

After cleaning up and putting on fresh clothes, we changed her jewelry to match her clean set of clothes. I also brushed her hair and put a different headband on her. I thought she had her crown on when I brought her into the restroom, but I couldn't find the crown anymore after getting her cleaned and changed. So if it doesn't show back up, I may need to go pick up another one. At least those are very inexpensive.

I also need to go in and do a sneak cleaning. Mom (like many others with dementia) hoards things, like silverware, napkins, cups, etc. I can't throw these things away or put them back in the kitchen if she is watching me. I must be in stealth ninja mode to clean her room. This usually only happens if Sheila is there to occupy her attention. I need to thin some things out in her closet, too, so that she doesn't have so many choices, BUT there is a fine balance of thinning things out yet make it still look like she has a lot. I'm sure this will change more and more as the disease progresses.

Mom Chronicles October 27, 2018
I couldn't attend the doggie event at the memory care center, so Jenni sent me these pics. Animal therapy is great for dementia patients!

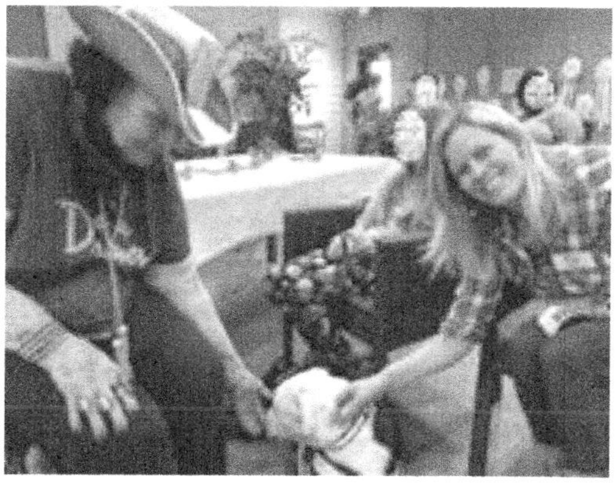

Mom Chronicles November 5, 2018
When I arrived at the center, it was close to dinner time. Mom was at the table, and she picked up the spoon and said, "this isn't good." I asked what was wrong, and she said it doesn't work. I told her it was a spoon. She didn't like it at all.

They brought the food out, and the chef forgot to cut up her food again. I will have to reach back out tomorrow to remind them to do this. I don't always get there by dinner time, but this is the 2nd time over the past couple of weeks that I was there at dinner and her food wasn't cut up. She had a baked potato last time, and she told me she didn't know what to do with it. She just doesn't remember how to cut up food with her fork. I cut up the meat for her, but she didn't want it tonight. It was a little too tough for her. After that, I took her into the middle room and worked on her nails. I put a different color on her, and she seemed to be happy. I also bought her some new makeup. She hasn't been wearing makeup the last several times I've been there, so I'm hoping it will spur her to put it on again. I don't care if she looks like Mimi from the Drew Carey show. I just want to see her put makeup on because I know it used to bring her so much joy. I also brought in some peanut M&Ms. When she thought I wasn't looking, she took the bag and hid it in her wheelchair near her back.

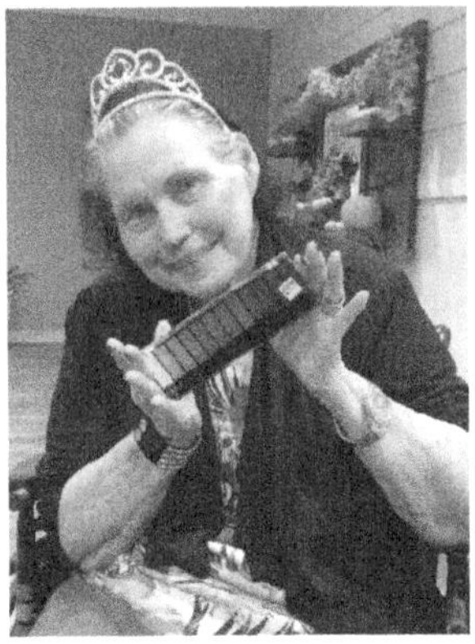

I took a video of her when I gave her the makeup. You would think she received a priceless treasure. Too cute. And notice she is still wearing her birthday crown.

Finally, Sheila and I Skyped for a few minutes so that they could see each other. At first, Mom didn't seem to comprehend that it was Sheila, but as soon as Sheila said, "Hi Mom," it clicked, and she recognized her. I think seeing her on the phone threw her off this time.

Mom Chronicles November 6, 2018
One of the beautiful ladies in Mom's "house" passed away on Friday. She was the same lady who poured juice on my head a while back, so I had a special connection to her. They held a Memorial Service for her today. Mom recognized her picture and started crying during "Amazing Grace." I'm not sure if she was connecting to the loss of Miss B, the song sung at a lot of funerals, or the idea of sadness associated with a loss. No matter the reason, it was a little tougher leaving her today. One - because she was sadder than normal and two - attending a memorial just makes me realize my time with her is getting shorter.

There were some other emotional decisions made today concerning Mom that I will share later. I need to talk to some family members first. Lots of coincidences fell into place, so I feel it's the right decision, but it will still be a little hard.

I'm ending this one short today because my eyes are starting to leak again.

Mom Chronicles November 6, 2018
I've had a chance to talk to the hubster, the sister, and the kiddo about today's events. Those three are the major players in my decision-making for Mom, so I wanted to share the info with them first.

We have decided to move Mom to a different memory care center. We have a good friend who is about to place her mother into memory care. During her research, she found a center very close to me when I'm at work that was purchased by another company and has gone through major remodeling and restructuring. The place is beautiful and has many amenities, plus they have a reduced rate special that is locked in for the entire time that Mom would be there. She would also have a private room. This move is going to save Bruce and me a significant amount of money.

I didn't go into making this decision lightly. Having Mom go through another transition period will be difficult, and we will miss the friends that we have made at the current memory care center. They have become like family to us. Mom and our friend's mother will have rooms next to each other, and there is a 50's soda shop-themed room right there by their rooms so that they can play dominoes together. Let me be perfectly clear... our current memory care center has been absolutely fantastic. They have done nothing wrong, and if I ever had an issue (which will happen anywhere we go), they fixed it or retrained staff immediately. That's why this decision has been so hard! And if this new place doesn't work out for whatever reason, I will take Mom back there immediately. But I am very optimistic that this new place is going to be a huge blessing.

I also love that it will be close enough to spend about 30 minutes during lunch with her.

We will move her in there on December 1. Send lots of prayers up during that time!!

And pray for my friend. I have had a year of being adjusted to Mom living in memory care. This move is brand new for my friend, and she's worried that her Mom will be angry and not transition well. However, we are hopeful that they both will do well living next door to each other.

Mom Chronicles November 8, 2018

I submitted all the paperwork for the new memory care center, and they answered all the questions that Jenni encouraged me to ask. She has grown to love my mom and only wants the best for her, so she told me some questions to ask that I didn't think to ask the other day. The new center answered them satisfactorily. There are a couple of things they need to work on, but I think it's all going to be okay.

Also, while helping my friend who will be moving her Mom into the same center go through this process, I found this blog site of the top 50 suggestions for moving a loved one into a memory care center. It has some great reminders for me to use with Mom on Dec 1.

www.seniorlink.com/blog/50-tips-on-transitioning-a-loved-one-to-memory-dementia-or-alzheimers-careyour-blog-post-title-here (Trowbridge, 2020)

I hope this helps others who are going through a similar journey.

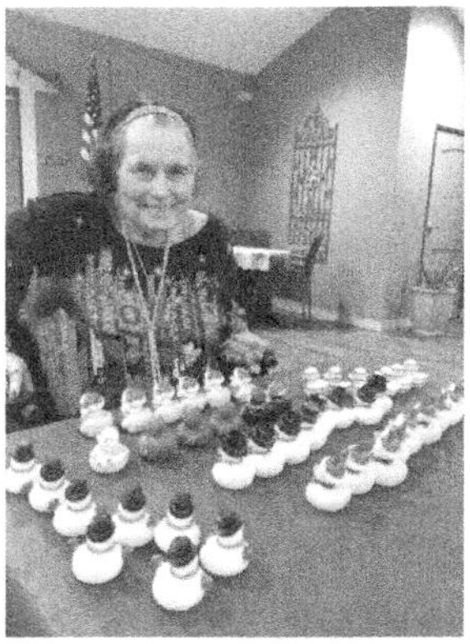

Mom Chronicles Nov 9, 2018

I stopped by for a short visit with Mom this afternoon. When I got there, the "three musketeers" were coloring. I do hate that I'm breaking them up in December. I have grown attached to these two other ladies. They always want a hug and kiss when I leave Mom each time.

After they were tired of coloring, the other two went back into the main house to watch TV. I kept Mom with me, and I brought out a bag of Christmas-themed ducks. I asked her to help me sort them. She did well and had fun while sorting.

Mom Chronicles November 10, 2018

I pulled some photos from the memory care center's Facebook post today so that I will always have them. It looks like they all had a great time! They were exercising without realizing it!!

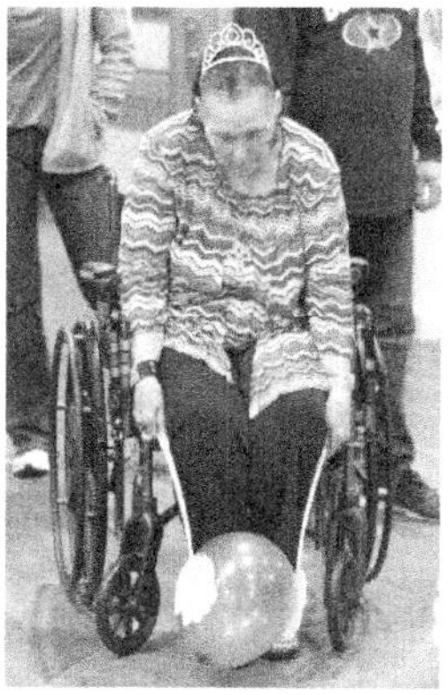

Mom Chronicles November 17, 2018
Sheila and I hadn't seen Mom since Monday, so it was good to see her. She was in a good mood today, but she was "different." It's like she didn't have the patience with us to make her laugh. We usually act silly with her to get her to laugh. She would laugh some, but more often than not, she would just look at us like she was saying, "behave."

Also, her words were very slurred today. I think there were only a couple of phrases that she said that made sense. Most of the words were just jumbled syllables. We think she may have just been more tired today than usual. Sheila will visit her tomorrow before heading home, so she will let me know how she is then.

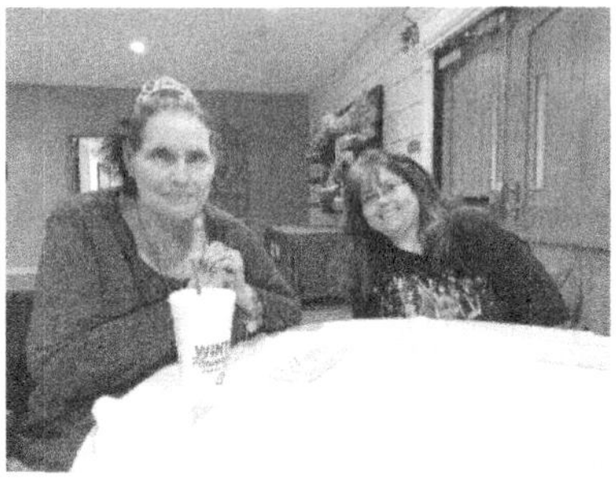

*I forgot to add that I need to get her hair colored again. We noticed that she tried to use her eyebrow pencil to darken the gray hair that has grown out.

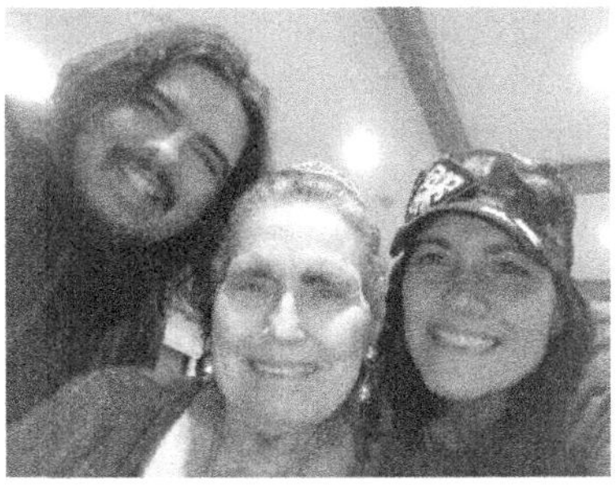

Mom Chronicles November 21, 2018
The munchkin and I visited Mom for a little while this afternoon. Josh made her laugh while wearing her crown and one of her earrings. It was a nice little visit.

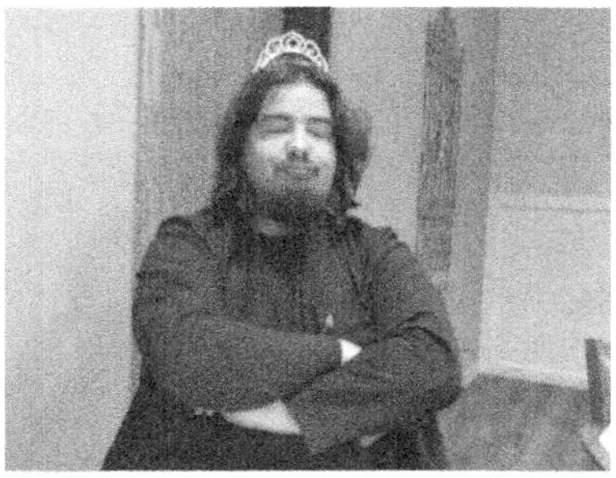

Mom Chronicles November 26, 2018
The most wonderful neighbor in the world met me at Mom's today for a visit. When Lynda Hart and I first walked into Mom's "house," Mom acted like she hadn't seen me in years. She hugged and hugged me and started tearing up a little. Then I showed her Lynda and asked if she remembered her. Mom acted like she recognized her and gave her a big hug. Lynda was one of the fabulous friends who would sit with Mom or check on her for me when I needed someone close to the house. It was just a short visit tonight, but that's okay. I'll go back in a few days. Lynda and I then went and had dinner together to catch up. I sure miss her and everyone on that block!! Love ya, Miss Lynda!!

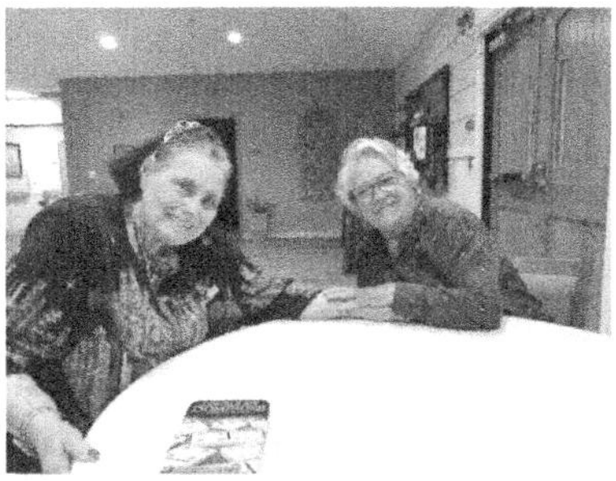

Mom Chronicles November 28, 2018
I took the morning off to meet the nurse from the new place who needed to evaluate Mom before admission.

She asked Mom some basic questions. She remembered her first name, but she couldn't remember her last name, her birthday, where she was born, etc. When I used the phrase we always used about our last name,

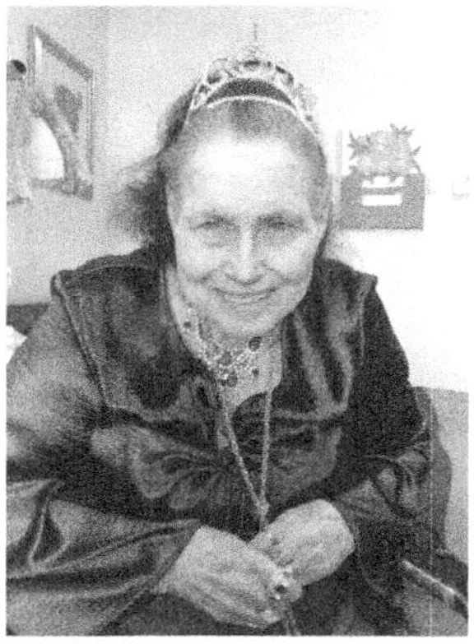

"Parsley - like the green stuff you put on mashed potatoes," she lit up remembering that phrase. During the evaluation, she kept looking at her fingernails and kept trying to tell me they "weren't good," which meant it was time for me to fix them again. So, I did as soon as the nurse left. She is now happily sitting at the dining table about to have lunch.

I still haven't told her we are moving her Saturday. There is no sense in worrying her about it now. On Saturday, I will just tell her she is going to a new place to get some more rehab for a little while and that she will be able to see her friend, Ms. Janet. Plus, I will have her room decked out very pretty to help in the transition. This was just another day in our Alzheimer's journey.

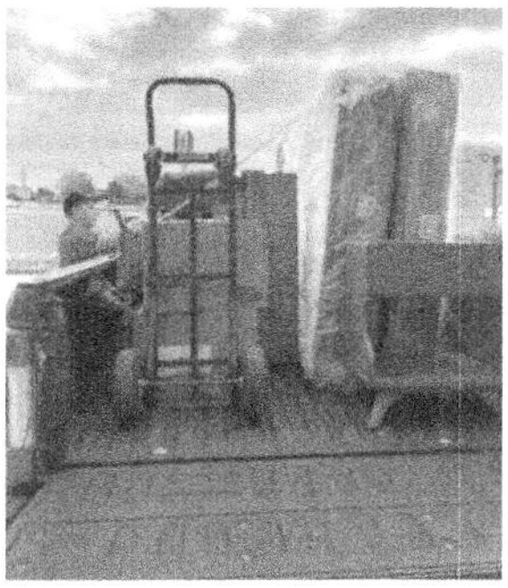

Mom Chronicles November 30, 2018
Phase 1 of the "Mom Move."

The hubster is helping me move Mom's furniture from storage to the new place today. She will be using the same furniture she used when she lived with us. It was also the same furniture at my grandparents' home that we would sleep on every time we visited. I think Uncle Quinton even used this set when he was younger.

It's also fun seeing the old gum dried behind the back of the bed. I wonder if it was hers, Uncle Quinton's, my brother's, Sheila's, or mine!

Mom Chronicles November 30, 2018
Phase 2 of the "Mom Move" is complete. Her furniture is set up in the new place. Phase 3 will be tomorrow when we get her things in her current room and use it to decorate. I will also get more of her photo albums for the shelves and wall photos to hang since there will be more room. I also was able to put the little curio cabinet with wood carvings from one of her grandpas. I don't know which grandpa. She said she carved one of the tiny chairs when he taught her how when she was little. I'm hoping, since it is a memory from her childhood, that she will remember these. And for the emergency "calm her down" scene that is possible tomorrow, I bought some chocolate-covered cherries. She always loves this candy every Christmas.

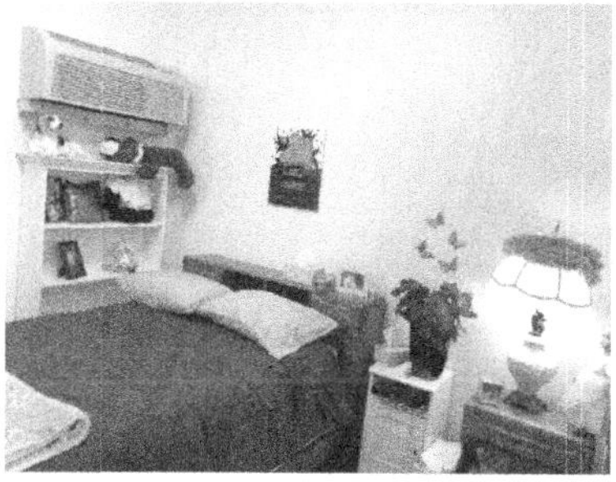

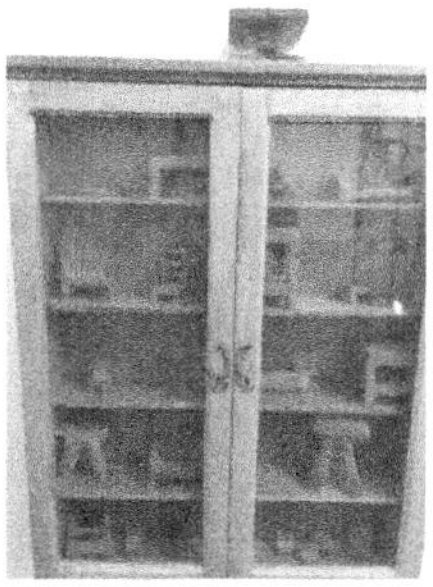

Mom Chronicles December 1, 2018
Phase 3 of the "Mom Move."

Today was a really, really long day. Sheila kept her busy in the middle room while Bruce and I packed. The other center was supposed to pick her up at 10 am, but they had issues with their van, and the Uber wheelchair assistance service was running behind. So, I suggested a wheelchair van from an ambulance service. I was getting concerned that the longer we waited, the more of a chance of Mom having an accident, and we had already packed everything up. Sure enough, she did have an accident, so we scrambled to find clean pants in the boxes already packed. The wheelchair van finally arrived at 11:30 am to pick her up. Mom was confused, but we told her we were taking her to a new place where she could have a private room and her big bed again. She sounded excited, but she wasn't comprehending everything. Many of the staff members hugged her and told her bye. Several promised to visit her at the new place. I learned that her nickname from one of the staff was "Sparkles." I love that nickname! It's perfect for her.

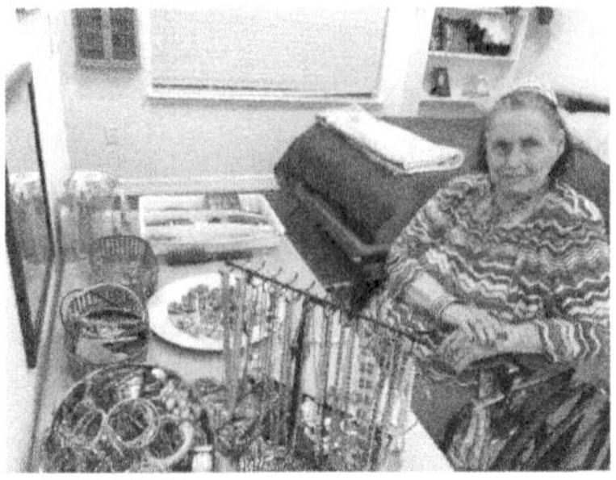

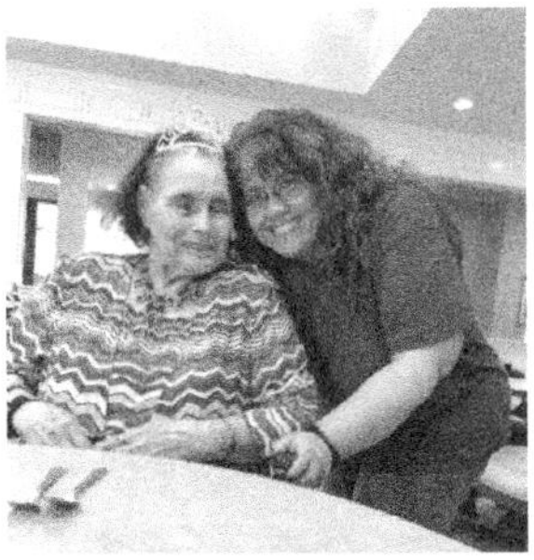

When we arrived at the new place, she was upset. She also seemed to be in more pain today. She was "moaning" with every breath most of the day. We figured the move just made this worse.

She went to the dining hall first but didn't eat much. We then took her to her room and showed her what we had done so far. She loved it. Sheila took her to the soda shop and worked on a door hanging craft with her. It will be sparkly and have her name on it.

Every time we took her back to her room, she acted like it was the first time she had seen it, and she ooohed and ahhhed over it.

Dinner time was rough. The kitchen staff had all three utensils on the table, and she just kept staring at the knife and picking it up like she didn't know what it was. The original memory care center where Mom lived never had a knife on the table (at least I never saw one), so she had forgotten what it was. They also have three courses which confused her too. She had some soup for the first course, and then for the second course, they brought out a menu for us to choose what she wanted. We picked something, and when they brought it out, she didn't want it. By this time of the afternoon, she was more stressed out, so she wasn't hungry. The aide said we could pick out the meals for her, or they could bring out both options on plates and let her choose. I think we will try the second option first. I just need to make sure they know her food must be cut up for her.

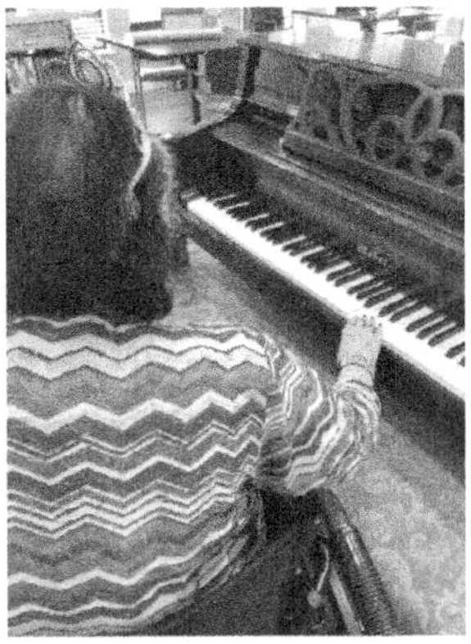

We showed her some of the places around the center, including a room with a piano. Then we took her back to her bedroom, and of course, she ooohed and ahhhed over it again like she hadn't seen it.

Sheila had to run an errand, so I asked her to pick up a shake for Mom on her way back. On a good note, she and Miss Janet visited each other for a little while, and they seemed so happy to see each other. Also, Miss Janet seemed to be okay so far with her move-in day. We had a few concerns with various things throughout the day, but I chatted with one of the directors, and most issues were resolved. I will say the staff treated her very well and with respect when they worked on changing her. They learned quickly this is not easy since she screams during this process. But they were very calm and tried to comfort her. Of course, they could have been doing this because I was there, but I don't think so. It's always so hard to hear her scream. She did this over at the other memory care center too, so it wasn't new, but it's hard to hear. I feel so sorry for her when she does this.

We stayed with Mom until she laid down for bedtime. I laid with her for about 10-15 minutes just to help her relax and get sleepy. She patted my face and told me she loves me and misses me. I told her the same back and reassured her I would be back in the morning. I know it's going to take a while for her to settle into the new place. So we will just take it one day at a time.

Mom Chronicles December 3, 2018

The last three days have been an emotional whirlwind of frustrations. I started a venting post last night that was really, really long, but before I could press "share," FB quit on me without saving it, so I figured that was God's way of saying, "sleep on this before posting."

As expected, Mom is emotional and disoriented at the new place. I expected this and just need to give her some time. She was actually good today when I got there by lunchtime. But as the day progressed, she got worse (probably due to sundowning). Last night, my sister had to FaceTime with me before she headed back to Huntsville to let me see Mom and help calm her down.

I am having some issues with things that are happening there. I won't go into everything but suffice it to say, the level of care is not good right now. They aren't checking on Mom throughout the day to change her. I had to go down to the front living room area and ask someone to come to her room and change her. It's unacceptable to make her stay in the same diaper all day long. They are supposed to check on her every 2-3 hours, but they haven't been. I was there from 11 am through 7 pm tonight, and again, no one changed her until bedtime. After the aide changed her and put her to bed, Mom immediately had another accident. I asked the aide to come back down and clean her as soon as possible, but she got ugly with me. I lost my cool with her. If you know me at all, you know this isn't the way I act. I am always calm and hold things in without confronting people. Because the aide wouldn't come back down right away, I helped freshen Mom up myself so that she could try to get some sleep. (Since she was already lying down, it was easier for me to change her myself. If she had still been in her wheelchair, I would not have been able to do so.)

There are some issues with mealtimes too, but we will get this resolved soon too.

They also didn't have her medications right – the medication aide said they didn't have orders in her file, but the new nurse called her Saturday night and told her where the orders were. Well, last night before Sheila left, she learned that they still weren't giving meds because the orders were missing. So I had to get the director involved to get her medicine administered. I was upset that she had gone the whole day without her meds.

I spoke to the new nurse today. She was very apologetic and promised to get things fixed. I like her, so I will give her some time to work her magic. The director also stopped by the table at lunchtime and said because of all the issues that happened this weekend, they will make a policy change and not allow admissions over the weekend. There just wasn't enough management on site on the weekends to help resolve problems.

In my opinion, this new management team grew things too fast with this low introductory care rate and made promises they couldn't keep right away. However, I do like the marketing director – she has been checking on me daily and contacting the various directors with the issues we have been having. I think the executive director wants things right, too - we will just have to see. And I do like the nurse. I also like MOST of the aides. They have been very friendly – they just need some training/retraining, and they need a care plan for Mom to follow.

I'm going to give it until the end of December to see if these changes are made. If not, I'm taking her back to the original memory care center immediately. At least there, I had peace of mind. Right now, I don't have that peace. I'm constantly worrying. Oh, and Jenni stopped by to visit Mom today because she knew how upset I was. I am so grateful she did this. Thank you, Jenni – if you are reading this. You and Olive made Mom smile and giggle, which was fantastic!

Mom Chronicles December 4, 2018
I try not to get on FB for personal posts during work hours as much as possible, but I just had to do one quick post.

One of the staff members just called me. She's been out the last three days and was reading Mom's chart. She wanted me to give her as much information about Mom as possible so that she can help her. So I explained all the problems we experienced this weekend.

She didn't have any issues with Mom being combative this morning, and neither did one of the aides the other morning. So she said she would do two things: 1) train the staff on how to approach Mom. They need to explain every single little thing they are about to do in short phrases. 2) They will also try showering in the morning instead of evenings to see if she isn't combative then.

She also asked about activities. She said Mom didn't want to go out of her room at first but then got her make-up all on and asked if she could leave her room now. I told her she participated in many activities at the other center but then there were many times all she wanted to do was sit in front of the TV. I mentioned that we either need to get cable in that back living area OR they needed to keep DVDs going on there so that she has a space to go to when she doesn't want to participate in activities. I could put a TV in her room, but she doesn't understand how to operate a remote control – not even the elderly kind of remote control that only has a few buttons.

We also talked about meals. The meals I have seen look wonderful. The problem is they give them too many choices. They want the residents to circle the items on a menu. Mom can't read or comprehend words anymore, so they let them look at demo trays they bring out to the table. Again - Mom doesn't seem to be able to handle this. It's too many choices. Alzheimer's patients can't comprehend, so as Jenni reminded me yesterday - it embarrasses them because they don't understand. They also serve three courses: soup, the main meal, and dessert. I told her it was confusing her to see the soup and then thinking that is all there is to the meal. She is going to try bringing all three courses out at the same time. I reminded them that all food needs cut up, that she doesn't like cheese, that she doesn't like sauce, and she definitely doesn't like food mixed up or touching. They must be compartmentalized. This is a big change from her "old self." I explained that she often doesn't understand what to do with her utensils and that they need to keep the knife away. I also explained how I saw one of the other patients walking out of the dining hall with a knife in his mouth. He is further along than Mom, so I got the attention of an aide to get the knife away from him safely.

So, if this person does what she says she's going to do, I think we will be okay. She is the first person to ask me about Mom to understand her specific needs.

We shall see... one day at a time. Keep the prayers going up that this facility will work out after all.

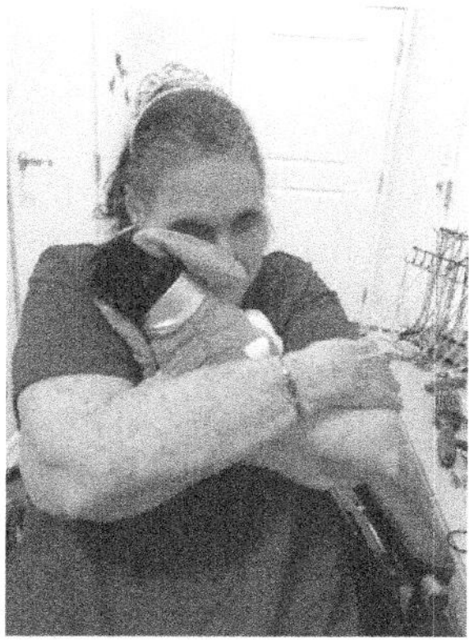

Mom Chronicles December 4, 2018
After having a rough few days, it was nice to see her smiling and laughing. Thank you, Beth Dolliver, for the singing Elvis doggie. It was a HUGE hit!! I have several videos because she kept being surprised each time.

I am crying tears of joy!!

Mom Chronicles December 4, 2018
You guys know I use my Mom Chronicles for both journaling to help me remember this journey, but I also use it to help others going through dementia with a loved one too.

The latest thing I want to talk about is getting my mom to bed. For the last three nights, as soon as the aides finished changing her diaper and putting on her pajamas, they put her straight to bed. She fights it and has been crying so hard. I know part (most) of this is because she's in a new place. The aides also don't know the tips and tricks on how to work with Mom. This has been breaking my heart, and I've been lying down with her to calm her down. Tonight, I used the small photo album and music. She was good after doing this for about 5 minutes or so.

Jenni, the director from the previous memory care center, has been a huge blessing to me. She has been patiently answering questions to prepare for a "come-to-Jesus" meeting I'm going to have with the directors tomorrow at the new facility about her care plan and one particular aide. She talked to her nighttime staff for me to ask what they had to do with Mom. For Mom, they had to tell her that her friend was about to go to her room to get ready for bed, so it was time for her to do so too. Then once they got her in her room, they changed her and got her to lay down. They had to use a "parent voice" (not yelling, but a stern directive as a parent.)

I learned that she did fight them verbally (cuss them out and call them a$&holes) most nights but would calm down within 5 minutes or so. Jenni said this is how dementia patients still voice their independence and believe that they are still in charge.

I would much rather she cussed them out rather than crying. The crying is breaking my heart. Of course, if there were any way to keep her from doing both, that would be even better, but that's just not how this disease works, unfortunately.

So tonight has been another whirlwind of emotions. She had incredible joy with the Elvis stuffed animal that sings, but bedtime was awful. I will be discussing this with the new place's staff tomorrow. We are still in the early stages of this transition, but things need to be fixed now, or they are just going to think I'm okay with this level of care. My mom has no voice. I do, though, and it will be heard.

Mom Chronicles December 5, 2018
Today was much better. I had a meeting with the new nurse and the Memory Care Director this afternoon. I also briefly talked to the Executive Director. They worked with me through many of my concerns, and we came up with suggestions and recommendations that were going to be carried out. I think many of them are

going to help the other residents as well. They still have a few processes that are being ironed out, but it's a step in the right direction.

When I went back to Mom's room, she was in her closet trying to get her teal dress on. She was ready to dress up. As far as I know, she hasn't worn it in over a year because it still had her Concordia Lutheran Church name badge clipped on it. It did my heart good to see this.

Tonight, the medication aide stopped by to talk to me for a few minutes about Mom and wanted to know more ways to help her. I told her that Mom doesn't like to go to bed early, so she said to bring her up to the front when I leave at night. She could hang out and watch movies until she was ready for bed. Well, Mom proved me a liar. When I was ready to leave, she said she was ready to go to bed. So, I took her to her room and helped her get her gown on. I told her I needed help changing her underpants, and at first, she balked. But I used the suggestion Jenni shared with me, and it worked. Two of the aides came down, and we all got Mom changed and in bed with no issues at all. No screaming. No crying. It was heaven.

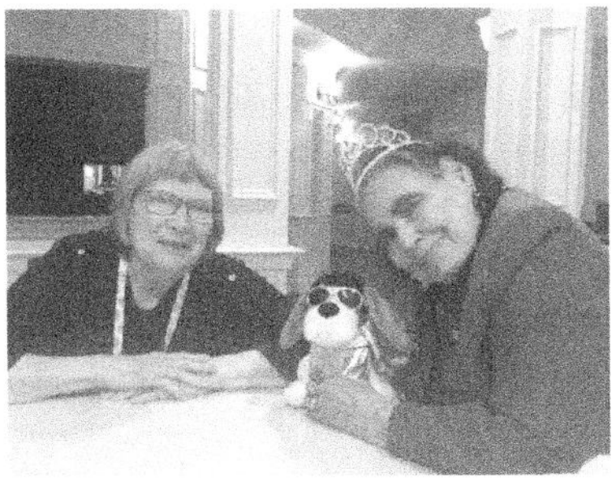

My takeaways? It was her choice to go to bed. She wasn't forced. We used calm talk and playful talk. We had her "dance" her feet apart before she stood up to be more stable. The aide promised me she would share this trick with the others so that they all knew one secret to help Mom. We know this may not work every time, but it worked tonight. She also played with the Elvis doggie again. She LOVES it! The aide that I had trouble with the last two nights said hello and was not rude tonight. So, all in all, it was a great day. I will be able to sleep tonight.

♥

Notice here that I said we had Mom "dance" her feet apart. By now, her leg/hip joints were starting to "freeze" - this is also called limb contractures. She is not limber anymore. She could still stand up (hunched over) with a lot of assistance but her legs are basically "frozen" together, so it made it hard to put the diaper on. Range of motion exercises are extremely important, so please consult your loved one's physician to learn how to do this safely. The center should also have a physical therapist who can help with these exercises. Mom, however, did fight this a lot because it is painful. She eventually ended up bedridden/chair-bound with her knees permanently bent at a 90-degree angle because she could no longer straighten out her legs. Pressure sores are a critical thing to watch for when you notice the limbs starting to freeze.

Mom Chronicles December 6, 2018

I have the BEST co-workers and friends in the world. Pastor Ken called me yesterday and checked on my mental and spiritual health because he could see how frazzled I was in my recent posts. Beth Dolliver gave the Singing Elvis stuffed doggie to Mom a couple of days ago. Many friends send cards to Mom frequently. Today, my co-worker Ligia Curtis brought this necklace to me during lunch to give to Mom. They have all been a huge blessing to my family and me. I will take this necklace with me tonight and give it to her then. She is going to LOVE it!!

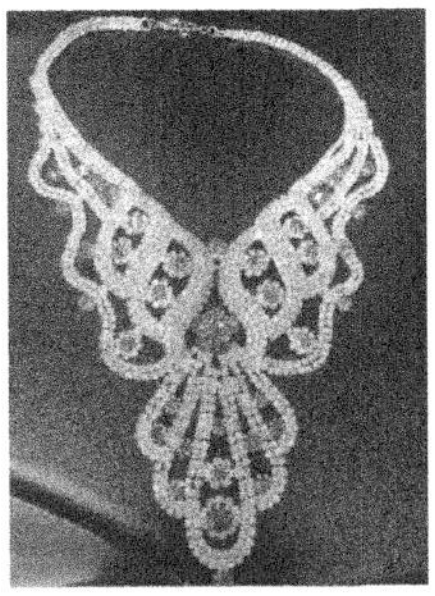

You all are the best, and I am grateful you all are in my life!!

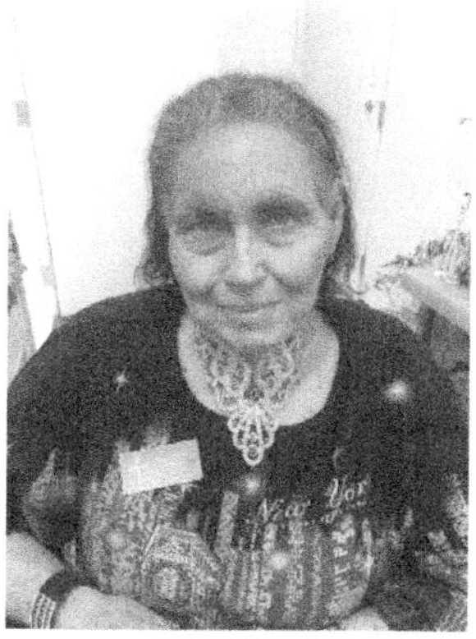

Mom Chronicles December 6, 2018
Today was another successful evening with Mom, for the most part.

She was in the dining hall when I arrived. The first thing I noticed is that she was wearing her Concordia Lutheran Church name tag.

She ate most of the dinner. They still haven't implemented the pre-chosen meals I picked out, and it wasn't cut up for her. I'm giving them a few more days since I just gave the chef the menu yesterday. He also needs an order from the doctor to cut up her food first. I'm not sure of the reasoning behind that. I think their mealtime routine still needs some considerable refinement.

[I later learned that a doctor must prescribe any mealtime change in how food is served to any resident in a residential care facility.]

Miss Janet, Mom's friend who is transitioning to living at the center as well, thinks she is in a hotel, and her car is out front in the parking lot. I said it is, but it is cold and raining, so she will need to stay another few nights until the rain clears up. Mom asked if her car was out there too. I said yes. She hasn't asked about her car in years!

We went to the "soda shop" and played dominoes for a while. Then we went to the family room across the hall and started watching a movie.

It was getting close to the time for me to go home, so I gently asked if she was getting tired and ready to go to bed since it was dark outside. She said yes. Whew. We have learned it needs to be her choice to go to bed. But, it doesn't mean I can't plant the seed!!

We were able to get her to bed calmly again tonight. She almost lost it a couple of times, but we redirected once and used the photo album the second time. At first, she pushed the album away from me, saying, "no!" But the moment I showed just one picture from it, she completely changed. It was like flipping a switch.

The bad part tonight is that she now has an open wound with blood. I had them slather the prescription cream on her and then sent an email to the head nurse as soon as I got home.

She had this happen several times at the previous memory care center, but they stayed on top of it and applied the cream heavily. This facility just needs to learn to do the same.

I plan on being there every evening for the next week or two to make sure they are doing what they need to do and that the wound does not get worse and starts to heal. I also want to make sure every single aide who meets Mom knows how to help her go to bed easily.

Finally, I gave her the new necklace tonight. She LOVED it. I need to get a necklace extender for it, though. Thank you, Ligia, for making my mom smile tonight. You are a blessing to us!!

One day at a time. One moment at a time.

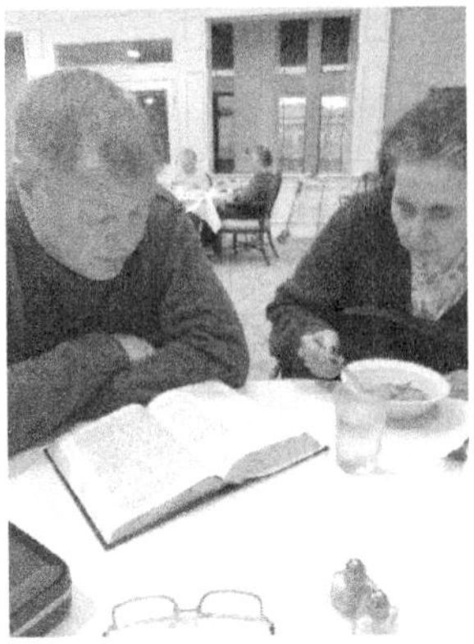

Mom Chronicles December 7, 2018
Pastor Ken came to visit my Mom today. She was so happy to see him. He was reading the Christmas story for Mom, and an aide heard him. He asked for a card so that he could call Pastor later. When Mom saw this, she asked for a card too.

We are watching the movie "Mrs. Doubtfire" now, and she couldn't understand what was happening when he was transforming into a woman. She was in shock!

That is one of the downfalls of Alzheimer's. They can't differentiate what is real and what isn't. News is the worst for them! Graphic movies and shows are bad, also.

We haven't done the nighttime routine yet, so hopefully, it goes smooth tonight. Fingers crossed!!

Mom Chronicles December 8, 2018
Small successes!! There were no knives in the dining hall tonight! I don't know if it was a one-time fluke or not, but I will take this as a small success for the memory care residents here!

I also chatted with the chef again this afternoon. Next week, he is hiring staff who will be responsible for preparing the right plates and serving all residents, keeping glasses refilled, providing a different meal if they don't like what is served, etc. That way, the aides can concentrate on helping the residents eat if they need assistance. He said to give him a week to work out the kinks and text him if something isn't right on her plate.

One day at a time. One moment at a time!!

Mom Chronicles December 8, 2018
Tonight was the BEST night so far, getting her to bed. She was completely helpful and in a good mood for the whole time the aides were helping her get ready for bed. She didn't panic, didn't cry, and told them thank you for the entire time. I didn't have to resort to using the photo album to calm her down. I kissed her good night, and she smiled and told me good night as well.

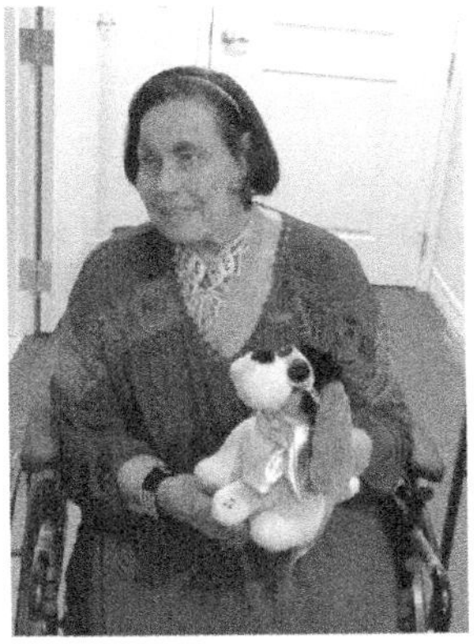

The aide that I had difficulty with several nights ago was the one helping her tonight. She was very friendly to both Mom and me.

I will continue to come to the center most nights over the next few weeks to make sure it continues to go well, especially until I can get a camera in there.

Oh... and two last things. The beautician colored, cut, and styled her hair today. Because I'm saving money on the rent, I can now put money towards this each week. Second, having her hair done will keep the aides from having to wash her hair during showers which will be less traumatic.

We also brought Simi up to see her. They were both so happy to see each other!!

Mom Chronicles December 10, 2018
I just ordered Mom an adult bib. It has embroidered pearls on it. I hope she likes it and will use it!! *Edit... teachable moment!!! Jenni just taught me a good term to use to maintain dignity. A bib should be called an

"adult garment protector, apron, or cover"!! Remember, our loved ones don't want to be treated like children.

Mom Chronicles December 10, 2018

Soooo... Mom had a major accident in the family room where we were watching TV after dinner. It got all over her and on the floor.

I took her back to her room because she was close to having a major meltdown (understandable), and then I went down to the front of the center to find an aide. I found the medication aide and asked her to send help. She said she would.

I waited about 20 minutes and asked her again. She said they are helping others right now and said I should just pull the help string. Okay. I did that. I waited another 20-25 minutes before they finally came to help. I had to keep Mom redirected from going full meltdown mode. That little photo album has been my lifesaver.

They are short-staffed. My friend Cathy is meeting with the directors tomorrow, and that is one of the things she will confront them about because they were not honest with us on the patient/staff ratio. We even asked twice about this to be sure we heard it right.

I fear that she would have tried to change herself and possibly would have fallen. How long would she have waited for assistance if I hadn't been there? She doesn't understand that she can pull the cord for help.

The previous person who changed her today also didn't do things correctly. I don't want this to be TMI (too much information), but she uses a diaper and a thick, wide incontinence liner to help catch it all. The liner was not there when they changed her this evening. I will have another chat with the nurse tomorrow.

Edit: another teachable moment from a friend!! Don't call adult diapers "diapers" in front of your loved one. Call them disposable underpants. With Mom, I call them "underpants" or "briefs." Soooo... if you have a loved one wearing diapers, don't call them diapers!!

When I left her, she was okay. I won't see her again until Wednesday, so I hate that I won't be there tomorrow night.

I'm praying God shows us the way this is all supposed to work out. There are several positives about the new place, but it's not worth it if it's just a glorified nursing home.

Mom Chronicles December 13, 2018

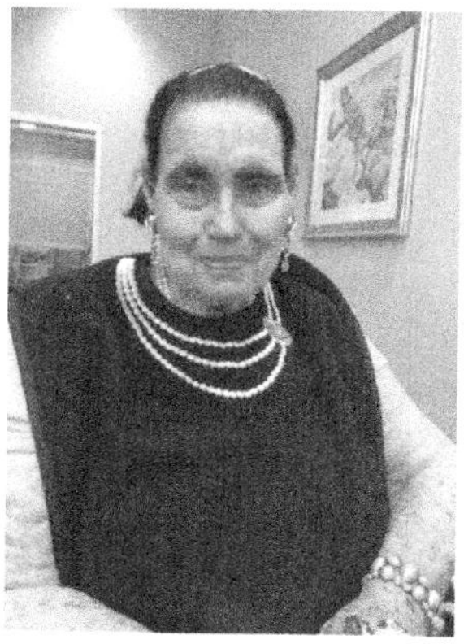

Mom got her new "apron" today. She loves it. If she likes wearing it, I may buy one for each day so that I can wash the others. I'm sure they will get dirty every day. It has a place to hold her tissues, so it would be great to wear all the time. We will see...

When I got here, she was at the dinner table and holding the Elvis doggie. She played it a couple of times for me.

We will see how the rest of the evening goes. I've been trying to stay until she goes to bed, just to make sure that process is going well.

Mom Chronicles December 13, 2018

You all know I try to find humor in this adventure. Well, here goes tonight's funny even though it was not very funny to me at the moment.

When I first walked into the center this evening, I smelled a powerful "aroma" near the family room back here by Mom and Miss Janet's room.

I thought maybe a toilet was clogged, or maybe a diaper wasn't thrown away. The aides are always good about taking soiled diapers out of the room, though.

After dinner, we came back to the family room so that I could put in a new DVD movie. The smell was horrible. I finally found the culprit. There was a "healthy size" bowel movement pile behind the table on the floor, probably the result of one of our "wanderers." I imagine he feels much better (and lighter) now, but oh man, it made my eyes water.

One of the aides cleaned it up and sprayed air freshener, but it seems like the "aroma" is embedded in the sofa fabric. I was texting Cathy about it, and she asked how it was affecting the "mommas." It wasn't phasing them one bit!!!

I'm dying over here, and they are completely oblivious!! Instead, they are engrossed in the movie "Jailhouse Rock." "Crappy" topic, but I thought you all would enjoy my misery!! Pun intended. 😊

Mom Chronicles December 14, 2018

Help me interpret this one. Mom doesn't like the soup because it's "running around and laying down."

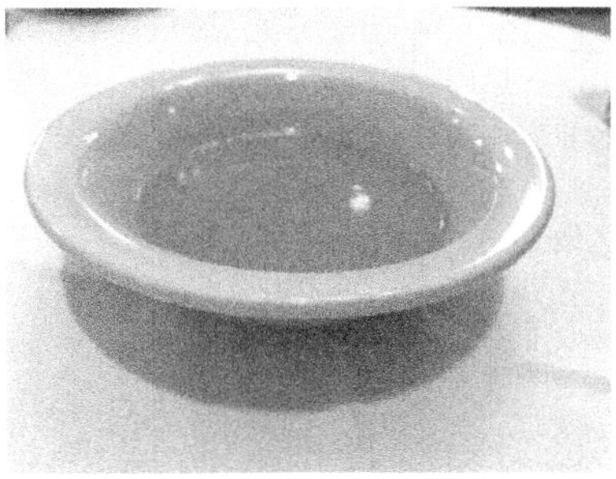

Oh, to be inside the mind of a dementia patient to figure out what she is trying to say. No, wait... I don't want that. Never mind.

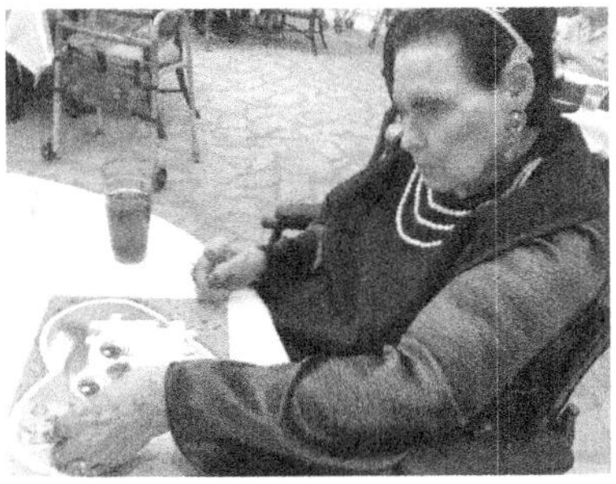

Mom Chronicles December 14, 2018

This lady is very impatient!!! Luckily, we had brought a puzzle down to the dining hall, so I have her working on it while the main course is prepared.

I did notice that she is now down to 24-piece puzzles. I don't think she can handle any more than that.

Mom Chronicles December 16, 2018

Two things today...

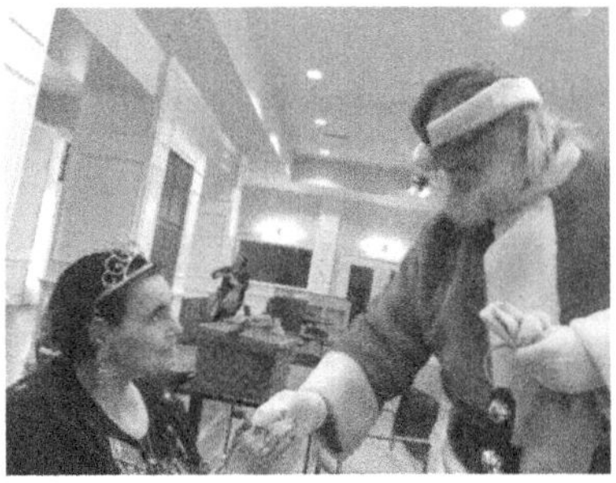

1) we are still trying to get mealtimes right for Mom. I spoke with the chef's assistant, and hopefully, we got more resolved. Time will tell.

2) John Sopko, aka Santa Claus, and several of the kiddos and parents from Concordia Lutheran (our home church) visited the center where Mom lives

and sang Christmas carols. She and the other residents enjoyed it. This short video clip is of her singing "Merry Christmas to you" in the tune of "Happy Birthday" to an ornament the kids gave her.

Mom Chronicles December 16, 2018
Apparently, Mom had a very rough time going to bed tonight. Bruce and I had gone home after the singing to get things done around the RV. As much as I want to be there every night to help, I just can't.

Cathy was still there with her mom, so they even tried having her help calm Mom down. It didn't work. She said it took three people to get Mom into bed. She was screaming and yelling at them. She screamed at Cathy too. Jenni said that she did that to them at the previous center as well sometimes.

I made up a couple of video clips that I just sent to Cathy if she is there when I'm not. I'm also going to try to get the aides' phone numbers too so that I can forward the video clips to them. I don't know if it will help, but we will try it.

I'm sure things will get better after she starts to realize this is her new home. I just need to be patient. And hopefully, they can give her anxiety meds sooner in the afternoon to give it time to work before bedtime.

I know I need to not worry about it, but I do. All we want is for our loved ones to be happy and feel safe. I imagine if I had known she fought them at the other center, I would have been worried there too. I also must remember this is the disease. She doesn't mean to be ugly or mean. That just isn't the "real her."

Cathy said she stood outside the door while Mom was yelling, and she said the aides stayed very calm with her. Have I mentioned lately that Alzheimer's bites??!!!

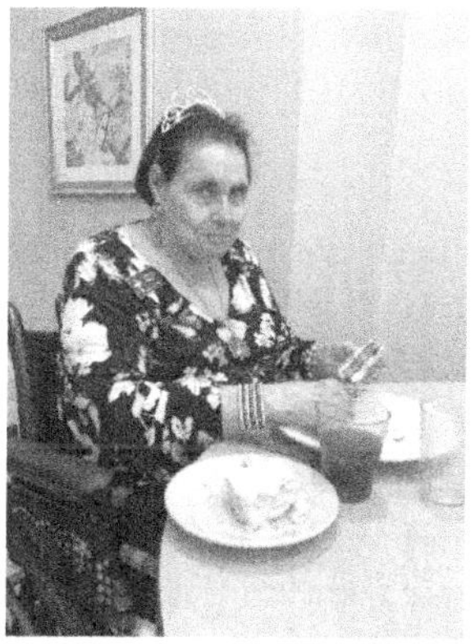

Mom Chronicles December 17, 2018
She's in a great mood and is eating her dinner. Blessed are those who can easily forget a rough evening. We will see how she does with bedtime tonight. Fingers and toes crossed!!

Mom Chronicles December 18, 2018
Well, we are still working on mealtime issues. They brought out her sandwich, all cut up. She refused to eat it that way. (Understandable.) I know it may be confusing that I asked for her food to be cut up, but I had hoped that they would understand that it is just foods that aren't finger foods that need cut up. That's my fault for "assuming." I had them take it back and bring out a whole sandwich. She ate it then. I've sent another message to the chef. I'm hoping they get this part of the care fixed.

She was upset and wanted to "leave this place." After getting dessert, she was better.

There was a group of kids with a music teacher playing the piano, so we stopped to listen for a few minutes. She had a sudden sharp pain, so I had to take her back to her room. I notified the medication aide to come and check on us but that I would work on redirecting her. I got her back to her room and put a movie on her TV. That worked—no more pains. I did end up buying her a small TV with a 5-button remote control. The center won't put cable TV in the back family room, and the aides don't always remember to keep DVDs going, so I wanted her to have something to keep her occupied when there aren't any activities. Otherwise, she is lost and doesn't know what to do. I want them to fix this, but I need to pick my most important battles to fight.

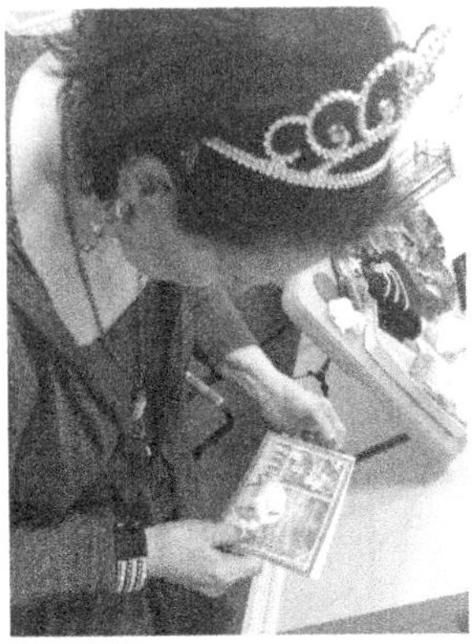

I helped her look at a few Christmas cards that came in. The video clip is of her looking at a card from our friends Brenda and Ron Selzer.

The only other thing memorable this evening is that she saw that it was dark and asked what she would do. I told her the aides would come to help her get ready for bed soon. She asked where I was going. I told her after we put her to bed that I was going home. She exclaimed, "home??!!). I said yes. She said, "you don't live here?" I said no. Then she settled down and said "oh."

So, we are watching a movie and just biding our time until it's her turn on the rotation to get ready for bed.

Mom Chronicles December 18, 2018

Well, tonight was the last straw. I won't share why but I have sent notice to this center to let them know I will be taking my mom out of their facility and moving her back to the previous center as soon as the notice period is up. If I could move her out tomorrow, I would.

Let's just say this daughter is fed up and will not deal with this any longer than I need to. Unfortunately, I will have to put up with the 30 days' notice, and believe me, it's killing me to do that. I want her out tomorrow.

I don't regret trying because if they had lived up to their promises, it would have been perfect. They just didn't have their act together yet.

I'm taking Mom back to the other center where she will be loved, respected, taken care of, and engaged.

Mom Chronicles December 19, 2018

God's hands are at work in all things. I am getting Mom moved back to the other center on Friday. I am just waiting on some logistics to be finalized.

I'm also meeting with the executives at this current center this afternoon to share my thoughts and experiences. They know they can't convince me to keep her there. I'm praying that I stay calm and professional when I talk to them.

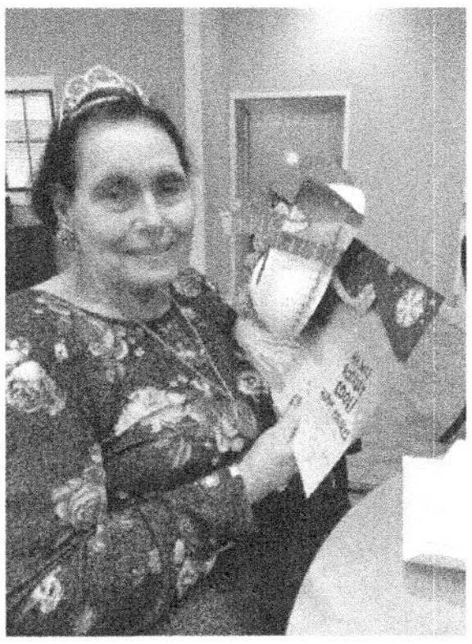

Mom Chronicles December 19, 2018

I had a meeting with the directors and expressed my concerns again. I offered suggestions for how things could be improved. I told them how the previous memory care center did things with their meals, activities and keeping their resident families in the loop so that we could see how they were engaged. I told them of the things that happened to Mom that were not excusable.

I expressed how I built a relationship with the director and the other staff members at the other center but never could get anyone but the sales director to respond to me here.

They tried to keep us here, and I appreciate that, but I just can't. They assured me they wanted to learn and make things better for the rest of the residents. I pray they do because my friend is still going to try keeping her mom here. She's conflicted, but this is the only option she has at the moment.

Hopefully, my words will make a difference for current and future residents.

To end this on a bright note, Mom received 2 Christmas cards today. She LOVES them!! Thanks for being my friends and supporting us with thoughts and prayers through this journey.

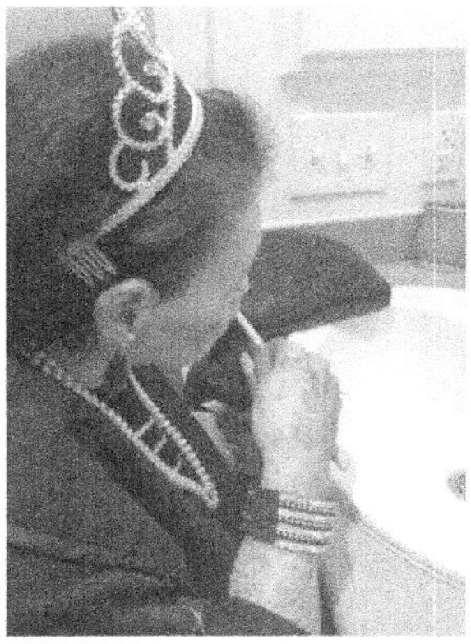

Mom Chronicles December 20, 2018

Mom's confusion level was off the charts tonight. When I first got there, she was at dinner. I noticed she had her toothbrush with her on the table. She did not eat much, was upset, and wanted to go back to her room. As soon as we got back to her room, she tried to brush her teeth. I helped her, and then we left the bathroom. Not even 5 minutes later, she wanted to brush her teeth again. Keep in mind over the last four years that she has been here with me in Texas, getting her to brush her teeth has been like "pulling teeth." Pun intended.

[After experiencing something a few years later in the nursing home, I now believe that Mom probably had something in between her teeth that she couldn't get out. That was probably why she was trying to brush her teeth. If I had thought this through more carefully on this visit, I would have tried flossing her teeth.]

After getting freshened up, we went to the family room to watch a movie. I could tell she was in pain, so I asked the medication aide to give her a pain pill. About 6:30 pm, she was still looking pretty upset, so I asked if she was ready to go to bed. She could only say, "I don't know."

I had the aides help me get her ready for bed, but she was yelling and not wanting any part of it. She kept crying out. One aide (the one I have had trouble with) was getting impatient and told the other aide that she didn't have time for this - right there in front of me! She had other patients to take care of at the moment. The other aide said she needs to be patient and let Mom do this on her own time. That made me happy because that aide showed compassion. Needless to say, the other aide ticked me off again. Oh - she DID have time for a smoke break immediately after helping Mom, but I won't get started on that!!

The photo album helped some with trying to calm her down, but it just got to the point where the aides had to lift her into bed without giving her a choice.

I laid down with Mom to try and calm her down. I tried the photo album again, but by this point, there were some pics of us she didn't recognize that she has recognized every day before today. Several were of me. She didn't recognize me. This was a dagger to the heart. I fear - is this the start of the phase where she starts going downhill faster?? It was probably because she was so stressed out and upset.

I just kept stroking her cheek and forehead, trying to reassure her and trying to encourage her to close her eyes and go to sleep. I could tell she was exhausted but fighting it. It reminded me of trying to help Josh go to sleep when he was a baby.

I am hoping the extra confusion is something that can be fixed, like a UTI (urinary tract infection). UTIs can cause massive confusion, according to all the Alzheimer's research and blogs I read. So I'll ask the nurse tomorrow back at the other center if the doctor can test her for a UTI if she is still experiencing confusion.

We will be starting the move back to the other center in the morning. Josh and I will be missing our work holiday luncheon tomorrow, so for all our co-workers, we wish you a wonderful holiday break. We will miss celebrating with you! My prayer buds, please lift one for my momma. She really needs it right now.

Mom Chronicles December 21, 2018

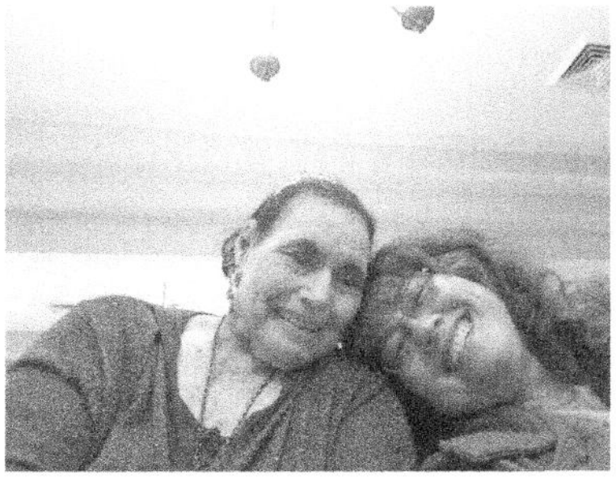

This update will be short and sweet tonight. It's been a long and crazy day. Mom did very well with the move back over to the other center. The staff hugged her when they saw her. Even her former roommate remembered her, which is amazing for a dementia patient!!

They also had several things going on today, like Christmas carols and some children who came to sing. My sister and I are happy. Thanks for the prayers!! If I haven't mentioned it lately, this memory care center is truly a fantastic place to let a loved one with dementia live!

Mom Chronicles December 26, 2018

Jenni just sent me a message saying Mom is back into her old routine and doing great. Sheila and I are so happy to hear this. The home health nurse was there visiting another patient and was surprised to see Mom. She said Mom looks so much better here.

Mom Chronicles December 28, 2018

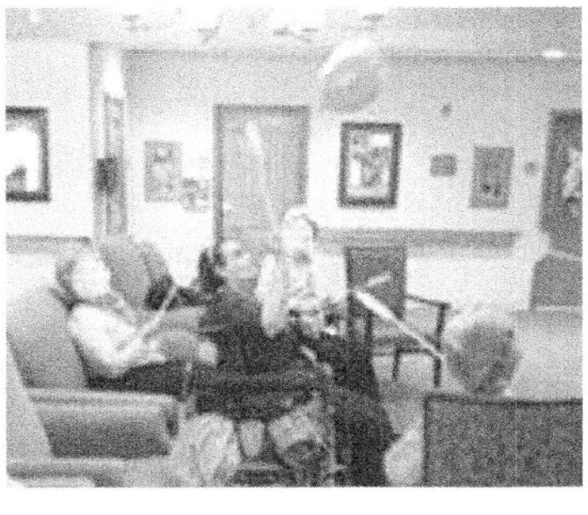

My beautiful friend Dani Gray went to visit Mom this morning. She sent me this photo – it looks like Mom was having fun batting the balloon with her friends!

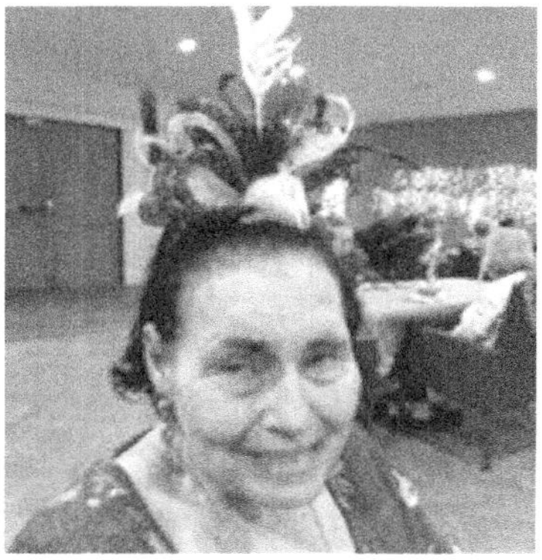

Mom Chronicles January 1, 2019

Look at my beautiful mom during a New Year's party at the center. They even gave her a special hat just because a regular New Year's crown wouldn't work for their princess.

Mom Chronicles January 4, 2019

I visited Mom for about an hour today. She was doing great. She's happy and content. I even got her to sing our little song (I love you a bushel and a peck.) She used to sing this with Ted all the time.

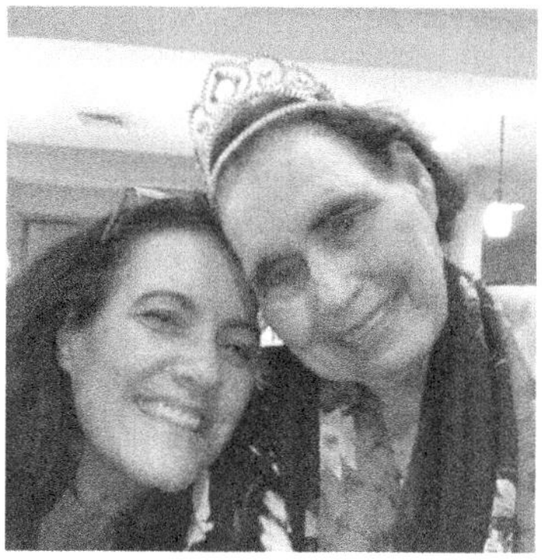

One of the residents wasn't acting like her usual self, though. The only reason I bring this up is because that is another reason why I love the people at this center so much. They recognized this change and made a phone call. Witnessing their attentiveness helps me know that when they notice any changes in Mom, they won't just let her sit there without being checked on. So, yes, she is back where she belongs. Safe and sound at "home."

Mom Chronicles January 7, 2019

Have I mentioned lately just how fantastic my friends are? I came back from lunch to find these beautiful jewelry pieces in my office to give to my mother. So I will spread them out over four visits to "spread the joy"!

Thank you, Ligia! I know you don't do this for public recognition, but you deserve heartfelt thanks for caring for a lady you have never even met. Thank you!!!! I can promise you that this will bring her a lot of joy!!!

Let's have a vote! Which set should I give her tonight?

1) turquoise coloring set
2) pink, green, blue, and yellow set
3) blue and coral set
4) multicolor - black, green, red, purple, yellow

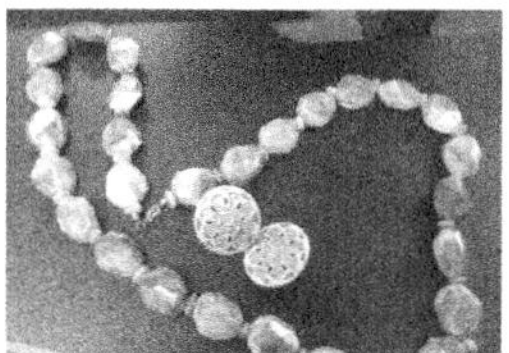
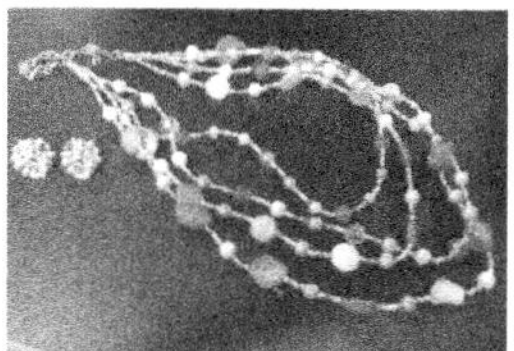
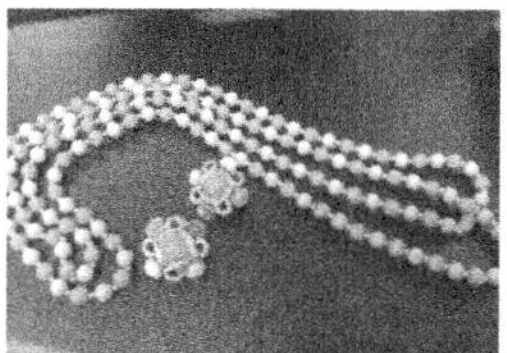
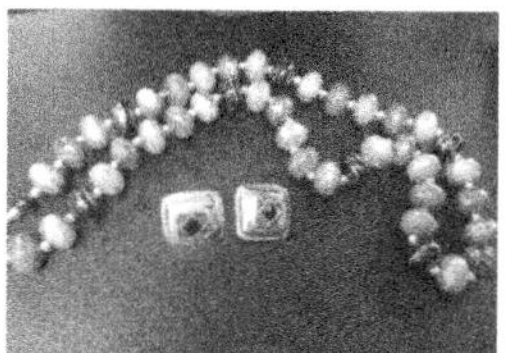

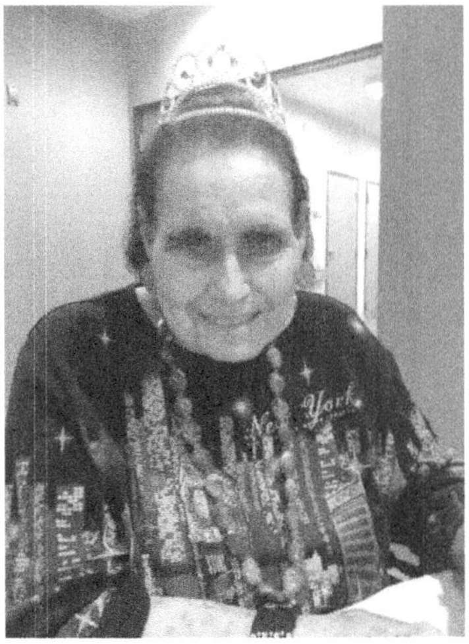

Mom Chronicles January 7, 2019

If you saw the post from earlier today, you know that I received four necklace/earring sets from a friend. After asking you all and some co-workers which one I should give first, the winner was the first set. She was thrilled to receive it!

She did seem more subdued tonight. It's like she was just very tired. She also kept shifting in her wheelchair, so she seemed uncomfortable too.

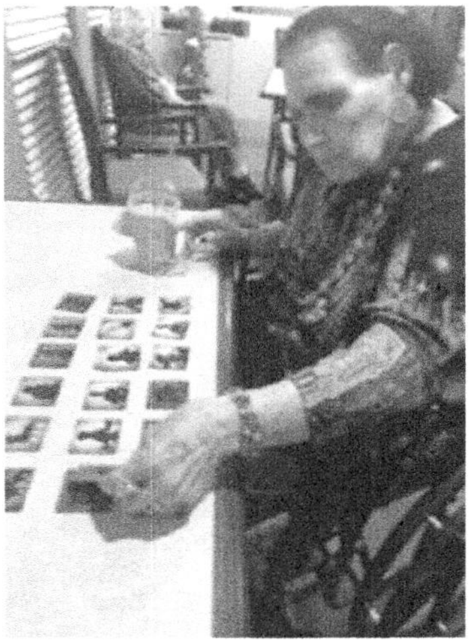

I worked on her nails and then did a matching game with her. I found this matching game on the sale aisle at a local department store after Christmas and thought I would try it with her. Sheila tried it first the other day, so she gave me a head's up on how she handled it.

I started first with just a few of the colored-only matches. Then I put out a few of the shadow-only matches. She did well with both. But then I put out several sets of the colored tiles plus a shadow match of them. She was able to get a few of them but not all.

Thank you again, Ligia, for the jewelry. We will give her set #2 in a few days.

Mom Chronicles January 17, 2019

It has been one week since I visited Mom. I don't normally go that long without seeing her, but my work trip threw my schedule off this week.

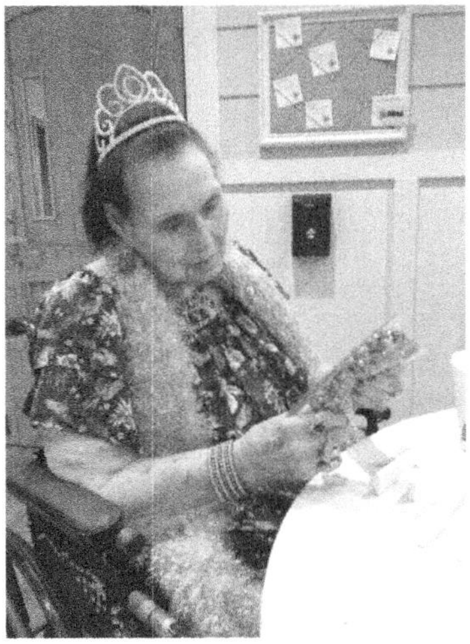

When I got there at 5:00 pm, she had already eaten and was in her room looking at her jewelry. She didn't eat much, though. It looks like she only ate some of the vegetables and dessert. She didn't touch the main course.

Like the last several visits, she just seems more subdued. You can see in the little video clip when I gave her the new necklace and earrings, she enjoyed them but was very quiet about it. Up until a few months ago, she would be giddy over any new piece. I'm not sure what's going on with her. Bruce said it could be because it's dark now when I visit her in the evenings. I even asked her if she knew me. She just quietly laughed. That's usually her "sign" that she doesn't know the answer and is confused. I think she knows me, but then I have seen her light up with total strangers and act as if she knows them, so that's hard to say. I think it comes and goes because she can tell people I'm her daughter most of the time. So, who knows? She could be just having a rough few weeks, or it could be the shorter days.

One day at a time. One moment at a time. And thank you again to my friend Ligia for the necklace and earrings. This is the 3rd set I've given to her from the last gift you dropped off. You will never just know how appreciative I am!!

Mom Chronicles January 20, 2019
I'm so thankful the center does its best to protect our families. Sheila stopped by to see Mom on her way out of Dallas to head back home and found out the center is closed to visitors for a few days due to a stomach bug. They are trying very hard to keep it from spreading.

I'm praying for the caregivers to keep them healthy and give them patience as they deal with this. You know the patients don't understand why they are sick, so I'm hoping those all affected heal soon!!

Mom Chronicles January 25, 2019
They had another resident who got sick yesterday, so I still can't visit Mom yet. They just sent me a message and said she has not gotten sick (thank the Good Lord) and that she is in great spirits.

I'll check on Sunday to see if they have given the all-clear yet for me to go inside to visit.

Update: Jenni called me to let me know that as a family, we have 24/7 access to Mom and apologized that we didn't understand that. It's just safer for everyone since this virus is bad around the area. We don't need to take a chance of a visitor bringing the virus in again and getting another resident sick. I also personally don't want to get ill and infect my co-workers. Soooo... I can see Mom anytime... it's just safer for all concerned until we see that the virus is gone.

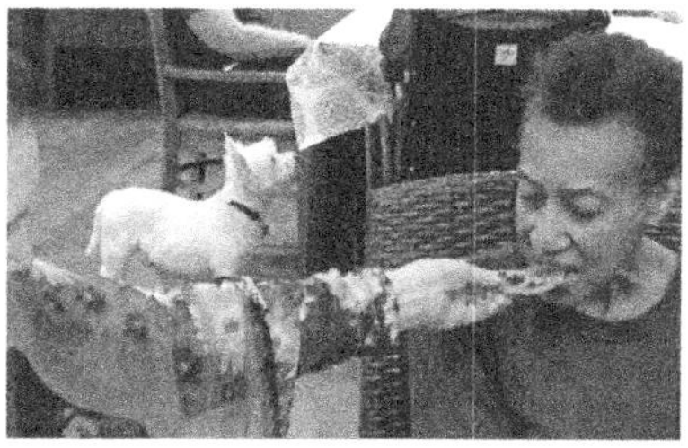

Mom Chronicles January 25, 2019
My momma... she still loves to help people!! Here she is helping Myra Hamilton-Brown's mom, Myrtle Hamilton, eat a cookie.

Mom Chronicles January 26, 2019
Jenni had the honor of meeting with the U.S. Representative in our area, the Executive Director for the Alzheimer's Association, and the VP of the Board of Directors for the Alzheimer's Association this morning.

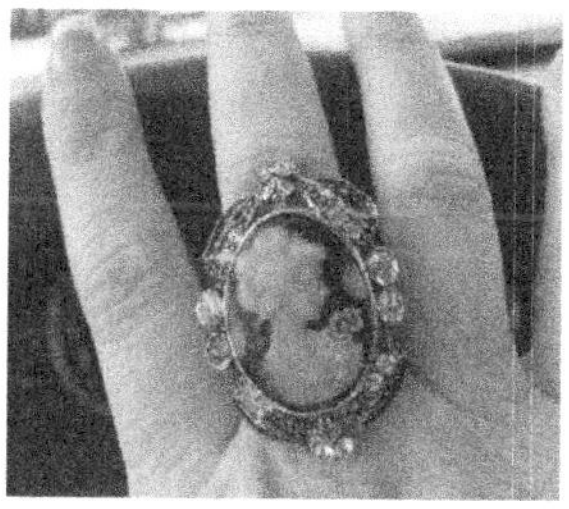

She wore this ring in honor of Mom to talk about how she has brought peace to her patients and how it is a tool caregivers can use to build trust with her. In addition, she was able to talk about the financial needs of caregivers briefly and shared a little about Mom. Thank you, Jenni Knutson, for being our voice!!!

Caregivers for dementia patients need huge financial support in this country. It is fast becoming a national crisis. Bruce and I are blessed with our careers to manage memory care fees for the most part, but there are so many people who don't have the luxury of placing a loved one placed in memory care and must try to take care of them at home without any support or training. They lose their jobs and put their lives on hold. It's a hard life. Dementia patients truly need memory care, especially in the beginning and middle stages. They also need Medicare or something to help pay for it. Nursing homes are NOT the answer unless they make some significant changes in how nursing homes are run.

Mom Chronicles January 27, 2019

The sign is still up for visitors to call first due to illness, but since Jenni said I have 24/7 access to Mom no matter what, I decided to visit her today since it's been over a week since I've seen her. So far, only two people have been sick in her house, so hopefully, she won't get it (nor me!).

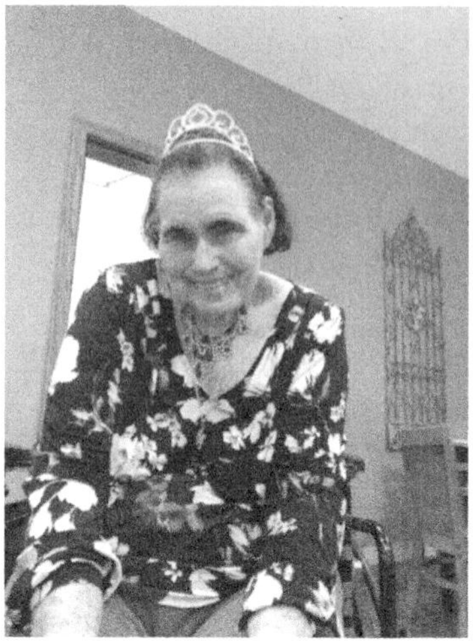

I gave Mom a mani/pedi. She is a happy camper!! She is in a good mood and dancing and singing to the music on her playlist. She's bouncing her feet, but I can't record it because it turns off the music when I try to record it. So, I had to go with still shots today.

I also gave her the last necklace set from Ligia. She is more responsive today and was able to show how happy she was to receive it. I did get to record this!!

Mom Chronicles January 29, 2019

I just thought my bad experience with "that other place" was over, but no... it's not.

Apparently, the medicine refill wasn't turned off at their pharmacy, so the pharmacy delivered Mom's meds to the other place on January 11, according to the pharmacy's records. Wellllllll, when our current center tried to order Mom's meds from their pharmacy, they couldn't because Medicare won't pay for the refills in the same month.

Our fantastic nurse tried to find out as much as she could but couldn't get anywhere. Finally, the other place told her they sent them back. Their pharmacy said they didn't receive them. It's a "he said, she said" deal now. Without those meds, their pharmacy can't put them back in the system to release the other pharmacy to fill them.

I left several messages with the other place asking for the paper trail of when they sent the medications back. More than likely, they threw them away. We will see if I get a response from their nurse and Memory Care Director. Hopefully, tomorrow I can get more answers. I may have to pay out of pocket for this month to make sure she has the medicine she needs. Our nurse is checking for me on meds we need right now and which ones can wait.

Fingers crossed they can find the meds in a corner somewhere at the other place or some kind of tracking documentation to verify they actually sent them back!!

Mom Chronicles January 30, 2019

Here is a follow-up from the medicine fiasco.

Fib #1 to me today from "the other place." The meds were destroyed on Jan 23, according to "our guidelines."

Fib #2 to me after asking for a receipt or documentation on this: The pharmacist destroyed the meds here at the center.

After asking the name of the pharmacist, I had nothing but radio silence. Next call? The other pharmacy. It took a couple of calls to finally get to an assistant manager, but they said they only destroy narcotics, and there would be three people signing off on it. She said no one has guidelines for destroying regular meds. They should have been given back to the family. She explained that no pharmacy destroys meds unless the person is deceased.

They reversed the meds on Mom's account and charged the "other memory care center" for the missing meds. The assistant manager told me that the memory care director over there said it was an "accident." Oh really? Then why lie to me and say the pharmacist is the one who destroyed them. I guess they didn't expect me to follow through with getting to the bottom of this.

So, Mom is getting her meds tonight, and thank goodness Medicare is paying for them because the cost to me was going to be $450 out of pocket for three weeks of meds. The Namzeric (Alzheimer's medication) alone was going to cost $388 by itself. I was seriously considering taking her off them.

So, to end this on a great note, Mom will have her medications tonight. And I have her back in a stand-up community that does everything by the book and out of love for their residents.

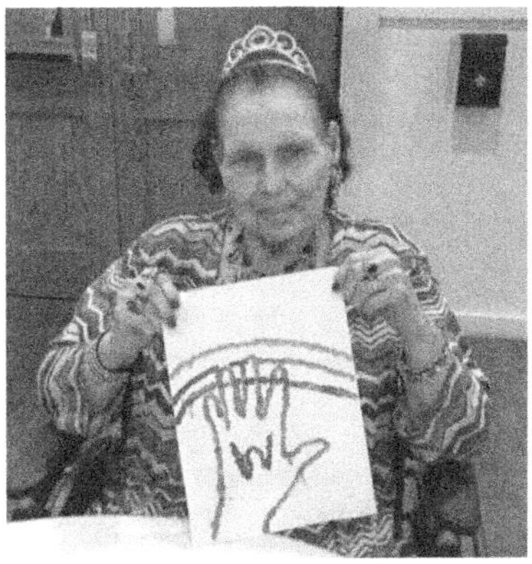

Mom Chronicles January 30, 2019
From Shauna... (thank you, Shauna, for always keeping me in the loop!)

"Aboriginal painting. She made it because it told about her life!"

Mom Chronicles February 4, 2019

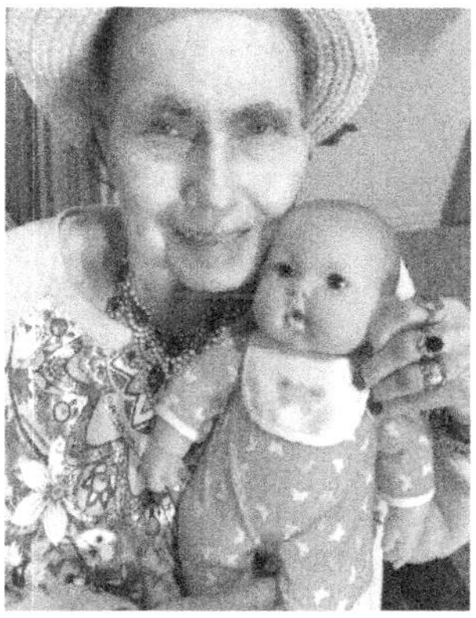

When I arrived at the center tonight, Mom was wearing a pretty spring hat and holding a baby doll. I think this doll belongs to one of the other residents, but she held it like it was her own. This is the first time that I'm aware of where she wanted to hold a baby doll. I know that many ladies in the later stages of Alzheimer's want to hold dolls like babies, so I've been expecting it. There are many realistic baby dolls out there, so I'll look for one for her so that she isn't taking this one away from the other resident.

I also was able to be with her at dinner time. The chef separated her food as we asked. She doesn't like food mixing or touching anymore. She still didn't eat the chicken strips, but she ate everything else.

She did appear to be hurting more tonight, so I asked the medication aide to give her a pain pill. Hopefully, she eases up soon. Finally, I gave her another new ring tonight. Yes, she was happy!!

Mom Chronicles February 7, 2019

Mom was in a good mood tonight. I brought her another new ring. She didn't have enough fingers, so she put it on her thumb.

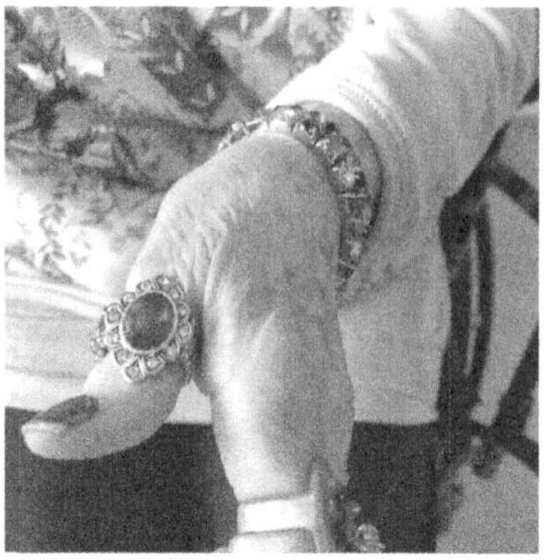

We played a few rounds of dominoes, and during one game, she decided to have two different spinners. I didn't stop her this time. All in all, it was a great visit.

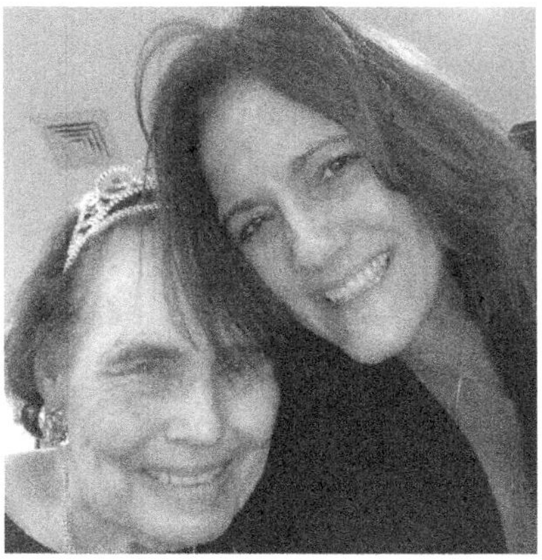

Mom Chronicles February 11, 2019

Mom was in a great mood tonight. Yes, we played dominoes. Yes, I gave her a new ring, and yes, I spoil her rotten.

When I left, I leaned down to hug and kiss her. Mom's best friends wanted a hug and kiss too. I love those sweet ladies!!

Mom Chronicles February 14, 2019

I surprised Mom with a card and a stuffed bear for Valentine's Day. She was happy to receive them.

She was in a good mood tonight except for once when I tried to correct her on not using two spinners. I usually just need to gauge reactions each time she does this. If she laughs, I will keep correcting her. If she gets persnickety, then I just let her have her way. Tonight, she got persnickety, so we had several rounds with more than one spinner. All I could do was smile at the fact that I have a 76-year-old toddler on my hands.

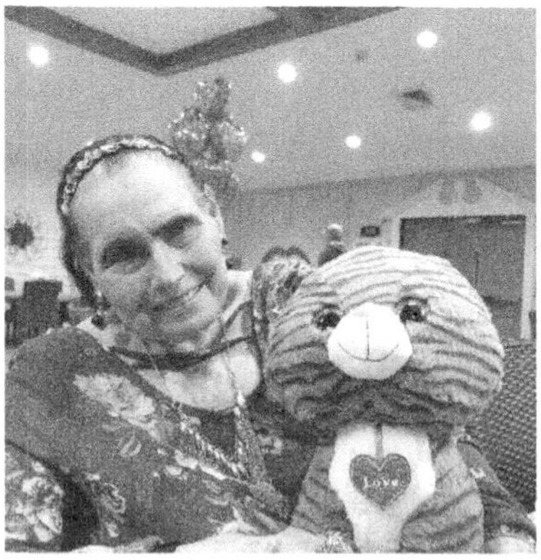

When I left, the TV was off in the main living area, so she thought it was bedtime. I told her it was still early and that she could just visit with her friends. So, I wheeled her out to sit with her best friend and pointed her towards her so that they could chat. I wish I was a fly on the wall to hear their conversations. Neither can make a complete sentence for the most part anymore. But they are friends, so I'm sure they have found a way to communicate that works for them.

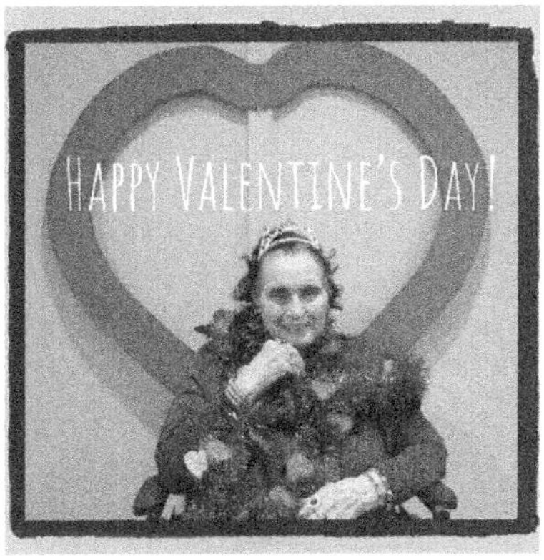

Mom Chronicles February 14, 2019
I love that the center keeps families in the loop with activities that they do with their residents. Today they had a Valentine's bingo game, and then they took some beautiful pics. Here is my sweet Momma.

Mom Chronicles February 18, 2019
Mom was in a good mood tonight. Our visits are basically the same every time. It either entails painting fingernails or playing dominoes.

Tonight, she played the double spinner technique lots of times. She loves to always start with double five as the leading spinner, and then if she can't figure out a good play, she makes the double six another spinner. Unfortunately, she got persnickety when I corrected her during the last visit, so I didn't even try to correct her tonight.

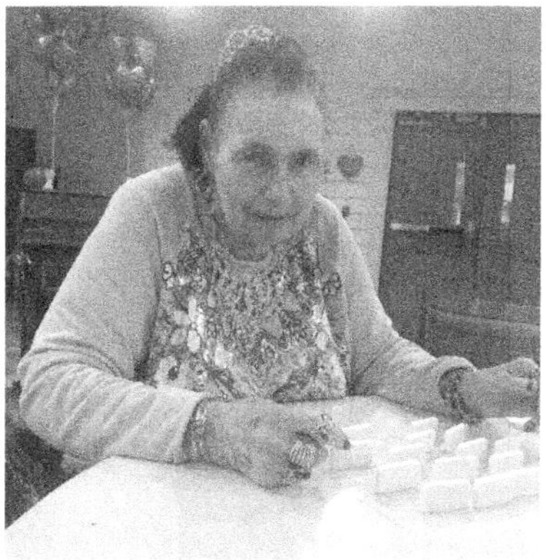

I also know how much she loves to have the double five to start the hand, so I have perfected the sleight-of-hand technique that Bruce learned from his Uncle Justice. I always make sure she ends up with it to start the game.

Finally, there were two hands where she played the domino on its edge instead of flat on the table. I just calmly laid it down flat so that she was none the wiser.

Mom Chronicles February 21, 2019
When I walked in tonight, Mom hugged and hugged me like she hadn't seen me in years. I just let her hold on to me until she decided to let go. In her mind, it may have been years, but in reality, it's only been three days.

I noticed that she was wearing no jewelry other than two rings; no earrings, necklace, or a million rings. She did have one bracelet on, but that's it. I took her into the middle room so that I could paint her nails. She was shifting in her seat a lot and grimacing, but she would either say no or just make a sound like "eh" when I asked if she was hurting. I asked her if she wanted me to get her a pain pill, but she said no. She didn't want me to leave her side. I finished her nails, and there were still 15 minutes left before the support group started, so I played music for her. Finally, she asked if we could go back into the other room. I said sure. I wheeled her to the TV area, and she was ready to tell me bye. She just seemed more out of it tonight, but if she was in pain, that might be causing it. I did ask the aide to make sure she gets a pain pill soon. He said he would let the medication aide know. In the support group, I was the only one who showed up. So, the leader and I just chatted about our lives and got to know each other a little more. I'll get back over to see Mom this weekend and take her some makeup. New makeup should make her a little happy.

Mom Chronicles February 24, 2019
We decided to visit Mom today after going to church. I knew she needed some makeup, so I picked up a few things for her. The video shows her excitement about it.

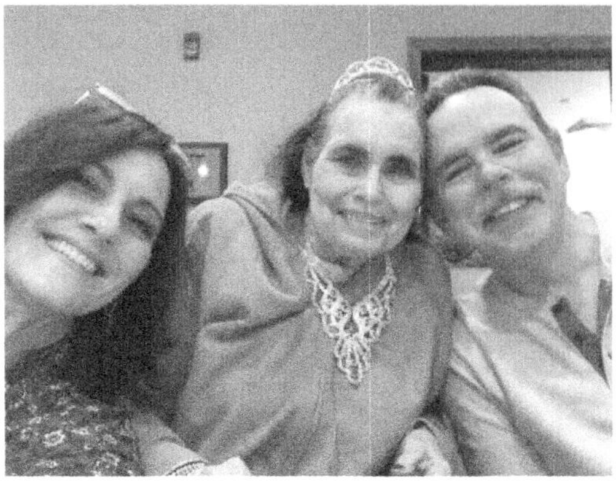

After that, we played a few rounds of dominoes - of course, doing the sleight-of-hand trick to make sure she always got the double five. Bruce loves practicing his Uncle Justice's trick.

She was hurting, so I asked the medication aide to give her a pain pill. Hopefully, she eased up soon after we left.

We tried to Skype Sheila in, but the connection wasn't that great today. She will be up next weekend, so she will see Mom then.

Mom Chronicles February 26, 2019
During tonight's visit, I tried some new things instead of playing dominoes. After painting her nails (which was hard to do because every little thing hurt her fingers tonight), I brought out a "Search and Find" book to see if she could find the matching images. She did okay but couldn't find all the ones I asked her to find. Then I pulled out a sticker book. She did OK if I gave her a sticker and told her where to put it. She didn't want to choose which sticker to pull or decide where to place it. I remember learning that Alzheimer's patients can't handle lots of choices. She seemed to enjoy the activity if I took the options away.

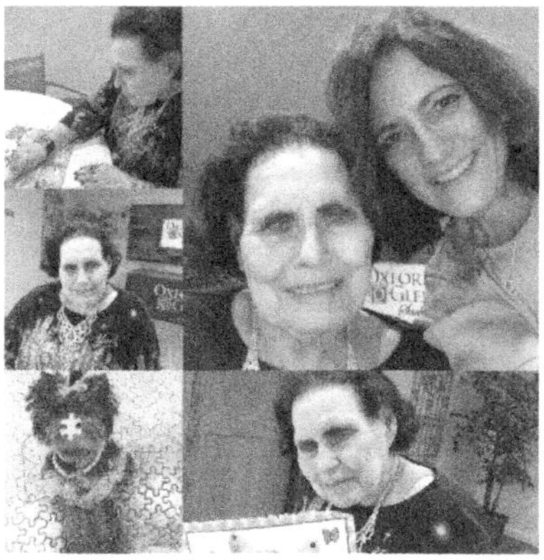

Then I pulled out a new puzzle that we hadn't put together yet. Once I got the border together, she did pretty well. The only bad thing about this BRAND NEW puzzle was that a piece was missing. Ugh! I looked in her lap and all over the floor to see if it fell. Nope. No missing piece anywhere. For someone who has developed a mild form of OCD on certain things, she didn't do well with that, so I redirected her real quick, took the puzzle apart, and threw it away!

Finally, the hairdresser colored and styled her hair today. She called me yesterday and asked me if I wanted her hair to be black and not dark brown. I had to explain that Mom's hair is naturally black (except for the gray), so yes, I wanted it to be colored black. Every hairdresser I've brought Mom to over the last four years has always wanted to dye it dark brown. Nope... it needs to be black. That's all I've ever known her hair color to be!! Other than the pain she was in today, the visit went well.

Mom Chronicles February 28, 2019
When I arrived at the center today, everyone was in the common room eating dinner and listening to someone playing music for them. Mom seemed to be enjoying herself. While she was in there, I went ahead and replenished all the supplies she needed for the month. That stuff adds up quickly! Not that I want her on hospice, but that will be one benefit when the time comes. Hospice will pay for most of these supplies. Once I got all this unloaded, I went and got her from the common room so that we could play dominoes. I also brought her a treat of soda and candy. That made her happy. The only other memorable thing tonight was that one of the residents just stripped down to her drawers right there in the dining room where we were

playing. Mom's favorite phrase when something like this happens is "oh my God." I told her to try and just ignore it and that the aides will help Miss E. get redressed soon. They were currently assisting another resident, so they hadn't seen her get undressed yet. For what it's worth, I tried to talk Miss E. into putting her pants back on by telling her it's cold, but she wasn't listening to me at all. The aides know what works best for her since they see her every day.

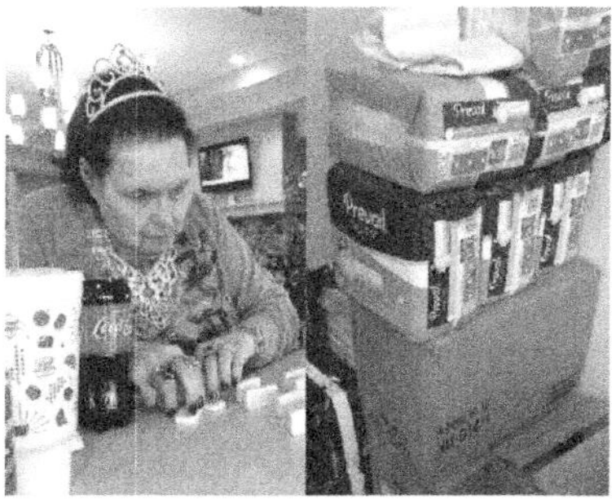

Mom Chronicles March 5, 2019

I arrived at the center at dinner time. Mom didn't eat much - just the green beans and a couple of pieces of chicken. She didn't even want to wait for dessert, which is unusual for her since she loves dessert. They also don't have her on her regularly scheduled pain meds yet, so Jenni will check on that for me. I'm guessing the pharmacy just hasn't delivered them yet.

We went into the common room, and I painted her fingernails. After they dried (after she painstakingly showed me every place that didn't look right so that I could fix it), we played dominoes. There was one point she got mad at me. And when I say "mad," I mean I got that "look" I used to get when I got in trouble as a kid. Well, it's more of the look that Sheila would always get when SHE got into trouble. (I was an angel. Cough cough.) I had played on a four, but she had wanted to play the double 4. I told her I didn't have another play, but that didn't stop "the look" and a mad "sigh." I promised her I would play something on the next turn that would let her play it. That appeased her. Once I played that domino, all was right in the world again.

When it was time to leave, she almost started crying. I fibbed a little and said I needed to get home to cook dinner for Bruce. (Okay - that was an outright lie since we meet halfway that late in the evening so that we can see each other for a couple of minutes before he goes to work) She calmed down then. I promised her I would be back in a couple of days. Like Sheila said yesterday, she just seems more emotional or different lately. It could be the pain she's been experiencing - there is no telling. Jenni said she would also check into this for us as well. They genuinely care about their residents.

Finally, she was very obsessive about how the jacket on her 2-piece jacket folded. She wanted the jacket flaps to line up perfectly so that her pretty necklace was sitting perfectly over it. It took her several minutes to get it the way she wanted. When I left, she smiled, so hopefully, the rest of her evening went well.

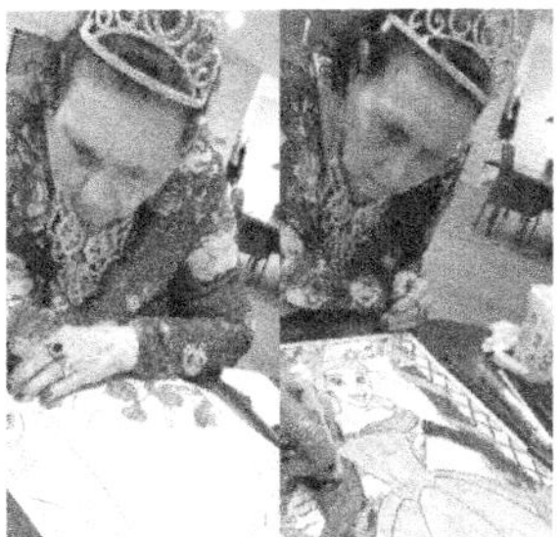

Mom Chronicles March 8, 2019

We had a simple visit tonight. I bought an oversized coloring book with Disney princesses, so we just sat and colored together while listening to music. There were a few songs she hummed to, and there were a few she tried to sing the chorus. She didn't get the words right, but she knew the tune. Since conversations are not an option, I'm just trying different things we can do together in comfortable silence. My "Mom's Playlist" gives us something to listen to every visit. Now and then, I'll get her to "dance" in her wheelchair to some of the songs. It just depends on how she's feeling that day. There was no dancing tonight. There was a minor issue about bedtime, but Jenni and I chatted about it, and I think it's going to be okay. We came up with some ideas to address it. She didn't cry or act sad when I left, so I left there on a happy note.

Mom Chronicles March 9, 2019

A few minutes ago, I got a call letting me know that they found Mom on the floor this morning around 4:30 am. The nurse said she's okay other than a little red mark on her face and that she's not complaining of any pain. They are monitoring her vitals, but everything seems to be okay.

Mom Chronicles March 10, 2019

Bruce and I decided to visit Mom after church just to do a follow-up on her fall. She seems to be okay. Her head only seems to be sore to the touch. She pointed to both sides of her hips as sore, but she didn't seem to be in pain like we have seen her in the past. She is on the regularly scheduled pain medication, so maybe that's keeping the big pain at bay. I know they are keeping an eye on her.

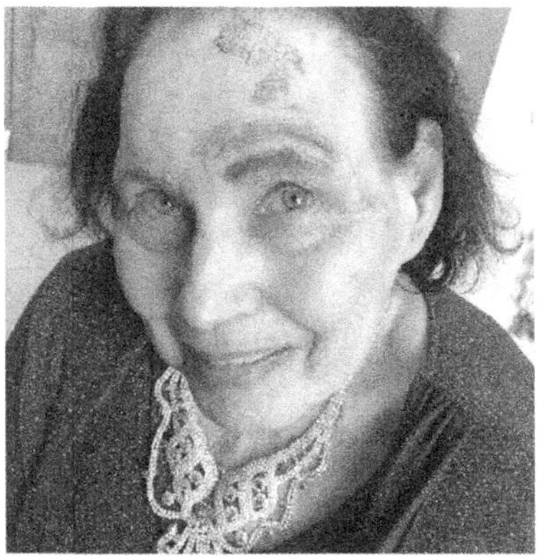

Mom Chronicles March 12, 2019

I visited Mom for a little while around lunchtime today. She was in a great mood and completely ate her lunch, which was good to see since I haven't seen her eat well in a while. She had her red cups with lids again, which she seemed to enjoy having again. (The other day, she had tried to drink her juice like it was soup again, so Jenni helped with getting the lidded cups started back up again.) I also helped her put on her clothes protector (the black adult bib with the embroidered pearl necklace). She seemed happy to have it again too. I don't think they have been using it since she has returned to the center. One of the aides said she would do her best to make sure it's being used. The bruise is looking better, and she didn't seem to be in pain. One of her friends kept asking her over and over what happened to her head. Mom never could answer. She just kept saying, "I don't know."

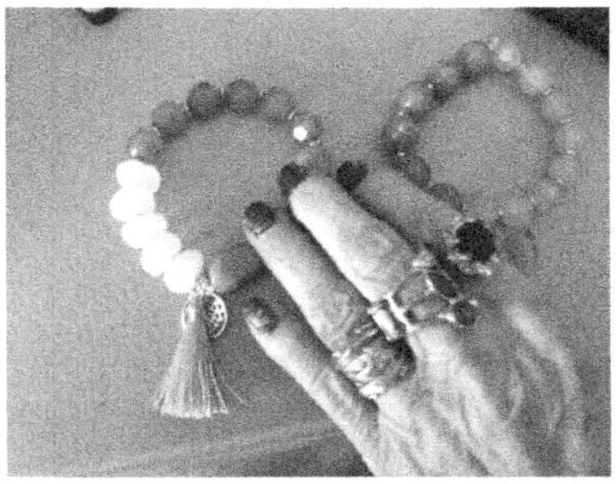

Mom Chronicles March 14, 2019

Thank you to Krista Manning for sending Mom a card and jewelry to help her feel better. The nurse told us the package came in yesterday.

That was such a sweet thing to do!

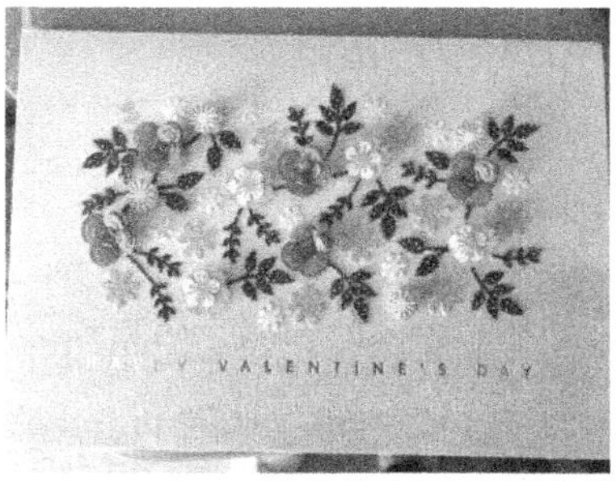

Mom Chronicles March 14, 2019

Mom is not feeling well tonight. They are doing a special art project with the families, so Sheila took a couple of days off work to participate tonight. Well... Mom wanted nothing to do with it. She started crying and saying "no." She just seems to be hurting more tonight, so we did ask for a stronger pain pill. We will try to take her in there again after she has had a chance to calm down. I hope she changes her mind since I think it would be special to do the art project together. We will see.

*Update: We were able to finally get her into the common area to do the family art project. The abstract part freaked her out, so she didn't like it, but Sheila and I had fun. Shauna thinks it may be because she used to paint when she was younger, so it wasn't her paint style. We got her to enjoy the snacks, and I think the pain pill is kicking in, so I think she will be better when we leave shortly.

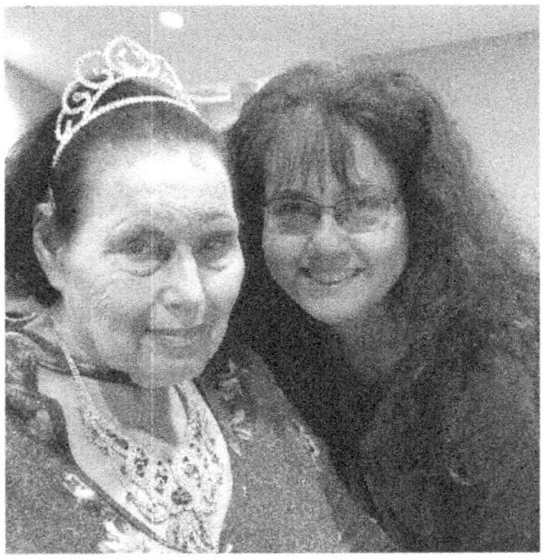

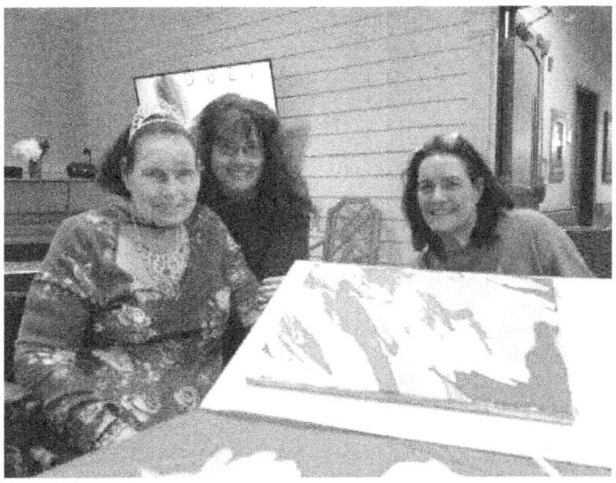

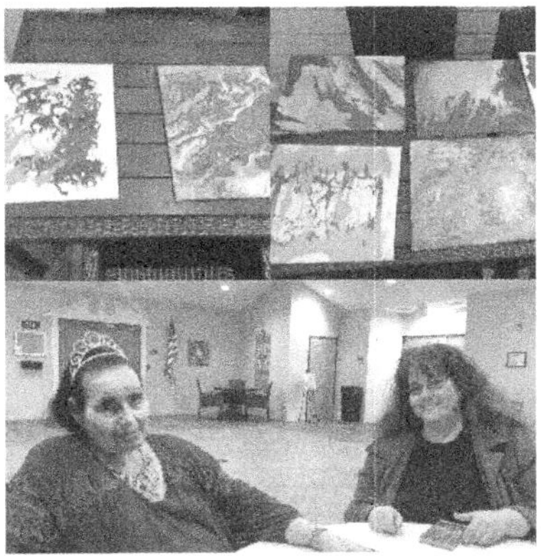

Mom Chronicles March 15, 2019
She is feeling much better today. The artwork from yesterday's project is dry for the most part. I think they all turned out pretty! All of the families will have something to treasure that they made with their loved ones.

Mom Chronicles March 19, 2019
We don't often visit Concordia Lutheran Church because of where we live now, but I'm thankful for the recorded sermons. This one is especially special since PK (Pastor Ken) shared about his recent visit with Mom. Thank you, PK, for visiting Mom even though she really can't communicate much anymore. You found a way to find her voice with hymns!

I think I need to add some hymns to her playlist that I always play when I visit her. Friends, what are some good ole Southern Baptist hymns that she may remember from her childhood?

www.vimeo.com/325089104?ref=fb-share&1
[I don't know how long the Vimeo recording will be available, but I wanted it shared in the book if it is still online. The part about Mom is at the 6:00-8:30 minute mark.]

Mom Chronicles March 21, 2019
Mom seemed like she was having a good day. I saw her shift in her wheelchair a few times, but she didn't seem to be in pain. The doctor prescribed some stronger pain meds earlier this week, so they appeared to be working today. Shauna said they took the residents outside today to enjoy the good weather. They also treated them to chicken nuggets, brownies, and other treats. This evening, there was a ladies' choral group there to sing to them. Mom really enjoyed that! We did play dominoes for a few rounds before the ladies started singing. She had a double spinner situation going on in a couple of hands. It doesn't do any good to tell her no. Tonight she just said, "these match." I couldn't argue with that logic. It was good to see her happy tonight. We ended with the song she and Ted always sang to each other: "I love you a bushel and a peck and a hug around the neck."

Mom Chronicles March 24, 2019
I bought some different color nail strips for Mom. She wanted to try the red and gold glitter version today. I only gave her two choices - any more than that would have overwhelmed her. I think they turned out pretty. We played "mominoes" - the new term I'm using for dominoes. My friend Terri suggested that word! Mominoes are basically dominoes according to Mom's rules:

1) she likes having the double 5 to start the game
2) she will play off more than one spinner
3) blanks don't exist, so we need to point them out to her; and
4) if you play on a domino that she wanted to play on, she pouts until you change your play. (This is my personal favorite rule.)

The last thing we did was Skype with Sheila. And on a final note, she seemed to be feeling well today.

Mom Chronicles March 29, 2019
I arrived at the Memory Care Center before dinner. Mom greeted me like she hadn't seen me in a year. It has been five days (since I was away at a conference), so it may have been a year in her mind. At dinner, she only used her fingers to eat the vegetables. She didn't like the chicken, so she wouldn't eat it. I tried it myself. The seasoning was good, but it was just a tad dry. They had sweet potatoes again on her plate, so I need to get word to the chef again about that. Mom has just gotten so picky. I don't know how much I should ask them for changes. I can only imagine the nightmare of making individual meals for everyone since everyone's taste buds are different - especially with this disease. I had half of my sandwich left from lunch, so I let her eat that. She loved it. I felt like a "momma" who always gives their last little bit to their kiddo (not that dads don't do this too!!) I didn't give her my cookie, though. There is only so much sharing I will do!! Besides - she did get a dessert at dinner, and she liked it.

The "mominoes" were in full effect tonight too. There were several rounds with double spinners, and then she did something tonight I had never seen her do before. We both were down to 2 dominoes each. She didn't like the plays she had left, so she pulled a domino from the table that had already been played a few plays before and put it back in her hand. Then she put down a domino that she wanted to play. All I could do was laugh. If you could have seen the determination or "stubbornness" on her face during that play, you would have laughed too. Finally, I gave her a new set of earrings. She seemed to like them. Sheila is coming up this weekend, so she will get a chance to visit Mom. It's hard for her to live so far away and not see Mom as much as I get to visit her. Maybe someday we can get her moved up here.

♥

Recall that Stage 6 patients can start to exhibit behavioral issues. Mom was more on the "defensive" type of behavioral issues in that she would yell, scratch, or hit at the caregivers if she didn't want to shower, or she would fuss at residents if they walked into her room. Her behavioral issues were not "offensive," as far as I know. I never heard reports of her instigating events at the center. Luckily, these behaviors can be addressed using medication which Jenni warned me about at the beginning when I had Mom admitted to the center. She did tell me it is a possibility that residents may need medication to help control behavioral issues. Luckily, Mom never had to be medicated for this, but I witnessed many patients at the memory care center who did experience this and had to be medicated.

Being medicated does NOT mean they have to become "zombies." Medication can help all kinds of issues and still allow the patient to function at the current level of the disease. However, it is important to monitor how the medication affects the patient and advocate for your loved one if you don't think something is right. In the next Chronicles post, a friend I met in an Alzheimer's Facebook group shared a scary experience with her precious mother due to medication. She graciously allowed me to share her family's story to warn others of this danger.

Mom Chronicles March 30, 2019

This post is not about Mom but about something to watch for if you have a loved one with dementia/Alzheimer's. I recently started following Venitra White-Dean, who often shares her Alzheimer's journey with her mother as I do. She posted this story and permitted me to share it. Medications can help control outbursts, but as she experienced, it ADVERSELY affected her mother. Luckily, a blessing in disguise helped them figure it out. Read what happened to Mama Frankie:

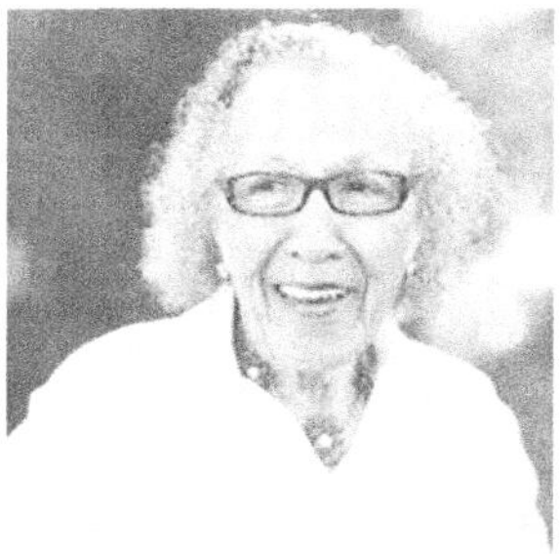

"Today is a great day! If you haven't been following our journey, we went through a big scare with Mama before her fall. At the end of November, Mama was put on a different medication to help stabilize her outbursts. We did not like the side effects and went back & forth with the doctor. Mama started losing muscle control (couldn't feed herself, needed help walking and toileting), lost weight, couldn't talk, and was in a 'zombie state' the majority of the time. We took her to the emergency room the 1st week in January to have her checked for a UTI. In older populations, and especially those with Alzheimer's, UTIs can have those symptoms. All of the medical tests came back normal. The ER doctor told us it was the progression of the disease. We brought her home and were at a loss as to 'what's next.' Nursing home? In-home care? The following week (January 10), she fell head first into the wall and fractured bones in her neck. The doctors in the hospital took her off of that one particular medicine. Within 2 days, she was talking, smiling, walking, and working on feeding herself. She was initially placed in a hard plastic neck brace. After 2 weeks, she transitioned into the softer foam brace. Today, March 30, we threw that softer foam brace in the trash can. I'm convinced that her fall was a blessing in disguise. If she continued on that medication, I have no doubt her body would have completely shut down. This whole ordeal has taught me more than ever, that we MUST advocate for those who can't do it for themselves."

♥

Our loved ones no longer have a voice. We need to be their advocate in all ways! Don't be afraid to speak up, to challenge something you think or know is wrong, and to ask questions from different people until you are satisfied that all that can be done has been done. Venitra didn't give up, and thankfully after still not getting the right answers, we believe that God intervened with a blessing in disguise to show the doctors what needed to be done in her mother's case. Mama Frankie went on to live another adventurous year and a half after her medication issue was corrected. It sure was fun (and heartbreaking) to watch her journey through Venitra's eyes. Mama Frankie and my Mom would have gotten along wonderfully if they had ever met!

Since behavioral issues are common in this stage, we can try to mitigate the aggression. For example, the National Institute on Aging (Coping with Agitation and Aggression in Alzheimer's Disease, n.d.) suggested these options for aggressive behavior:

- Try to find the root cause. Are they:
    - In pain
    - Sleepy
    - Constipated
    - In a soiled diaper or underwear (in later stages)
    - Depressed
    - Feeling loss (of freedom, not living in her home anymore, etc.)
    - Hearing too much noise in the room or confused
    - Around too many people in the room
    - Being pushed by others to do something (like bathe) or remember something
    - Feeling lonely
    - Experiencing medicine interactions

- Ideas for coping with this behavior:
  - Talk to the doctor for medication to reduce anxiety or pain.
  - Reassure the loved one. Speak calmly. Let them know you are trying to understand.
  - Allow them to keep as much control of their life as safely as possible.
  - Keep a daily routine.
  - Try gentle touches, soothing music, walks, or reading.
  - Reduce noise, clutter, and the number of people in the room.
  - Redirect with a favorite object, snack, or activity.
  - Limit the amount of caffeine, sugar, and junk food.
  - Take time for yourself away from caregiving.

Mom Chronicles April 2, 2019
Thank you, Theresa Alexander, for bringing a smile to my Mom's face tonight. I showed her the card you sent. She loves the kitty with the crown! Love you, my friend!

Mom Chronicles April 4, 2019
When I got to the center today, Mom was in her room. She needed help putting on an article of clothing and with getting her crown back on. Something was upsetting her. She was pointing to her hair and then to her lips. I figured it out. She needed lipstick. I couldn't find her lipstick, so I redirected her away from the mirror and asked if she was ready for dinner. (Note to self - I need to buy more lipstick!!)

Once we got to the table, one of the aides informed me that Mom and another resident got into a tussle earlier today. She said Mom was in her room and the other lady (a "wanderer") came into the room. They heard them yelling, and when they got there, the other lady had her hands on Mom, and Mom had apparently scratched her significantly. They don't know who started the "physical" altercation, but they were going to need to write it up. Mom doesn't like it when others walk into her room, but that is just a fact of life with these settings. At the previous care center, we had the option of getting a locked door, but that doesn't do any good when the resident doesn't know how to operate a lock!!

After dinner, Mom and one of her best friends went into the middle room with me. I played music which they LOVED. Both sang and "danced" a little in their chairs. We also worked on a kitten puzzle together. Towards the end of the visit, Mom was closing her eyes and nodding off a little. She seemed very tired today. Before I left, I gave her the new bracelet I bought the other day. She loved it as we knew she would!

Mom Chronicles April 9, 2019
When I arrived at the center, Mom was sitting at the dining table. They were getting ready to serve dinner. Miss A., her friend, told me, "oh good, you are here. She's been in a bad mood." Her friend can communicate much better than Mom.

Mom did light up some when she saw me and then showed me her nails. Miss Shauna said her nails were bothering her a lot today. She kept trying to redirect her, but it didn't work. I promised her I would fix her nails after dinner. I had to tell her that several times. Dinner was good tonight. She ate most of it. It was vegetables, mashed potatoes, and Salisbury steak. There was a small cup of gravy on the plate that she didn't want on her potatoes or steak. Instead, she ate it like soup then licked it clean once she couldn't get more out of the cup with her spoon. She treated it like dessert. It never ceases to amaze me how her eating habits have changed with this disease. After dinner, I worked on her nails. I put a different color of Color Street nail strips on this time. She loved them. They are gold and black and are stunning and perfect for her. I will order more of these in the future for her. She didn't want me to leave, but I promised I would be back soon. Oh, I FaceTimed with Josh so that he could say hi to her. She lit up when she saw her grandson. She loves him so much. She still remembers him but just doesn't know his name. Of course, she doesn't know our names either, so he knew to expect it.

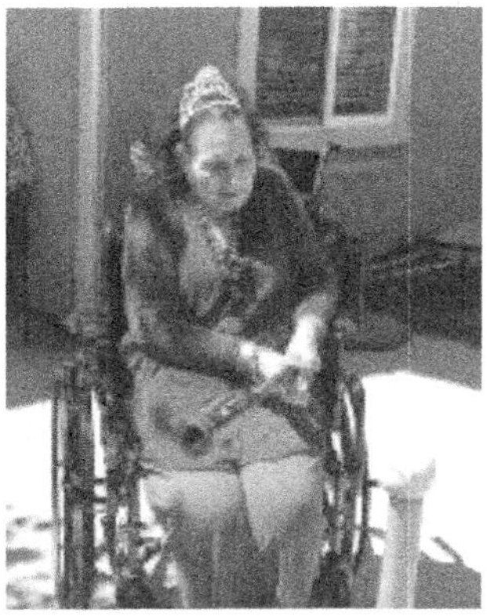

Mom Chronicles April 9, 2019

This. This right here is why I have Mom in the right place. I am at total peace knowing Mom is taken care of mentally and physically every single day.

Mom Chronicles April 10, 2019

It takes a lot of supplies each month to keep a loved one with Alzheimer's comfortable and taken care of physically. Thank goodness my UPS store peeps are so friendly and help me get these to the car each time!! I tip them like the folks I tip at the airport with luggage. It lets them know I appreciate them!!

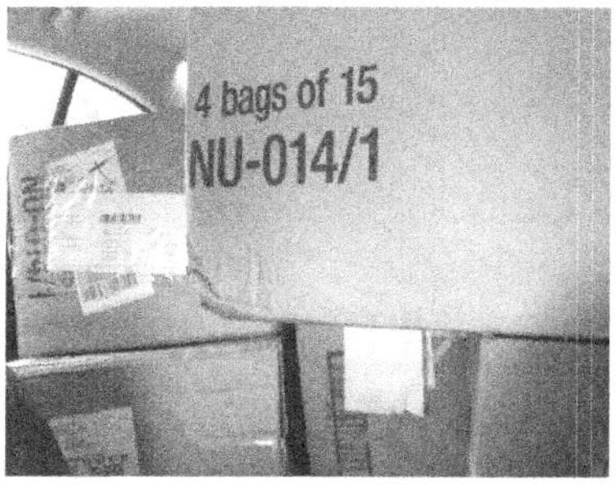

Mom Chronicles April 11, 2019

This was a simple visit tonight. We played "mominoes," and I Skyped with Sheila so that she could say hi. She kept saying the phrase "I love you" over and over. The rest of the conversation was jumbled. At one point, she pointed at me and told Sheila that she loves her "mommy." I don't think she really meant that she thought I was her mom. I think she just didn't know the word for "daughter."

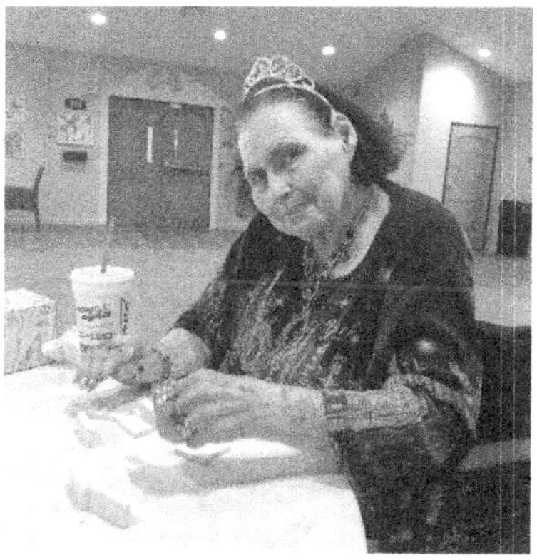

The only other thing that is sad to report is that one of her best friends at the center passed away the night before last. Jenni called and asked how I would like to handle it. I don't think Mom will remember being told, so I deferred the decision back to her. I think Mom's other friend, Miss A., will have a tougher time with it because she does a little better with her memory than Mom. A year ago, I didn't tell Mom that Ted passed away, and it worked well. She wouldn't have handled it well last year. This year, she is more advanced. I haven't heard anything concerning it yet, so I think she will be fine.

Mom Chronicles April 15, 2019

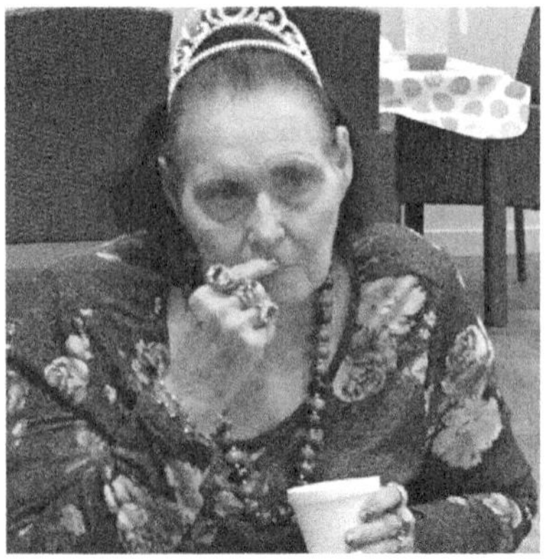

Look at the concentration on her face! From Shauna: "Brag time! We listened to classical music today. I had written the composers on the dry erase board. I said the names out loud as we listened to the music, and she would gesture when it was the one! Your mom got 4 out of 5 composers right. I was so impressed. She was very precise. She told me when I was pointing to the right one. Too funny." It could have been lucky guessing, or she may have just remembered some of the composers from her piano playing days as a teen. Who knows!!

Mom Chronicles April 15, 2019

Soooo... at dinner, she uttered the phrase (Oh Sh&t!) several times. Miss A. looked at me and said, "that's her favorite word!! She can be in another part of the room and hear that word and know exactly who said it!" Sheila and I can confirm that this was her favorite phrase even when she wasn't affected with Alzheimer's. It just cracks us all up when she says it. Unfortunately, she can't communicate much with us anymore, and I believe this will probably be the last phrase she forgets.

I allowed my mind to wander a little bit and started thinking that I would LOVE to be a fly on the pearly gates when she gets there. I can just imagine all the husbands standing there waiting for her when she arrives. All she is going to be able to say is "oh sh$t"!!!

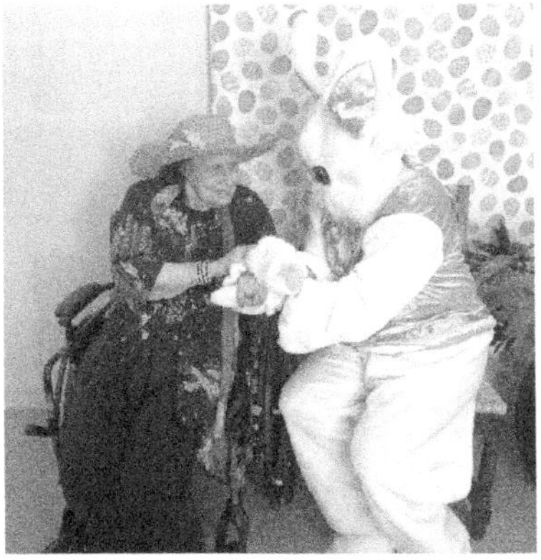

Mom Chronicles April 19, 2019

I had a little visit with Mom today. I was able to stay long enough to play a few rounds of "mominoes," did a short Skype session with Sheila, and then get some pics with the Easter bunny. I think they turned out cute.

Mom Chronicles April 22, 2019

There are no pics of Mom tonight. It was just a normal visit with fixing her fingernails and letting her Skype with Sheila. The only clear phrase we could get out of her was, "I love you." All other words were slurred or jumbled, so we had to pretend we understood what she was saying. We can generally get the context of what she's trying to say. I mentioned that her brother, my Uncle Quinton, will be visiting in a few weeks. She said, "who?" I showed her a photo of him taken with her a few years ago, and she seemed to recognize him. Or at least she pretended to recognize him. Unc knows that she may not know him when he visits, especially since he has a beard now. I am going to pull out some photos of when they were younger and then keep showing her his current pics so that maybe it connects when he does visit. It may not, but it's worth a try.

On a final note, I wanted to reiterate just how special the staff is at this center. They were a little short-staffed tonight, so the Enrichment Director was in Mom's "house," helping serve dinner and feeding a few of the residents who needed help. And then the Executive Director of the whole center was sitting with one of the residents, just holding his hand when I was leaving. He needed that extra level of care tonight. It was way past time for them to go home, but they were still there, showing just how much they care for their residents and giving that extra support their staff needed. My Mom is in the right place.

Mom Chronicles April 26, 2019
I have the best co-workers and friends in the world. Thank you, Jennifer Becerra, for the cards for Mom. I have something to brighten her day in my next four visits!!

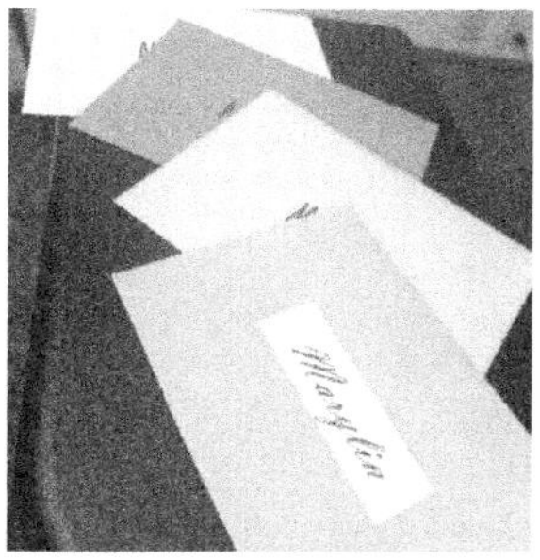

Mom Chronicles April 29, 2019
I didn't visit Mom today because I plan to go to the event tomorrow at the center to meet the owners. A few minutes ago, I got a call from Jenni. The first thing she always says is, "your Mom is okay." She knows my heart drops whenever I see a call from the center. She wanted to share a special moment with Mom today. One of the residents was in the atrium playing the piano, and Jenni and the others were in there placing tables and flowers for tomorrow's event. Mom made her way to the door and started banging to be let into the atrium. From what I understand, this is something she never does. They let her in, and when she saw Jenni, she held her arms out with tears in her eyes and wanted a hug. She acted like she hadn't seen her in years. We aren't sure who she was "seeing" in her mind, but she was truly happy and ecstatic to see her. She loved pointing at all the flowers (Mom LOVED gardening her whole life) and just held on to Jenni's hand while listening to the piano. Thank you, Jenni, for sharing this with me and for caring for my Mom.

Mom Chronicles April 30, 2019
When I arrived at the center, she was sound asleep holding a baby doll. When I woke her up, she needed to clear the cobwebs before she realized it was me. I sat with her while she had dinner, and then we went into one of the other "houses" at the center that is empty so that I could work on her nails. (She decided on sparkling purple tonight.) The atrium was packed with the "meet the owners" party. When I took her to the other house, she was amazed at how it looked like her house. All 3 "houses" have the same floor plan.

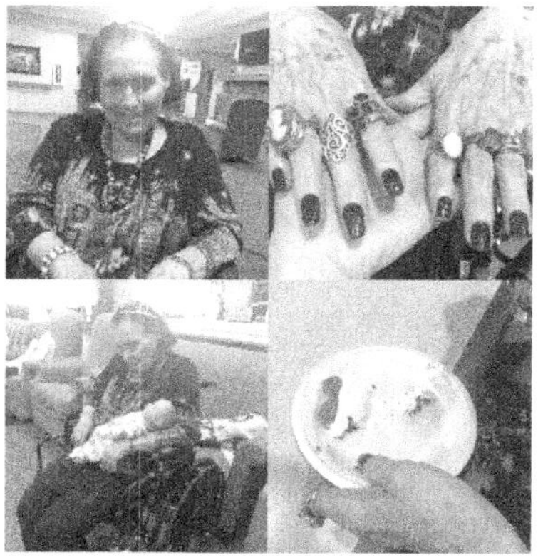

Another couple of events tonight were that we briefly Skyped with Josh and FaceTimed with Robin. Robin is Ted's daughter. She didn't recognize Ted's name or Robin's name, but she says she recognized her face afterward. We will never know for sure, but the simple fact that it brought Mom joy for a few minutes is all that is important.

Finally, she and I both had a piece of cake from the party. I was going to throw away the last little bit of icing from my cake, but she wouldn't let me. Instead, she wanted to lick that plate clean!! It was a good visit.

Mom Chronicles May 2, 2019

I have an interview with a newspaper reporter this morning. She wants to do an article on Alzheimer's moms and daughters. She wants some pictures of when Sheila and I were little with Mom. All my photo albums are in storage, but Sheila found this gem. This photo was from a family beach vacation visit down in Galveston when we were little.

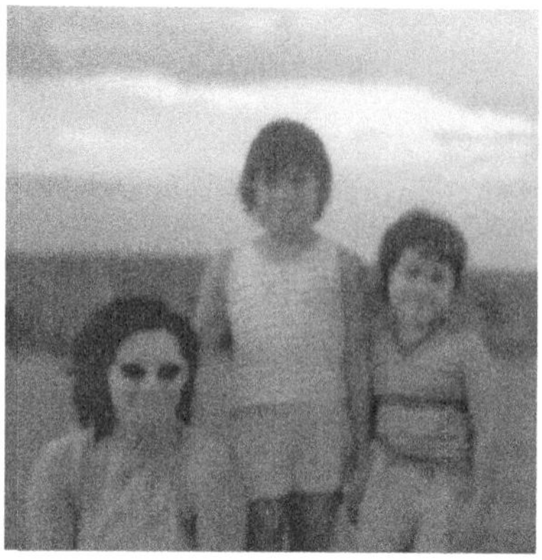

Mom Chronicles May 2, 2019

This video has Mom opening several cards and a new necklace. I love the faces that Mom makes on this video pretending to be a dog.

Mom Chronicles May 6, 2019

There are several things to post about tonight. First, she received several cards and nail strips from friends. She loved them all!

Second, my uncle Quinton is here for a couple of days, so he met us at the center to visit Mom. We were afraid she wouldn't recognize him because it's been two years since they have seen each other and because he has a beard. He has never had a beard before, so she has never seen him with one. But, we think she knew him. She was a little unsure at first, but she seemed to know him. While waiting for her dinner, she held his hand. I love that pic.

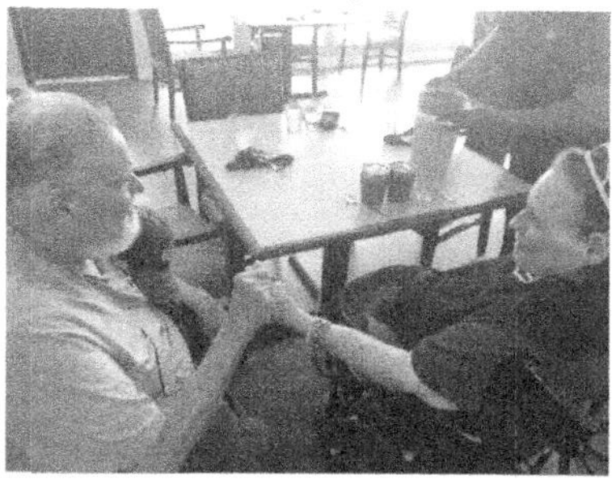

After dinner, we played "mominoes." Uncle Quinton said he hadn't played dominoes in 40 years, so he was totally fine with her rules.

We are going to visit again tomorrow before he heads back to Colorado. I'm so glad he was able to see her again before she progresses further in this disease. I love you, Unc!

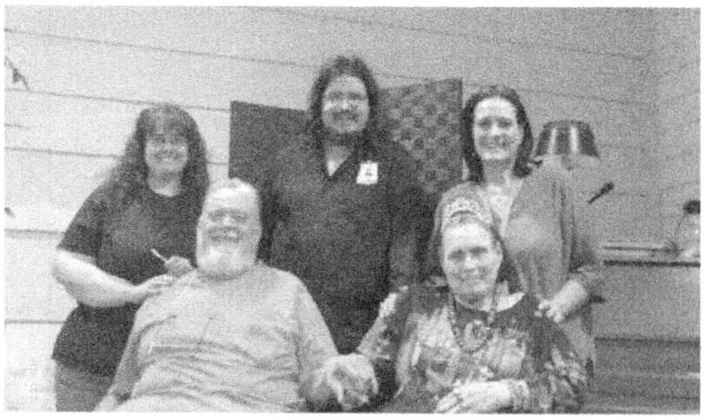

Mom Chronicles May 7, 2019

We were able to visit with Uncle Quinton one more night before he heads back to Colorado tomorrow. We are thankful that we think Mom knew who he was. She enjoyed his visit no matter what. Joshua also joined us tonight, so Mom was VERY happy. She loves her grandson!!

I changed her Color Street nails out with one of the sets mailed to me the other day by my new friend, Venitra White-Dean. She loved the color and the little hearts on them. Thank you, Venitra! Mom's friend, Miss A., was in the atrium with us so that she could enjoy the music and company. Sheila and I are familiar with her repetitive questions, but Uncle Quinton and Josh experienced it tonight. They both were very patient with answering the same question repeatedly for an hour. They were troopers!!

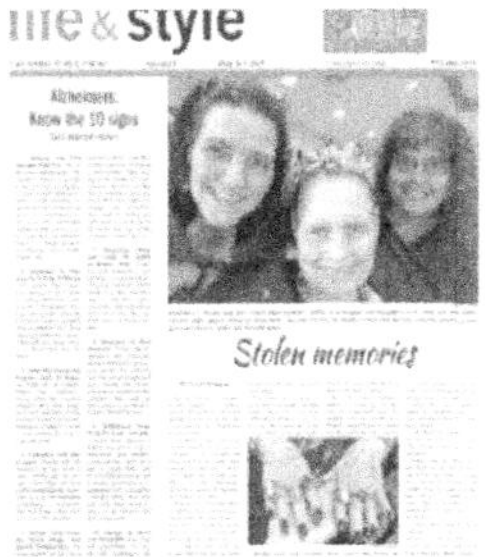
style

Stolen memories

Mom Chronicles May 8, 2019
I was permitted to post the newspaper article about our family. Thank you, Sonia Duggan, at Wylie News (C&S Media Publications) for sharing our story. Enjoy!!

www.bit.ly/3fW4HK2 (Duggan, 2019)

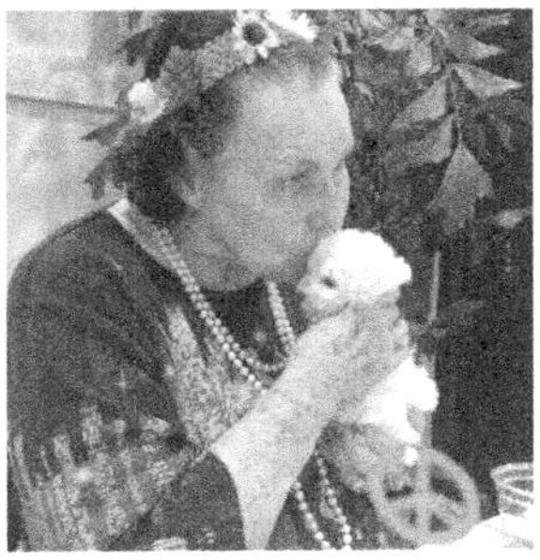

Mom Chronicles May 9, 2019
Tonight, the center celebrated Moms with a 60s themed Mother's Day Party. Lots of great food, music, and dancing. And someone brought a teensy, tiny puppy for the residents to enjoy holding!

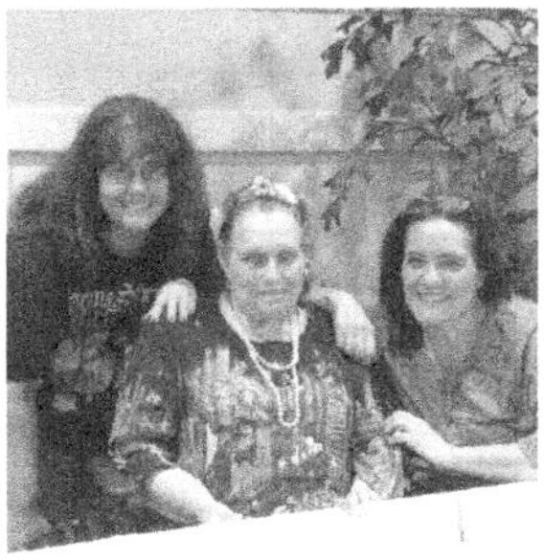

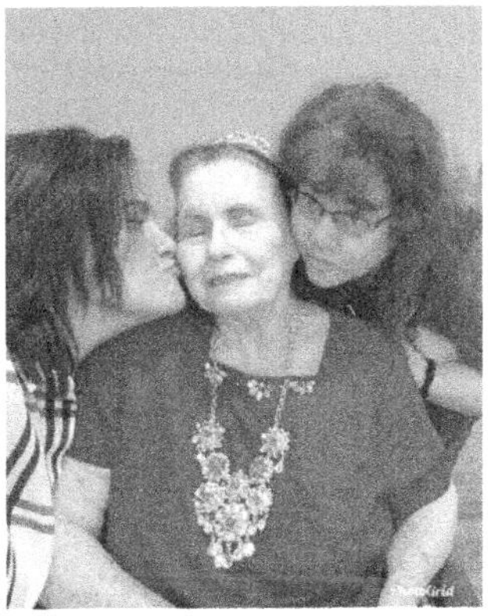

Mom Chronicles May 11, 2019
Mother's Day. I just love her face!

[This was our last Mother's Day to be with her face-to-face. In 2020, the COVID 19 pandemic hit, so we could not visit with her on Mother's Day.]

Mom Chronicles May 14, 2019
I finally bought some baby dolls for Mom. You be the judge on whether they made her happy or not. Enjoy the video!

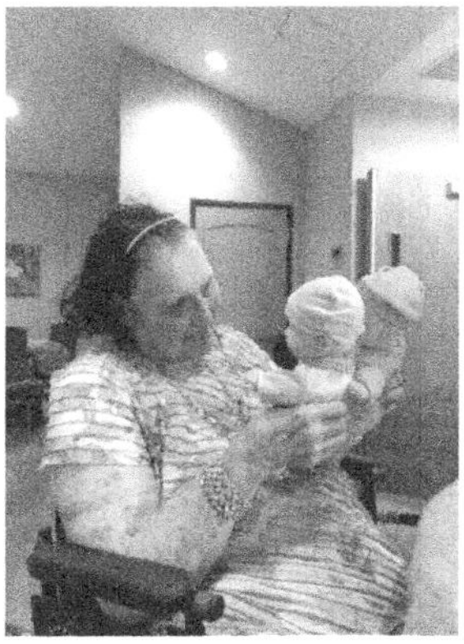

Mom Chronicles May 17, 2019
This evening, I took both Mom and Miss A. into the atrium to spend time with them. Another resident was a bit cantankerous tonight with some very colorful language, so I needed to get them both away from that

behavior for just a little while. When Miss A. isn't depressed, she's not a flight risk, so I will try to shower some love on her too. The atrium has an exit to the front door, so I need to be careful when I take her in there. Mom is not a flight risk. I am extremely thankful I never had to worry about her wandering off and getting lost on foot.

Anyways... tonight I fixed both of their nails. Mom chose shiny blue and silver Color Street strips, and Mom's friend wanted hers painted a soft pink. She was soooooo happy. It's so good to bring joy into their lives in such a small way.

We also played dominoes with a new set I bought. They have baby animal pictures instead of dots. They both did pretty well. I had to help a few times with matching some of the animals.

When I was leaving, I noticed a bowl of popcorn and several greeting cards behind Mom's back in the wheelchair. Yes, popcorn spilled all over the floor when I removed it. We opened one card, and I took the rest of the cards to surprise her with one each visit. It looks like this card was from Rita. Thank you, Rita!!! All in all, it was a nice visit.

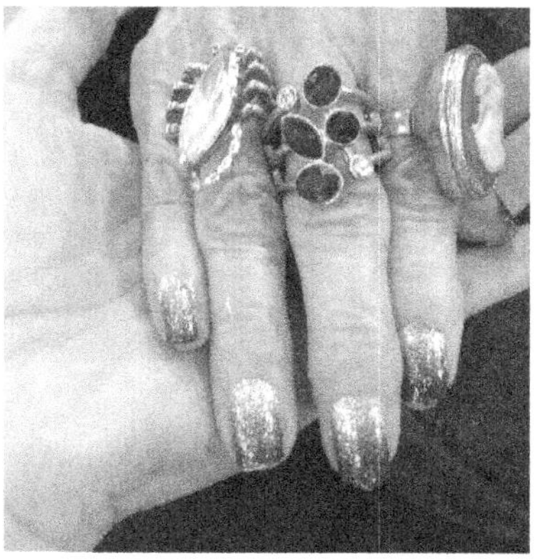
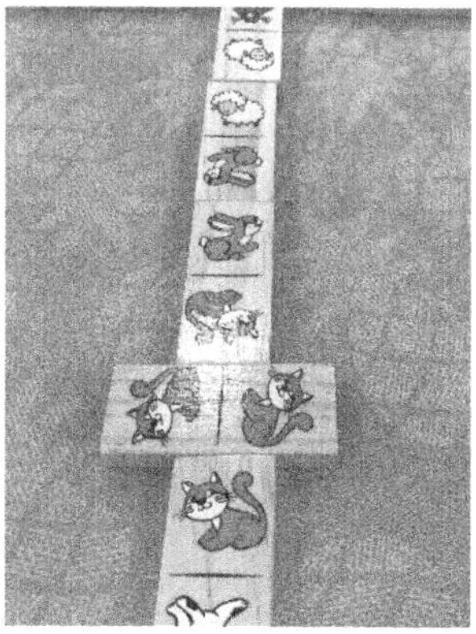
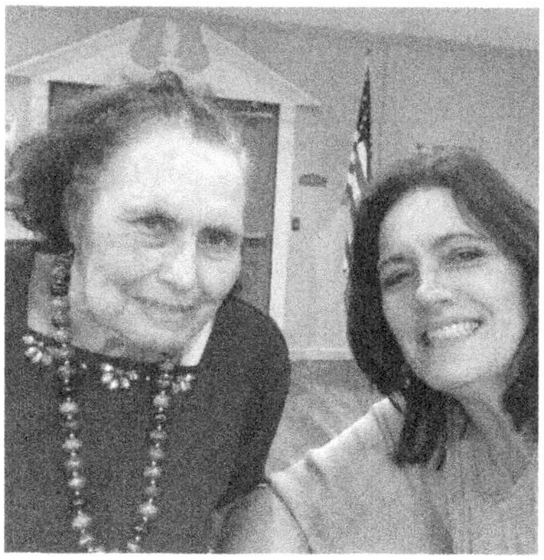

Mom Chronicles May 19, 2019

I visited Mom after church today. The aide said she didn't want to eat lunch. They tried a hamburger patty also, but she didn't want it. She did eat her cake for dessert, though.

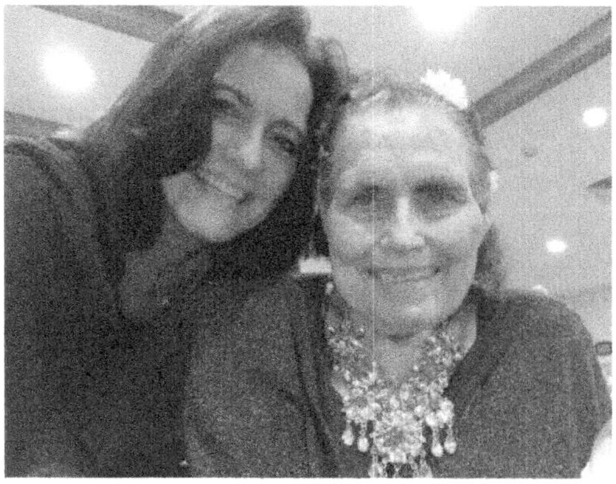

I took her to the atrium to play the new animal dominoes. She did well with them today. She was in a good mood but did seem to be in a lot of pain. I asked the medication aide to give her a pain pill. She enjoyed the strawberry shake, so hopefully, that will tide her over until dinner. Hopefully, she will eat her dinner.

I showed her a postcard from a friend and a sparkly card from one of my co-workers. A church friend also dropped off several cards. They brightened her day! I need to come up with something cute to display her cards. Maybe a photo album for her to flip through and look at the covers?

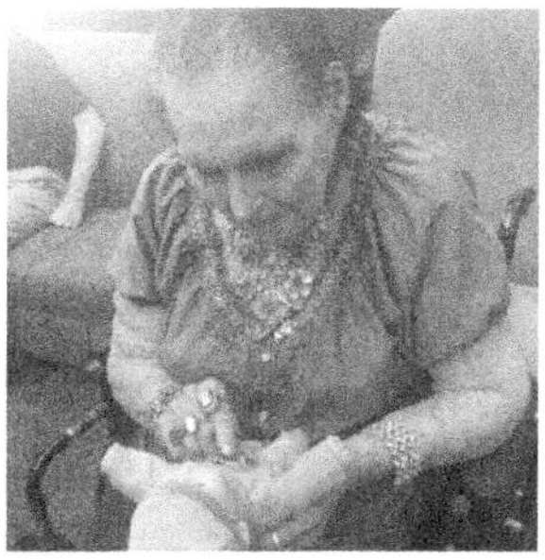

Mom Chronicles May 20, 2019

I am going painting with co-workers/friends tonight, so I had a short visit with Mom tonight. We put together a puzzle first; then I showed a card to her from Jennifer Becerra. She kissed the card… so cute!

I also Skyped with Sheila for a few minutes so that she could say hi to Mom.

While we were in the atrium, an elderly man wheeled his wife into the atrium from the other house. She looks further along than Mom. He had his arm around her shoulders and read a book to her. It was such a touching moment. I wanted to take a photo but thought that was too intrusive of their time together. I love that some folks still realize that even though our loved ones may not realize who we are, we still know who they were/are and will still take the time to let them know they are loved.

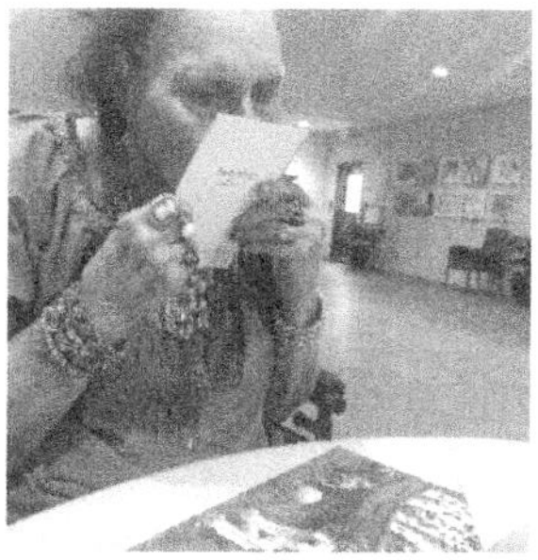

After that, I took Mom back into her house and gave her doll to her. She was happy.

Mom Chronicles May 22, 2019

I may ruffle a few feathers with this post. I believe it is very selfish not to visit a loved one because you "want to remember them the way they were before the disease." They are still the same person… they are just ill, and they NEED love. Even if they don't remember you, you show this person you care, and you can bring a little joy into their lives, whether they can show this or not. Like the man reading to his wife the other day, there was no indication she understood who he was or what he was reading to her, but she may have been able to hear him and be joyful inside.

And if you have a family member taking care of a loved one with dementia (or anything else for that matter), offer to sit with the loved one. Let them have a break away from caregiving. They need it. Trust me. **I will add that I was blessed with this. My sister, kiddo, and several friends gave Bruce and me breaks when Mom lived with us. We were very blessed!! I'm off my soapbox now and getting back to work.

Mom Chronicles May 28, 2019

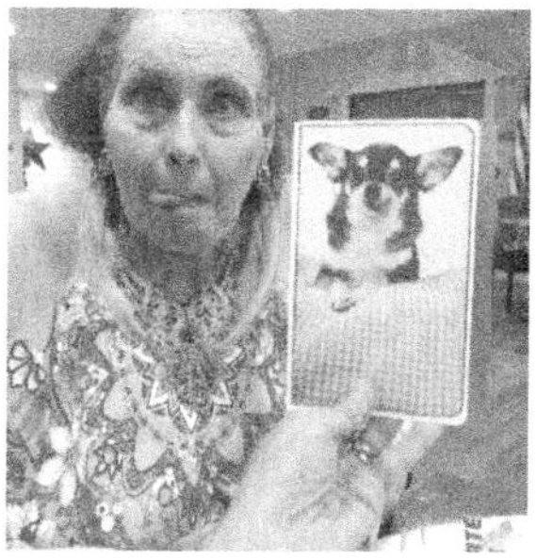

The costume jewelry I ordered came in today, and instead of giving her just one piece a visit, I gave her all four new pieces. I love her reaction at the end. If you have ever read "The Five Love Languages," you would probably guess that her love language is "gifts." I also gave two cards to her that came in. One from a church friend, Rita, and the other from a Huntsville friend, Theresa. Thank you both!! I got a good pic of her being silly and imitating the dog on the front of one of the cards. After that, we Skyped with Sheila for a few minutes, and then we played the animal dominoes. Other than her hips hurting, we had a good visit.

Mom Chronicles May 31, 2019

Tomorrow I will get a chance to tell our story in 2-3 minutes to our area's Congressman from the House of Representatives. I've been practicing with a stopwatch, and I'm still having a hard time getting my main thoughts down that I want to share. It will be a very stripped-down plea for more assistance for families needing financial resources for memory care placement. I'm just thankful our representative is willing to listen and that Jenni worked on getting this town hall meeting at the center. I know change won't happen fast enough to help us, but maybe it will help others down the road. It just takes that first step.

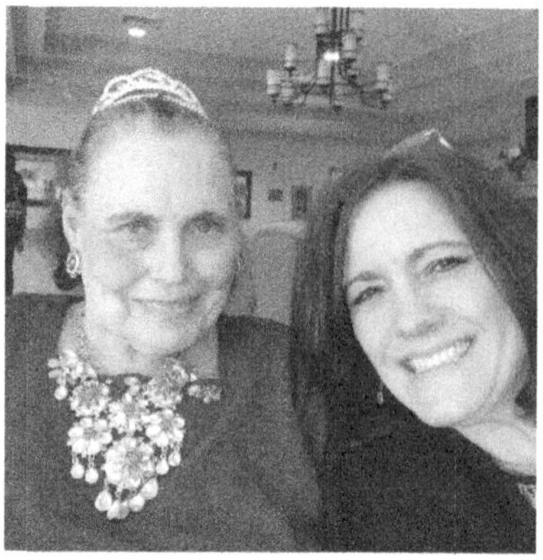

Mom Chronicles June 1, 2019

I'm visiting with Mom for a little bit before the event with the congressman. I learned that there are 2 of us speaking on behalf of families at the center. Until then, we are playing "mominoes" in the other empty house and eating trail mix.

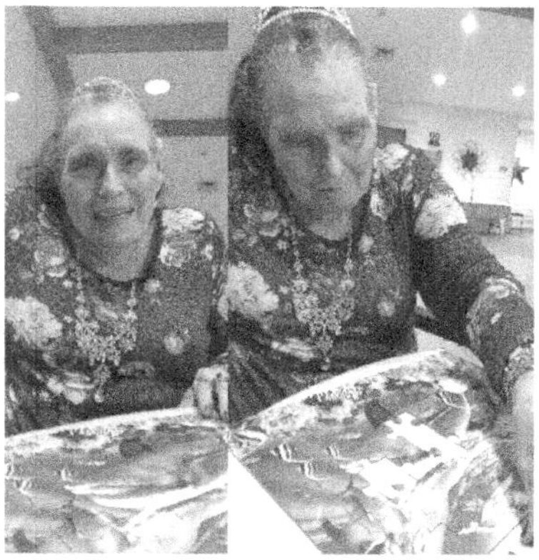

Mom Chronicles June 3, 2019

We just had a short visit tonight. The look of joy on her face as she puts the last piece of the puzzle in place is priceless.

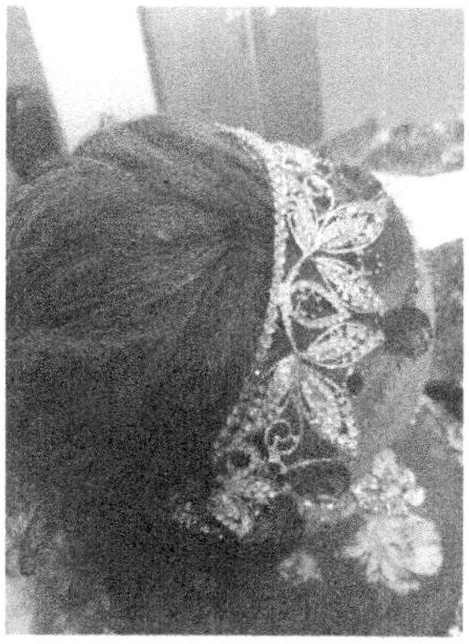

Mom Chronicles June 6, 2019

The first thing I noticed with our visit tonight is that she is wearing one of her crowns like a headband along with a second headband. I think that actually kind of works!

The second thing I noticed is that she had a baby doll tucked in by her side in the wheelchair. It wasn't the baby doll I had bought her.

I wheeled her into the atrium to fix her nails. We went with a sparkly pink shade tonight. Shauna stopped by and said that particular baby doll was a great thing for her today. Apparently, she held onto it all day and talked to it. It's the type that coos and cries when you squeeze the tummy. She didn't want to let it go. This one belongs to another resident, so I asked Shauna if it was worth buying a doll similar to that one, and she said definitely since it helped keep her engaged today. Soooo, as soon as I post my Chronicles, I will be searching online for a talking, crying, cooing doll.

After fixing her nails, I gave her a card from Tommy and Jennifer Tomlinson. She loved the puppies on the front and then LOVED the new nail strips that were inside. I think she wanted me to change out the ones I had just applied with one of the new sets, but I

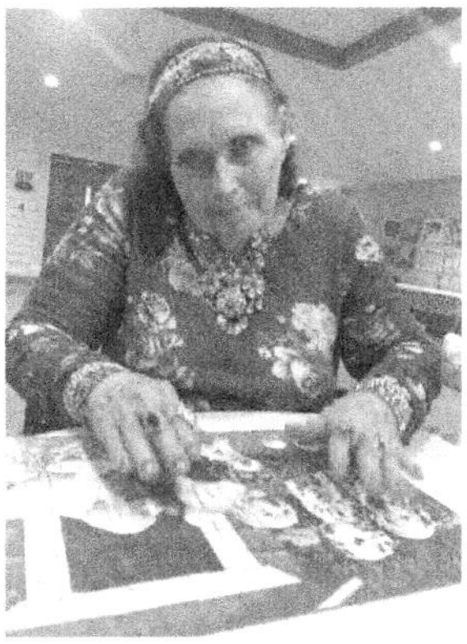

convinced her we would use them next week. (THANK YOU, Tommy and Jennifer! You helped make her happy today!!)

Next, we put a puzzle together. I had her do most of it. She needed some guidance, so I just kind of put the correct puzzle piece in the correct vicinity of where it belonged. I also had to have the jigsaw piece positioned in the right way to line up. She was having difficulty understanding she could turn the piece to get it to lock into place.

Finally, Bruce FaceTimed tonight since I wasn't going to see him before he went to work. He chatted with Mom for a few minutes. She was able to get the phrase "I love you" out.

Her hips still seem to be causing a lot of pain. I need to check on how much pain medication the doctor has prescribed and see if it can be increased some. I don't want her catatonic, but I also don't want her in pain.

When it was time to leave, Mom's friend was having a bad night again. She was sitting by the door, trying to leave. The aides were doing their best to distract her. I felt bad that I didn't take her into the atrium with Mom and me when I saw that she was distressed. She was fine when I first arrived at the center. I'll take her with Mom and me next time to see if it helps prevent her from having a bad night. I had to sneak out the back way (which goes through the atrium and the front door) since she and the aides had the door blocked.

Mom Chronicles June 12, 2019

Mom was in a good mood tonight. She had received a rose from the staff today. I also bought a new doll that "speaks and cries." She loved it. I put her name on it because the first couple of dolls I purchased aren't in her room. I'm sure they all are moved around with the residents. I know Mom even had a doll one day that wasn't hers.

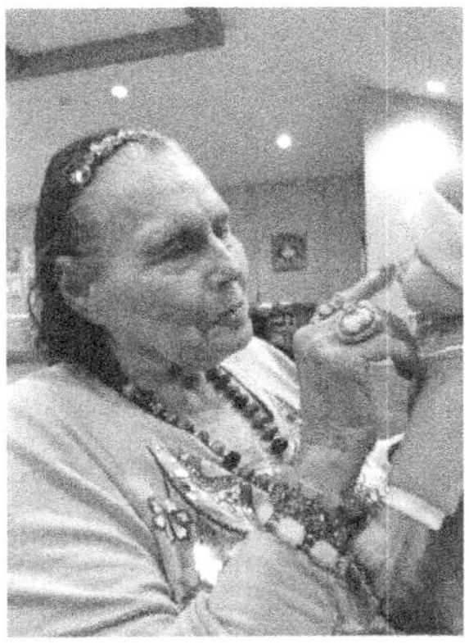

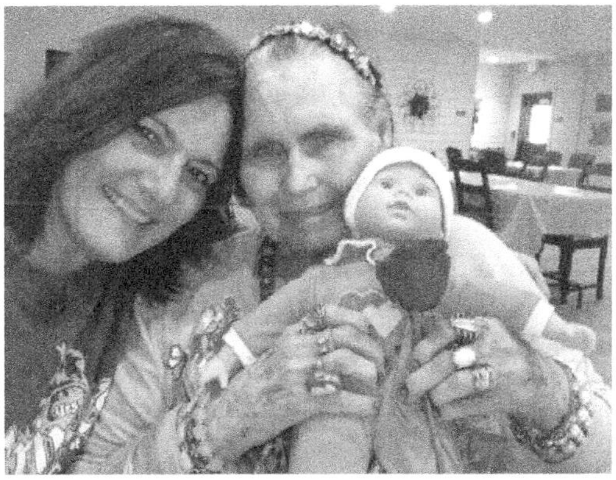

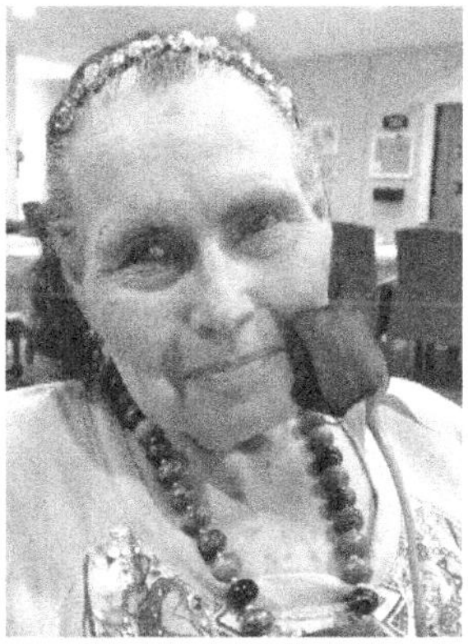

Mom Chronicles June 15, 2019

While Bruce slept, I drove over to see Mom today. When I arrived, they were mixing the ingredients for sugar cookies. Yum!! I didn't stay long enough, though, to reap the rewards. I just think it's so cool that the staff does little things like this to keep them engaged. Mom loved cooking and baking, so I'm sure this brought some joy to her. I brought Simi along today so that Mom could see her baby. Because one of the residents doesn't like dogs too much, I took Mom and Mom's friend into the atrium for some 50s music and a few rounds of mominoes. Before leaving, I let Simi get up on the table so that she could get to Mom's eye level. I wouldn't normally do this, but because I know they always put tablecloths on before serving folks, I did it this time. (Forgive me, Jenni!! I'll remember to bring some cleanser next time I bring Simi!!) That look on Mom's face is priceless.

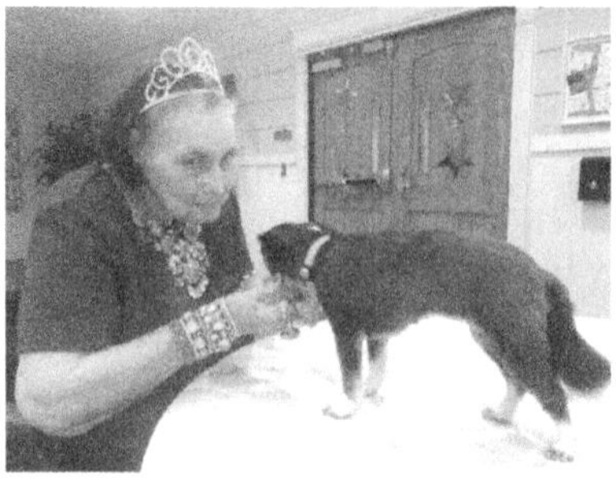

And boy, was she loaded down with the bracelets today!!

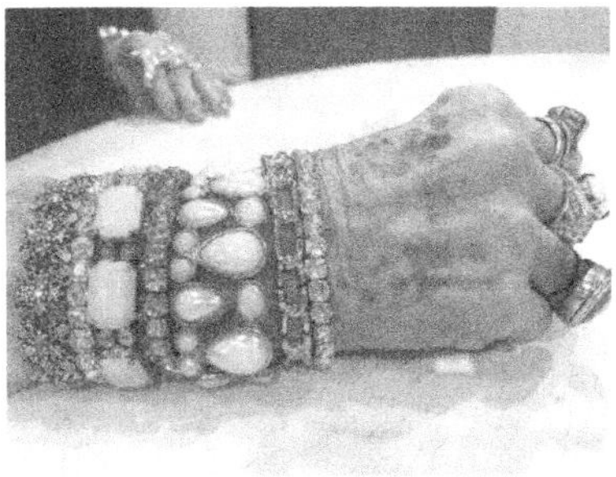

The only other thing worth noting was that the only clear phrase I got out of her today was "I love you." Everything else was sound effects. She uses sounds like woohoo, zoom zoom, etc., when she can't find the words. It seems like that's all I get from her now. But I guess if one of the last clear phrases that I get from her is "I love you," then that is pretty cool. I'll take it!! I love you too, Mom. I love you too.

Mom Chronicles June 17, 2019

I didn't take a picture today. When I got there, Mom wasn't in the 100-house where she lives. The aide told me she was in the 200-house with a few others doing a trial run during the day. They may be moving her and the others into that house within a few weeks. They were eating dinner. Mom was doing fine. I did have to help her with the last few bites because she had a hard time getting the rice on her spoon, AND she wanted to make sure the red pepper pieces were not in her rice. She has become a very picky eater.

Mom's friend, on the other hand, was not doing as well. She couldn't understand why she was over there. Mom doesn't know better... she thinks she is still in the same house because it looks the same. But, mom's friend is a little more with it and knows it's different.

After Mom finished dinner, a new aide walked over and started talking to Mom. She was engaging her and asking her to show her all her rings. Well, we looked down and didn't see any rings or bracelets at all. I asked if she didn't put them on today, and the aide said no, they were on earlier. She went to look on the couch, and I leaned over to see if Mom had placed them to her side in the wheelchair. They weren't there, but my forearm brushed up against her tummy, and I could feel them there. She had taken all her jewelry off (no earthly idea why) and slid them under the waistband of her pants. I'm guessing she thought that was her pocket. We pulled them all out of her waistband, and she was happy as a lark to put them all back on. But, again... we have no idea why she even took them off and hid them.

I will say I am very happy with the new aide. She showed that she knew how to engage Mom.

After that, I took Mom to the atrium. We Skyped with Sheila for a few minutes, played music, and played dominoes until it was time for me to leave. She could get a few more phrases out today that made sense, so that was good.

Mom Chronicles June 20, 2019

Mom was doing well tonight. She was in the 200-house with four others who were trying it out for a few weeks. She was finishing up dinner. She ate her dessert and then licked the gravy bowl dry like it was a dessert. She still had water and juice in her 2 cups. I started to take away her plate since it was empty, but she got upset. The new aide said she doesn't like anything to be taken away until everything, drinks included, were finished. So, note taken... leave the empty plate!!!

After that, we Skyped with Robin for a few minutes. Mom was able to get several phrases out that made sense. She loved to show Robin her rings. Robin went right along with it by ooohing and aaahing!

After the call, I explained to the aide that Robin is Ted's daughter and that Ted was Mom's husband. I pulled up pics. At first, she didn't recognize the picture of Ted by himself, but when I showed a pic of them together, she said, "oh, yes."

Mom's friend then asked if he was still alive. I should have lied, but I didn't and said no; he passed away about a year and a half ago. Mom looked at me sharply and asked, "He did?" I said, "yes, ma'am." He was very ill. The aide and I jumped on this quickly and redirected her to her jewelry to keep her from getting upset. I felt horrible for upsetting her for that few seconds!!

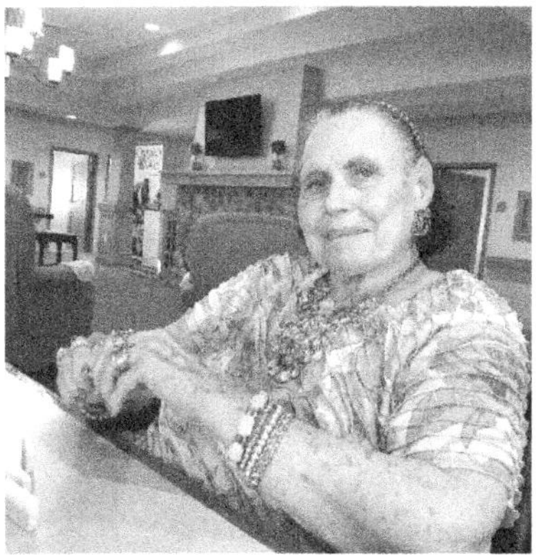

We then put a puzzle together and played "mominoes." She tried to do a double spinner again. I made the mistake of correcting her this time since Mom's friend was playing with us. I got the "go-to h-e-double-hockey-sticks" look (where my sister learned it from so well, by the way), so we played with a double spinner!! If she wants a double spinner, then by golly, we are playing with a double spinner!!

We ended with Skyping Sheila.

Mom Chronicles June 22, 2019

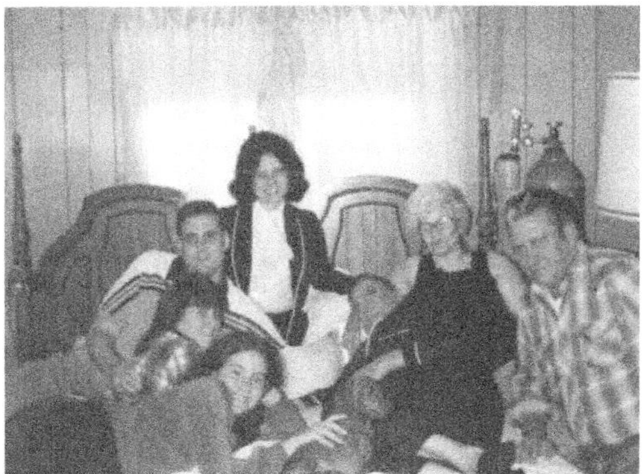

All my photo albums are in storage, so I miss looking through all the family photos. Uncle Quinton just sent this to Sheila and me. My Mom (isn't she beautiful in her suit), my Uncle Quinton, my sister, me, my dad, and my wonderful grandparents, TM and Daphne. Billy, the dachshund, was Grandpa's buddy. My grandpa had health problems most of the time that I knew him. We had many wonderful memories just laying on that huge king-size bed with him, watching TV or listening to him tell us the same old stories over and over. I would love to hear them just one more time!! Thanks, Unc, for sending the pic to us!!

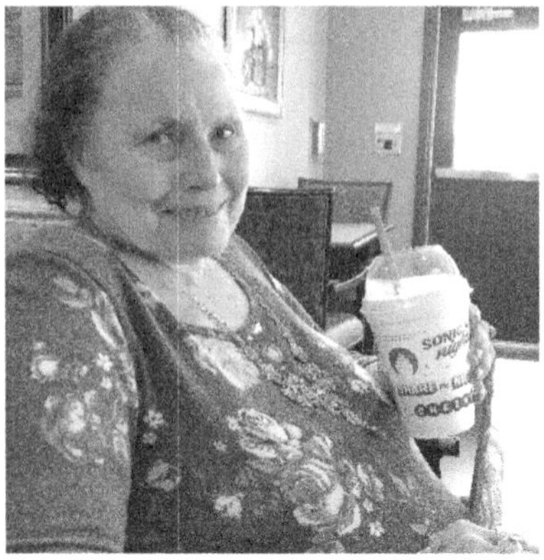

Mom Chronicles June 24, 2019
There was no crown on her head today, but I treated her and her friend to one of the new cake batter shakes from a local fast-food place. They both loved it!! We worked a puzzle and then were about to start a game of mominoes when her friend, Miss A., started getting upset with her phone. (Her family has it set up to go to voicemail, or else she would call them all day and night.) The aide tried to get her to go back to the other house because she didn't want to leave me alone with both of them while she was upset, but Miss A. wasn't happy with that decision. So, I stepped in and said I was taking Mom back over to their house too, so we could all go together. That appeased her. Luckily, once we got to their house, her daughter happened to be there to visit her. That brightened her up. Perfect timing!!

Mom and I then got to play a couple of rounds of dominoes. She was a little more off tonight with not matching a couple of her dominoes. I ended our visit with the song that she and Ted used to sing to each other: "I love you a bushel and a peck and a hug around the neck." She and I sing it to each other at the end of every visit now. It makes her smile.

Mom Chronicles June 29, 2019
Here are some notes from an event Jenni went to about Alzheimer's:

- Heart Health = Brain Health!
- 20% of heart function supports the brain.
- Cardio exercise is a must.
- Maintain good blood pressure and cholesterol levels.
- Nutrition plays a big role in prevention. The best diet for the brain is a Mediterranean diet low in fat and high in fiber.
- Diabetes can put you at a higher risk, so look for the best management options for this or options to reverse diabetes if you have it.

These are the best tools right now for trying to prevent Alzheimer's or dementia, but there is still no way to guarantee 100% that they will completely prevent it!

Dr. Grammas is currently starting research on the blood vessels in the brain as most studies have focused on plaques and tangles and have not made a lot of headway.

When asked about recent breakthroughs in the news about vaccines, etc., she didn't know the specifics of the trials. However, she recommended that we read the results to determine if they were from studies in mice. For example, she said Alzheimer's had been cured 40 times in mice, but because they only have a 2-year life expectancy, most of their findings haven't correlated to human Alzheimer's and dementia in the way of a cure.

Mom Chronicles July 1, 2019
I had a short visit with Mom tonight. I fixed her nails. She picked purple out of the 3 Color Street choices I gave her - surprise surprise!!

Mom's friend was having a tough night. She did not want to go back to her "house," so she became very upset. She cursed and hit the two aides. She even called 911 from her phone. I'm not sure what all came from that, but I can only imagine the police department understands the situation. The aides all handled it like professionals. The people who do this type of work daily deserve a medal and so much more.

Back to Mom, she was in a very happy mood tonight but was not wearing her crown. She couldn't talk much. Mostly gibberish and slurred words. "I love you" was clear, though, so I'll take it.

Bruce FaceTimed in for a few minutes so that he could show her Simi. She loved seeing them both but then kept switching back to showing Bruce her nails and jewelry.

She also wanted to hold her baby doll towards the end of the visit. No games tonight. It was just a "nail" night.

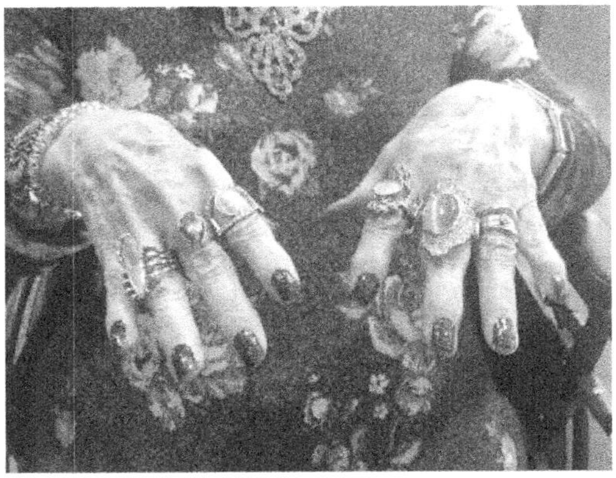

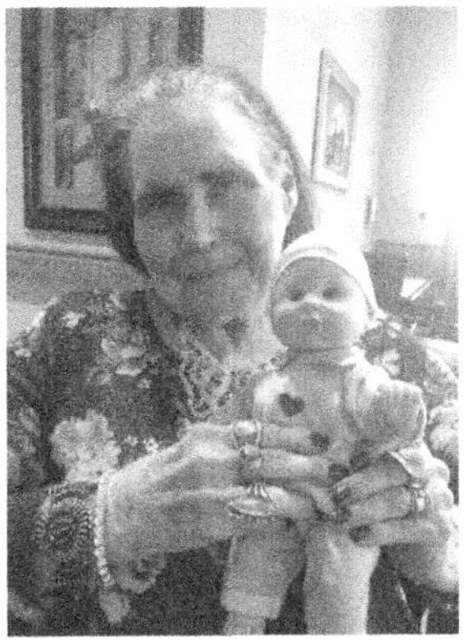

♥

At this point in our journey, I lost one of my adjunct teaching gigs. The department I worked part-time for decided to switch teaching responsibilities to teaching assistants instead of using adjuncts. I had to make the hard decision to go ahead and move Mom to a nursing home to use Medicaid funds to pay for her care. This was not an easy decision because I knew her level of care and engagement would not be the same as what she was getting at the current memory care center.

I visited several nursing homes. At one nursing home, the person giving me the tour told me they were a 5-star nursing home, according to the medicare.gov website. I had never heard of this rating system, so I looked it up. This center had a 4-star, not a 5-star rating, but I liked what I saw and had left a message for them to call me back to start the paperwork. Well, they never called back, so I took that as a sign not to place Mom there.

I started looking at other nursing homes. One had a horrible urine smell, so I did not want Mom living there. I settled on one that was located halfway between where I worked and where I lived. I checked the government site, and it had a 5-star rating and only had a couple of issues that weren't related to direct care of the residents. Here is the site if you want to look at the ratings and reports that the auditors file each year on the nursing home:

www.medicare.gov/care-compare/?providerType=NursingHome&redirect=true

Medicare.gov provides a list of questions to ask when looking for a nursing home. The pdf can be found at this link:

www.medicare.gov/sites/default/files/2019-10/NursingHomeChecklist.pdf

I have also shared these questions at the end of the book in the "Resources" section.

Mom Chronicles July 3, 2019
Long story short... I have to move my mom in a few weeks to a nursing home with Medicaid pending beds. It breaks my heart to leave this center because they are amazing, but one of my income streams (one of my adjunct teaching gigs) isn't going to be available in the fall. It has taken five income streams to personally pay for Mom's care at the memory care center. (Medicare nor Medicaid will pay for care in a memory care facility.) I found a nursing home with 4 and 5 stars across all categories, and I liked what I saw when I did a surprise visit.

I did have a short visit with Mom today. I noticed she wasn't wearing any rings today. I also noticed she still has congestion, and I heard her cough once. Jenni had contacted me yesterday to tell me the doctor prescribed something to try and get ahead of it. She was in a good mood, so I left her with our little song and a smile.

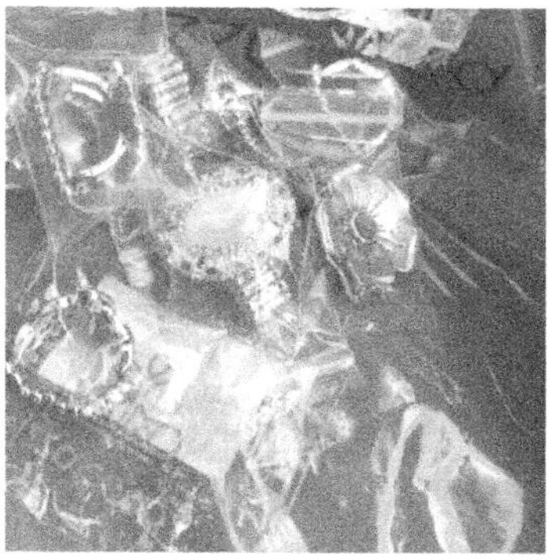

Mom Chronicles July 9, 2019
Phase 1 of "Operation Redirection during the Transition" is complete. Six new costume jewelry rings came in and are ready to go for next week. We will move Mom on Monday morning. I have the week off next week for vacation, so I will be there every day to help her get settled. Sheila will be here for the first couple of days. We are praying she adjusts very fast, but I'm realistic and know it will take time. I also talked to the lawyer today about Medicaid, and I have all my ducks in a row in that regard.

Mom Chronicles July 9, 2019
When I arrived at the center tonight, it was a little bit of a madhouse. One resident was at the door, so I had to walk around through the main entrance and enter through the back. It wasn't a big deal - I needed the steps.

The current house where Mom lives has more challenging patients. One resident kept trying to climb over the kitchen area gates. Another resident kept trying to take his pants off. Another patient decided to pour her drink on the floor. Another one didn't want to take her meds, so she poured her juice on her dinner plate. Another one didn't want to eat. The aides had their hands full tonight.

I stepped in to help get the juice poured for everyone - it was the very least I could do. Mom ate slow tonight. I had to help cue her some. I also helped cue another resident at the table who didn't want to eat. I was able to get that resident to eat some mashed potatoes, but that was it. Mom ate most of her dinner. They had pot roast, so she was getting meat stuck in between her teeth. I told her I would help floss her teeth when she finished eating. We finally finished dinner and went into the atrium.

Her nails needed fixing badly - Shauna said she was obsessing over them lately. So I put the gold and red nail strips on her tonight. While in the atrium, one of the residents kept trying to come through the door the whole time. I wasn't going to get Mom back into the house until we lost his attention so that he would leave the door. So... I took her into one of the little side rooms. She ooohed and awwwed over the art on the walls and the landscaping outside the window. She kept saying "it's beautiful" over and over. I posted a couple of these pics. It was a joy to see her happy like this.

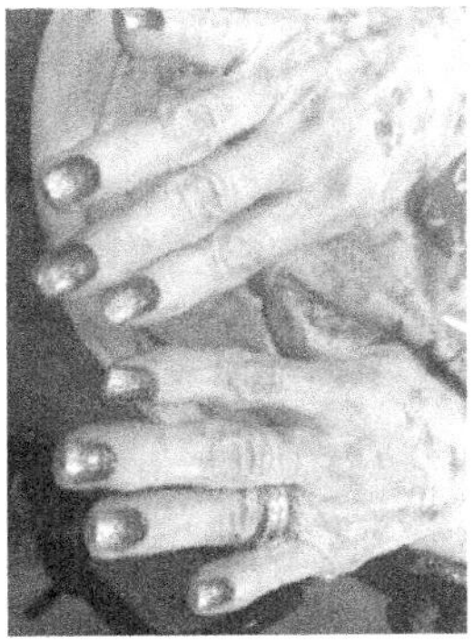

I also flossed her teeth to get the pot roast out that was stuck. I'm sure that is not what you all wanted to hear. The things I do for my Mom!! I kept opening my mouth and was saying "ahhh" like a doctor to get her to open her mouth wider, and she kept getting the giggles. We laughed and laughed about flossing her teeth!! I would never have thought that flossing would lead to one of my favorite memories, but it did!!

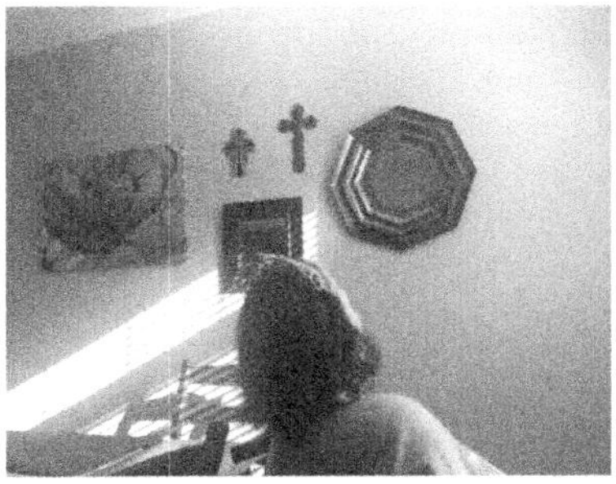

The resident finally left the door since he couldn't see us anymore, so I was able to take Mom back into the house. The madhouse from an hour before had calmed down in there. I was about to leave when she had a momentary look of panic in her eyes, asking what she should do. I pointed to the door to her room and said she's home. She's fine. She saw that and calmed down immediately. She recognized it as home. We sang our "bushel and a peck" song, and then I left promising to see her in a few days.

♥

Notice I mentioned "cueing" at dinner time in this post. I'll share more at the end of this chapter on how to do this, but it means helping your loved one remember to take a bite to eat. The longer you can have your loved ones eat by themselves, the better. Allow muscle memory to work. But at this stage, cueing is helpful to allow that muscle memory to work.

Mom Chronicles July 12, 2019
I just wanted to shout out to my co-worker and friend, Beth Dolliver. She knows that next week will be challenging, so she brought me a "survival bag" full of chocolate, a stress ball, and a little flower that lights up with different colors to help me redirect Mom when needed. I have the best co-workers and friends, period. Thank you, Beth!

Mom Chronicles July 12, 2019
I just did another quick visit to the new facility where I'm moving Mom to on Monday morning, and I am feeling better and better about the move. I saw the room where she will go, and it has a lady with late-stage Alzheimer's as well. Her husband comes every day from 5:30 in the morning and stays until 6:00 every night. This will ensure that if Mom needs help, he can push the call button for most of the day if she is in her room. I just LOVE the devotion this man is showing his wife!! I also liked the interactions I was witnessing with the aides, nurses, etc.

Also, they decorated the roommate's side of the room very bright and festive. It gave me ideas on how to display her stuffed animals. I was afraid I wasn't going to be able to bring them.

I'm feeling better and better about this. As Jenni has been encouraging me about this... I'm trying to be at peace with this decision.

Mom Chronicles July 12, 2019
Today was a half-day at work, so after stopping by the new center at lunch for a surprise visit, I visited Mom for a few hours.

We went into the atrium to play dominoes, and then Shauna and her crew came in there with the other residents to make ice cream. Mom didn't want to help shake the bag, but she ate every drop of the ice cream!

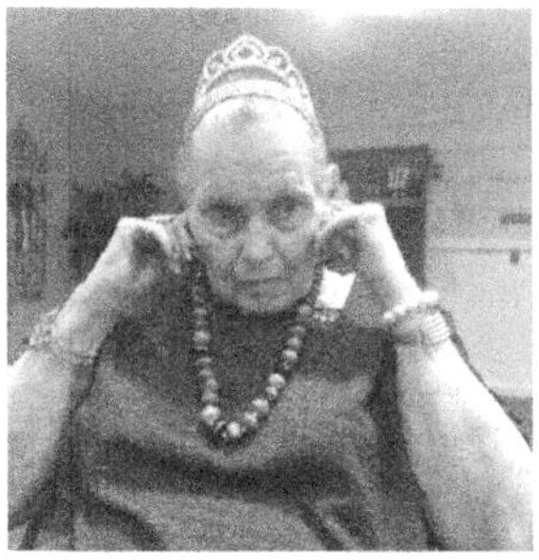

At one point, the fire alarm went off several times. It was great to see that the staff had a system in place, and everyone did their role during the alarm. The fire department showed up and helped get the alarm fixed.

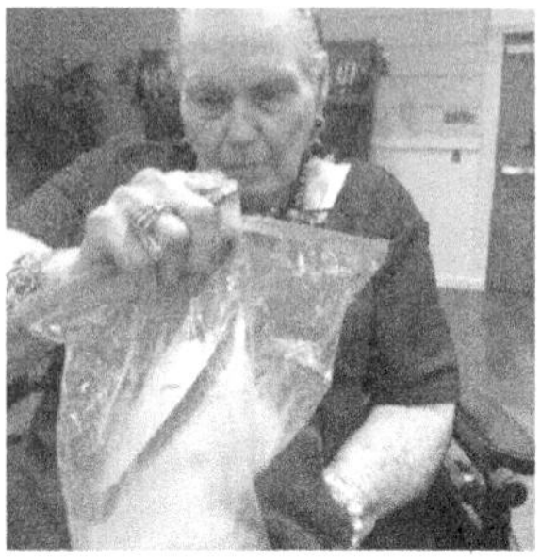

I was getting ready to leave, but Mom had that deer in the headlights look and held onto me. She was confused and didn't know what to do. I asked if she wanted to stay in the atrium with her friends and the music, but she said no. So, I took her back into her "house." As soon as she saw her room, she started to settle down a little more. She still wasn't quite calm yet, so I went to get her baby doll. That was the magic trick that worked. As soon as she had the baby to take care of, she was back to normal. I was able to leave without any issues then.

I also talked to one of the aides to find out what all has been working with Mom lately, so she gave me tips to share with the new staff next week.

The main things:
1. She needs to see her room/ her things. That is her "home"- her safe place.
2. When getting changed, she is afraid of falling. So the aides try to reassure her over and over that she's not going to fall.

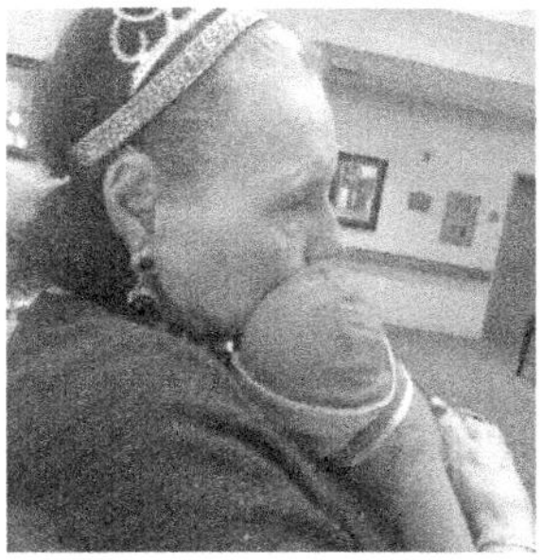

And then, of course, there are the redirection things that work for us:
1. Have her show us her jewelry and fingernails
2. Baby doll
3. Photo album book

♥

Stage 6 and Stage 7 are comparable to the last stage of Alzheimer's that the Alzheimer's Association calls "Late Stage." I share Mom's final stage in the next chapter, but I'm going to list the Late-Stage Caregiving tips here that I learned from Alz.org.

At this stage, our role switches to maintaining our loved one's quality of life. Alz.org shares that research shows that "some core of the person's self may remain." For me, that helps Mom's phrase that she uttered a while back, "I remember me," ring true. It's important to connect to your loved one in various ways. Communication verbally is now pretty much over other than some simple yes/no responses or the elusive "I love you." You can still communicate using the senses of touch, sound, sight, taste, and smell. Here are some examples:

- Play her favorite music (I chose music from Mom's teenage years.)
- Read meaningful book passages (Remember the story of the elderly man who read bible passages to his wife?)
- Look at old photos together (My sister used an online service to create small hand-size books full of photos - these books were lifesavers when we needed to redirect Mom. I recommend adding more pictures of your loved one because he now recognizes himself more than he recognizes family members.)
- Prepare a favorite food. (If she is in a memory care or nursing home facility now, bring in a favorite meal. Check with the home's caregivers to ensure it doesn't need to be prepared a certain way first. There may be swallowing issues, so find out if a regular diet is okay or does the food need to be chopped, pureed, etc.

For Mom, she loved when I brought in strawberry shakes and hamburgers.)

- Rub lotion that has a favorite scent into the skin. A scented lotion for women or aftershave for men should do the trick. If my dad had made it to this stage, he would have loved "Old Spice."
- Brush your loved one's hair. Mom loved it when I did this for her.
- Sit outside when the weather is nice. Let her breathe in the fresh air, see the birds flying and chirping, smell the flowers, and so on.

Care at this stage becomes extensive. Do your research on whether she will remain home with you or will move into a facility. Don't second guess your decisions. If you do your research, you can be at peace knowing you did all you could do. That doesn't mean things will always work out, as witnessed by our story. We researched until we were blue in the face about one facility, and you noticed it didn't work out. But we had a Plan B in place if it didn't work out. The important thing is that your loved one will get the needed care at this stage in whatever way that works for your family's unique situation. And don't forget that Hospice is an option as you get to a stage where the physician believes she has six months or less left to live. In our case, the pandemic in 2020 forced nursing homes to not allow hospice workers inside the facility to care for residents in that stage of life. As a result, she missed out on that extra level of care that she desperately needed.

Food and fluids are harder to control during this phase. Your loved one will eat and drink less. This is due partially to less movement, so therefore the body doesn't need the extra energy. It is also due to that part of the brain slowly dying. As a result, he will not be hungry or thirsty as the disease progresses. Dehydration is a common symptom when he is not drinking enough. Swallowing also becomes more difficult and eventually stops towards the end. Do you have end-of-life decisions in place? Does your loved one want a feeding tube when she gets to the stage where she can't swallow? Sweet foods will become popular since the sense of taste is one of the last senses to go. Nutrition shakes become invaluable in this stage to help your loved one get nutrients. Suggestions for mealtimes are as follows:

- Ensure your loved one is sitting upright comfortably to aid in digestion for at least 30 minutes after a meal.
- Adapt foods when swallowing becomes an issue. Soft foods can be chewed and swallowed easily. Liquids like water, juice, milk, and soup can be thickened by adding cornstarch or unflavored gelatin. Pudding, ice cream, and plain yogurt can also help.
- Encourage self-feeding as much as possible. Give her cues by putting food on a spoon or putting a chicken strip in her hands. Finger foods will help when they forget how to use a spoon or fork. Watch for things she is avoiding eating. For example, mom didn't like visible pepper flakes on her food anymore. We guessed she thought it was dirt.
- Assist your loved one with feeding. Try alternating small bites with liquids. Remind him to chew or swallow if needed. Make sure all food is swallowed before moving to the next bite. (Towards the very end, your loved one may pocket food in her cheek like a chipmunk because she doesn't remember how to swallow.)
- Shauna shared with me one time to always look your loved one in the eyes when helping feed her. It's so demeaning when shoving food into a mouth to get the dinner process done. Be patient. It could take Mom an hour or more to eat a full meal with cueing. She ate very slowly.
- Encourage fluids as much as possible. Try fruit juices, gelatin, sherbet, or soup. Don't forget to check the temperature of foods first before serving warm or hot liquids. If she has trouble swallowing, thickened liquids tend to help. The memory care center Mom lived at for a while would serve both water and juice. Watch for things that make her worried such as ice. Mom started believing that ice was something that didn't belong in her water or juice.
- Monitor his weight. Weight loss towards the end can be expected, but it is also a sign of inadequate nutrition, illness, or medication side effects. Don't forget to keep the doctor involved in this stage.

Toileting at this stage is more difficult. Depending on whether your loved one is still mobile or not, these ideas may need to be modified:

- Keep a toileting schedule. Keep a written record of how often your loved one goes to the bathroom and how much she eats or drinks. Bedside commodes can be used. When Mom lived with us, I purchased the liners from local stores in the pharmacy departments so that I wouldn't have to wash the pot afterward. These liners had an absorbency product similar to what is in a diaper to soak up liquids. It was easy just to tie the bag and throw it away. Keep the Lysol spray handy! This is NOT a pleasant experience, but the liners helped make it easier!

- As she gets closer to the end of her life, she may not have the strength to use a bedside commode. She may need her diapers changed in the bed. Hospice usually can help provide a hospital bed, and the hospice staff can teach you how to change and bathe your loved one. We used washable "chucks" to keep under Mom in case of leakage to protect sheets.
- Limit but don't eliminate liquids about two hours before bedtime.
- Use absorbent and protective products. Please remember not to call them diapers in front of your loved one to help retain dignity. Instead, use words like briefs or underpants when helping her get changed.
- Monitor bowel movements to avoid constipation. Use natural laxatives in the diet, such as prunes or fiber-rich foods, and consult the doctor if constipation continues.

Skin and body issues become more prevalent at this stage. He may become bedridden or wheelchair-bound. Skin can break down, creating pressure sores and joint freezing. These suggestions can help:

- Change the loved one's position at least every two hours to relieve pressure and help with blood circulation. (This was a struggle at some of the facilities Mom lived in, so I advise keeping a camera in your loved one's room to monitor how often they are turned.)
- Ensure your loved one is sitting up straight in the wheelchair to avoid pressure on her lower back. I don't know how many times I would get to the nursing home and need to ask them to help me straighten her in her wheelchair. She was not strong enough to shift herself in the seat anymore. Consider pillows to support arms and legs as well. Learn how to lift your loved one without hurting yourself. Nursing home staff have been trained but if your loved one is home with you, have home health nursing staff teach you how to lift your loved one safely. Don't lift by pulling on your loved one's arms or shoulders.
- Keep skin clean and dry. Skin starts to get thinner as your loved one ages and can tear and bruise easily. Avoid friction and use gentle motions when cleansing with a mild soap. Blot dry. Check daily for rashes, sores, or breakdowns. They will come up quickly.
- Protect bony areas by using pillows or pads. They would put pillows between Mom's legs and feet to cut down on the pressure of her legs and feet pressing against each other. If using a skin moisturizer, apply it gently. Don't massage it into her skin on those areas.
- To prevent freezing joints known as limb contractures, try to do range-of-motion exercises at least two to three times a day or as much as possible. Make it fun by having them kick at balloons. Get ideas from a physical therapist. These exercises will be easier to do after bathing when their limbs are warm.

Infections and pneumonia are risks at this stage.

- Keep the teeth and mouth clean to reduce the risk of bacteria in the mouth that can lead to pneumonia. I will tell you that this is difficult if your loved one is in a facility. They concentrate on keeping the loved one dry and fed, but teeth brushing was the last thing I noticed ever being attempted. The loved one may fight this too, so choose your battles. Keeping Mom dry was the main thing I wanted for her, so I didn't push the teeth brushing. Every family will be unique. Choose your battles. Other ideas from alz.org are to remove dentures every night to have them cleaned and to use soft toothbrushes or moistened gauze pads to clean gums and the tongue.
- Treat any cuts and scrapes immediately with warm soapy water and apply an antibiotic ointment. A deep cut may need a physician's assistance.
- Vaccinate for the flu every year and pneumonia every five years to reduce the risk. With COVID in our lives now, this may also be a yearly or semi-annual vaccine added to the recommendations. Check with your physician for advice concerning these vaccines.

Monitor your loved ones for signs of pain or illness. Because communication is limited now, you can monitor in these ways:

- Look for physical signs such as pale or flushed skin tone, dry gums, mouth sores, vomiting, fever, or swelling.
- Watch for nonverbal signs such as gestures, sounds, and facial expressions like wincing.

- Monitor changes in behavior. Is your loved one anxious, agitated, trembling, shouting, or having issues sleeping? These could be signs of pain.

Source: Alz.org, Late-Stage Caregiving
www.alz.org/help-support/caregiving/stages-behaviors/late-stage

CHAPTER 5: ALZHEIMER'S STAGE 7 ♥ THE LATE STAGE

We moved Mom to a nursing home, and I now know she only had one year left to live. She is still partially in Stage 6 and moving into Stage 7, the final stage at this point. Stage 7 is where the loved one may show some or all of these signs:

- lose the ability to communicate or respond (Mom has had difficulty with this for a while)
- need help with every activity such as eating, toileting, walking, and sitting up
- lose the ability to smile and may only grimace
- physical rigidity; joint deformities known as contractures
- neurological reflexes mimicking an infant emerge such as the grasping reflex and the sucking reflex
- pneumonia, aspiration, and infected decubital ulcerations are frequent causes of death at this stage
- lose their ability to swallow.

She has had trouble for a while with food or liquid going down the wrong "pipe" or swallowing too much and choking. The Social Care Institute of Excellence states: "As dementia progresses, it affects the area of the brain that controls swallowing. In advanced dementia, the person may have a weak swallow or lose the ability to swallow safely. For example, they may cough or choke after swallowing food or drinks." (Dementia: Eating and drinking at the end of life, n.d.) At the end of this stage, the Alzheimer's patient will truly forget how to swallow. For Mom, "forgetting how to swallow" happened during the last week or two of her life. I'll share more about this when we get to the last few "Mom Chronicles" posts in this chapter. (VISN 21 MIRECC, n.d.)

Mom Chronicles July 15, 2019

So far, so good. Mom's roommate's husband and daughter are here all day. They have a TV, so Mom is going to be happy watching it. We also had a chance to play some Bingo. She's not quite sure how to play it, but I made sure the activity director knows to get Mom for activities since she isn't going to know to come down and play.

I tried to decorate her room to make it cheery. She seems to like it so far. I have also talked to several of the aides and nurses. I just need to make sure I speak to each one on different shifts throughout the week.

I'll post more later. Keep the prayers coming for a smooth transition.

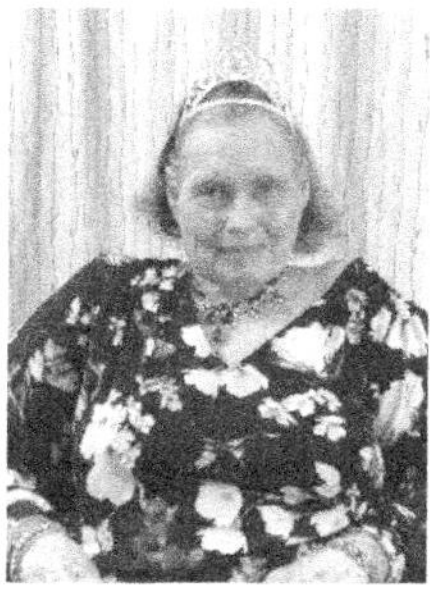
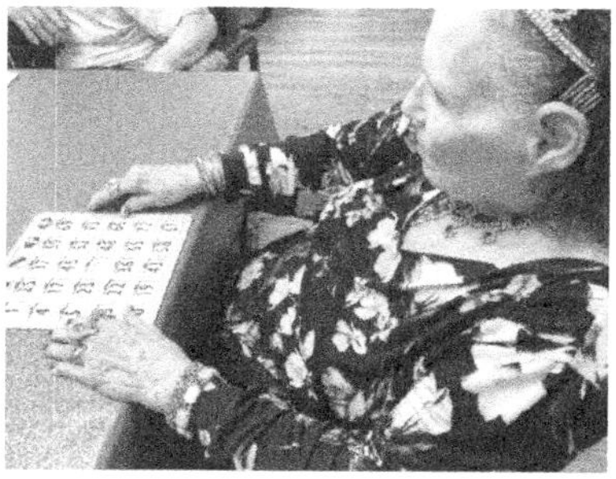
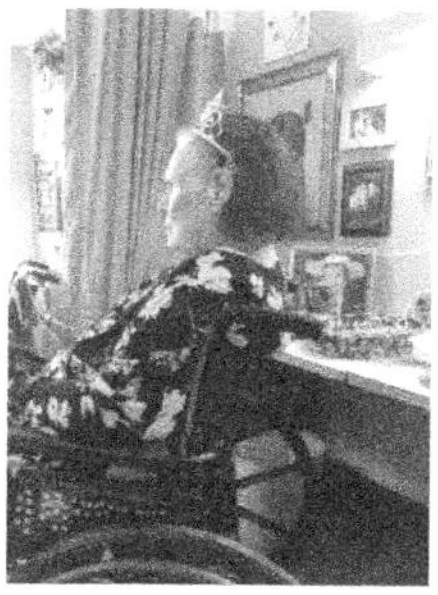
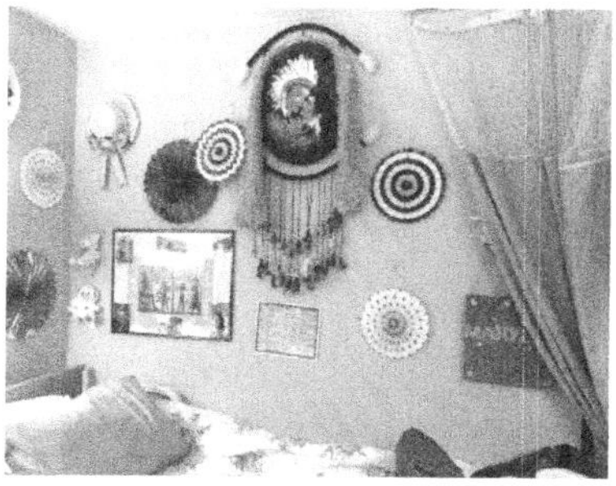

Mom Chronicles July 15, 2019
Lord grant me patience. And give Mom's roommate's family patience. With Alzheimer's, she has NO filter anymore. None. Nada. Zilch. Oy!!!!!

Mom Chronicles July 15, 2019
The day was good until dinner. Dinner went well until the very end. She choked, and it scared her. They do have her at one of the front tables that have aides to help. They weren't there this time because Sheila and I were there helping. They did come very fast because we were close to having to do the Heimlich maneuver. It scared Sheila and me too.

While going back to the room, she started saying no, and she wanted to leave. She's sundowning and in a new place. And she just went through a scary situation. It breaks our heart to hear that she wants to leave, but we were expecting it. All I can do is know that I have done the best research I could do to find a place to take care of her.

She's nodding off in her wheelchair now. They will be coming in soon to help get her to bed. We won't leave until then.

Mom Chronicles July 16, 2019
If there is a shiny side of Alzheimer's, it is that one forgets the "trauma" or bad experience that just happened. I arrived at the new center this morning, but she wasn't in her room. The roommate's husband gave me an update from the morning and said they had come in earlier to draw blood. She screamed bloody murder. I found her in the family room watching TV, so I sneaked by to talk to the food service manager. The manager was fantastic. She took all kinds of notes and said she would do everything she could to make sure Mom was eating what she liked.

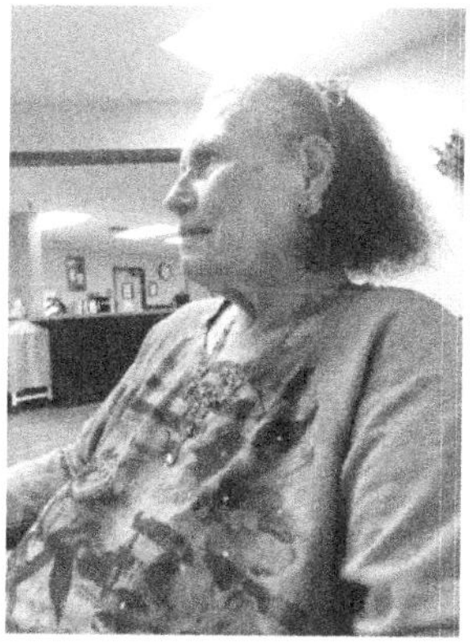

When I went into the family room to see Mom, she was in a great mood. I could see where they drew blood on her hand. The nurse said Mom wasn't happy with her right now because of the blood draw, but Mom had already forgotten about it. She just smiled and was very nice to the nurse.

She forgets something terrible (like getting changed) within a minute or two, which is a total blessing. She's in a great mood this morning, and I am extremely happy with all the staff I have met so far. They truly care.

Also, the physical therapist just came in to introduce himself and get to know Mom a little more. I explained how she fights therapy because of her pain level, so I encouraged him to think of ways outside of the box to get her to get some exercise. He said he would put his thinking cap on. I shared the balloon volleyball that

Shauna would do, but she also needs some activities to flex her legs again. Sitting in a wheelchair has "locked" up her muscles and joints. She's very rigid. I am signing off for now and hoping for a great day! We are off to a great start so far!

Mom Chronicles July 16, 2019
The dietary manager is trying something new with Mom. We will see if it works. She doesn't like her food to touch, so she put Mom's food in separate bowls. The thing to watch for is if she gets upset that she's "different" from others in the dining room. So far, it's working.

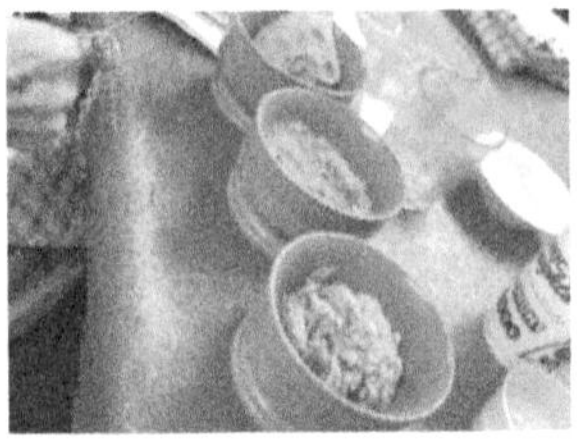

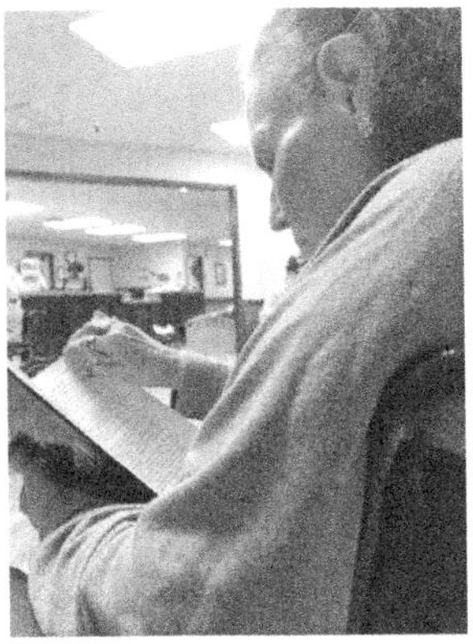

Mom Chronicles July 16, 2019
A deep memory is trying to come back. Mom used to LOVE reading Danielle Steel. She can't read anymore, BUT she saw this book in the family room bookcase and wanted it. She recognized Danielle Steel's very distinct book cover. She's opening the pages and just looking at them so intently. And she's humming. She's happy!

Mom Chronicles July 17, 2019
The morning went well. She's clinging to the baby doll - it brings her tremendous comfort.

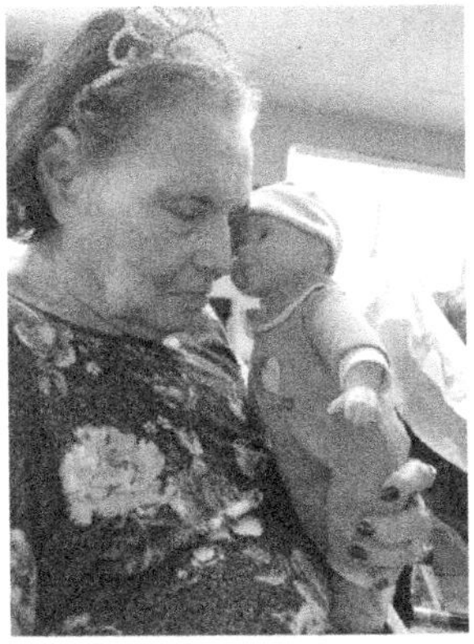

I redid her nails in sparkly purple and gave her two new rings.

The lab work from yesterday shows she is borderline diabetic. I'm waiting to hear back from the doctor on what that means. I'm guessing we will need to cut out bringing her shakes and treats.

Lunchtime was good. She had a hamburger, French fries, strawberries, and banana pudding. At one point, she forgot to use her spoon and used a French fry instead to scoop her banana pudding. She still seems happy, and that's what is important!

Mom Chronicles July 17, 2019
We are having a rough afternoon. She's not feeling well at all. The aides are still getting used to Mom and bless her heart; one aide just cried when changing Mom. Mom screams in pain but more so from fear when being changed. The aide felt so horrible. I tried to make sure she understood that Mom would forget the experience after a few minutes. I told her I so appreciated her compassion but not to let it get to her. It's just the disease. Another nurse came down a few minutes later because she could still hear mom whimpering. She asked if she could bring a little treat down to try and redirect her. I said sure. It makes my heart happy that the staff wants her to be okay.

I also just met the doctor. He's going to work on her pain management, and he said the X-ray of her lungs shows a little infiltration (pneumonia), so he has put her on antibiotics. So say a little prayer that she starts feeling better soon. I'm sure it's just a combination of the new place, the new people, the usual pain she experiences every day, the lung infection, and the disease.

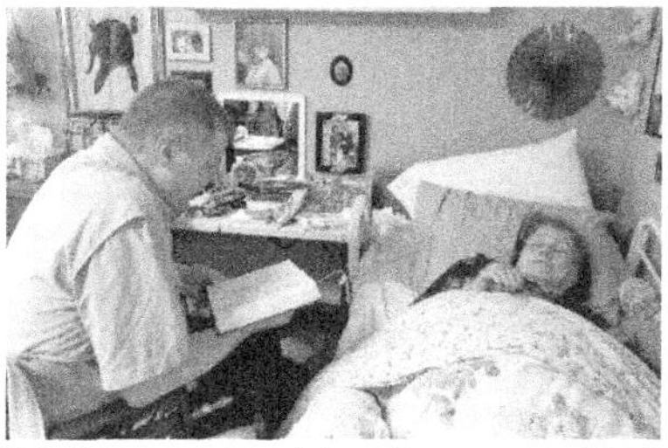

Mom Chronicles July 17, 2019

Thank you to PK (Pastor Ken) from our home church, Concordia Lutheran. I had left the nursing home about 30 minutes prior, but he arrived while Sheila was still there. She received permission from him to allow me to post the photos and video. Faith was/is important to Mom, and I know this helped lift her spirits this afternoon. She's not usually laying down - she just wasn't feeling good today. Thank you for showing your heart and compassion for my Mom, PK. Our family loves you!! It was beautiful to see her praying with you and trying to sing Amazing Grace. I'm sorry I missed the visit, but glad Sheila recorded this for us to keep the memory forever.

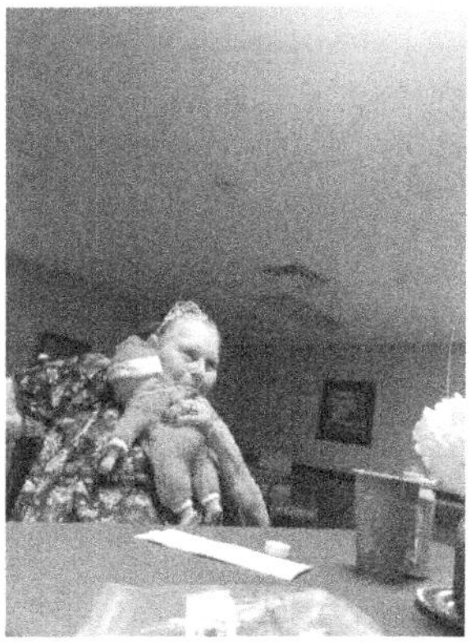

Mom Chronicles July 18, 2019

Mom did pretty well today. She is still in a lot of pain, but they just started the new pain regimen today. The activities director had a popcorn and movie hour. She showed several episodes of "I Love Lucy." Mom and the others loved it. Mom did hold on to her baby a lot today. I think that is going to be a regular thing now. I downloaded a pre-K game app on my iPad, and we tried a few rounds of matching colors and shapes. Unfortunately, she didn't do very well. It's so sad. The last thing is something that happened at dinner time. Another resident didn't like her dinner, so she asked for a cheese sandwich. Both guys working the dining hall said it's not on the menu. I asked about the menu at the front of the room that said it's ALWAYS on the menu. They got it made for her real quick. The reasons I fought for this lady who I don't even know are that 1) she couldn't fight for herself 2) I want to know that if I'm not here and Mom is not eating that they would at least try to get her something to try and eat instead of letting her go hungry. I usually am very passive, but I've seen myself become a "mama bear" when it comes to my Mama and others who can't speak for themselves. I will be chatting with the dietary manager tomorrow. She can't solve a problem if she doesn't know about it.

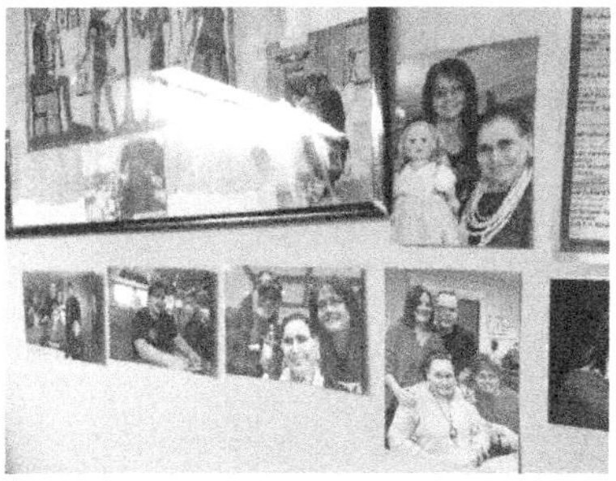

Mom Chronicles July 18, 2019

The little photos we put on the wall next to her bed have been a lifesaver! They keep her occupied. She's trying to tell me about them, but I can't understand anything she is saying. It's all gibberish.

Mom Chronicles July 18, 2019

Mom is no longer at the other memory care center, but everyone from there has become family to us. Shauna Sweetser saw my post about the photos on Mom's wall and how I couldn't understand a word Mom was saying. So she sent a text message to give me a tip: tell Mom that I appreciate how hard she's trying. That way, she will keep trying to find her words. For those of you on this journey as well, I hope this tip helps you as well.

Mom Chronicles July 19, 2019
I have three short notes for now.
1) When I arrived at the center, they were playing Uno. She enjoyed herself even though the activities' director was helping her and most of the others play the game. The hairdresser came in and was ready to color her hair. Mom didn't want to stop playing. The director was quick!! She said the game was over and all the other residents played along went along with it. I was able to get her away from the table. 2) She usually loves to have her hair colored, but her face is scrunching up in pain. It's like she can barely handle being touched anymore. She will be happy once she sees the final result, so hopefully, she can make it through the appointment. I have a cherry limeade drink that I'm giving sips to her to redirect.

Since I'm saving money, I'll be able to get her hair done more frequently now at this new place.
As I type this, she is settling down. I think the sensation of having her hair done is coming back. Her face is relaxing. Every girl knows how wonderful it feels to have her hair worked on. I don't know how many times I nearly fall asleep at the beauty salon when my hairdresser works on my hair. It's so relaxing!

3) I had a quick chat with the food director about yesterday. I promised her I wasn't a pain in the arsky, but I needed to make sure my mom and the others had a voice. She understood.

We will see how the day goes! I go back to work next week, so I need to make sure all concerns are addressed this week.

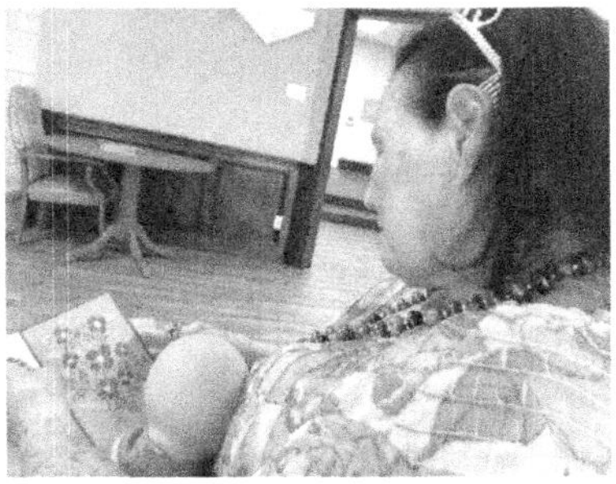

Mom Chronicles July 19, 2019
Thank you, Theresa Alexander! She hummed "jingle bells" while looking at the card!!

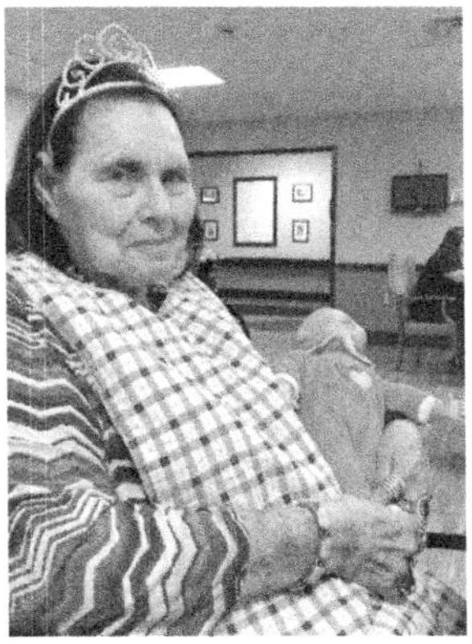

Mom Chronicles July 20, 2019
We are just waiting for lunch to be served... no words for me yet. She is just smiling and pointing to things like her baby doll or the drinks. Maybe I can get a few words out of her this afternoon.

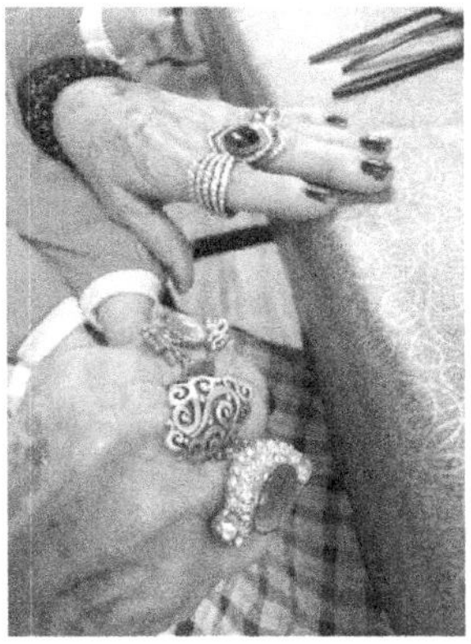

Mom Chronicles July 21, 2019
I was chatting with a new friend on the phone who is dealing with her mom, who has dementia, when I noticed the Director of Nursing (DON) called. Mom is safe but was being very combative this afternoon when it was time to change her. She was drawing blood on the aides this time.

Remember, I want to preserve Mom's dignity, but at the same time, I am also wanting to help others going through this.

The DON put me on the speakerphone with Mom. I said a white lie by saying I would be coming up there to visit her in a few minutes and to let them help her get freshened up with new underpants. (I remembered not to call them diapers!) She went from crying to being calm and saying okay. Mom won't remember that I told her I was coming up there, but it was needed to help her calm down. I needed a break today by getting errands done before going back to work tomorrow. I will be visiting her every day after work this week to continue helping her adjust to the new place.

The DON texted me and said Mom is changed now and that she is staying in her room with her until Mom calms down completely. It's still a traumatic thing for her to be changed most of the time because of her pain level, and well, nobody wants to be touched in that manner. I'm being honest here. It's just so personal. I told the nurse to show Mom the small photo book and to have Mom show off her jewelry.

I am very appreciative that the DON is taking the time to help redirect her instead of just leaving her in her room to cry it out. Have I mentioned lately that Alzheimer's sucks?

Mom Chronicles July 22, 2019

Mom was at dinner when I finally got there this evening. She did not have her crown on tonight, but she was wearing a purple headband. She was fine and ate most of her dinner. I learned she still loves tuna fish sandwiches.

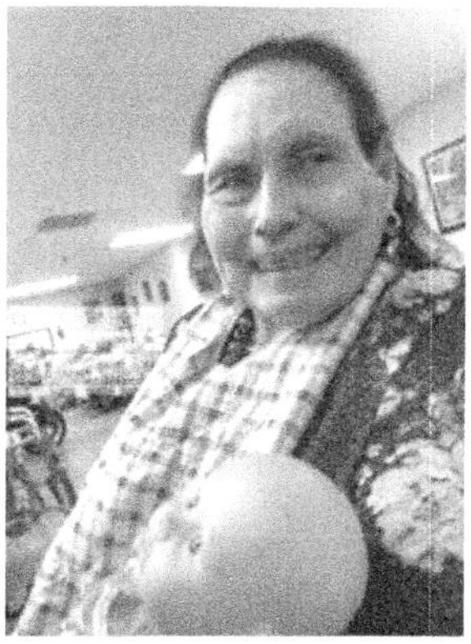

When I started wheeling her out of the dining room towards the TV room, she started panicking. She asked if she could go with me. Sheila wasn't available, so I had to FaceTime Bruce two different times to get her redirected. She was scared and kept saying she didn't know what to do. I know this will get better over time. She's only been there one week. I kept repeating slowly and repeatedly that she is safe and that the nurses would help her get ready for bedtime soon. I remember the previous memory care staff telling me to use short phrases and repeat them slowly to allow her brain time to process the words.

I was finally able to leave. I left my number with the nurse and told him that she's sundowning pretty hard tonight. So far, I haven't received a call, so maybe she is cooperating tonight.

Oh, the last thing I forgot to add on Saturday was that I had to take down her mirror. She was panicking every time she saw herself in the mirror. She didn't like her gray eyebrows and kept pointing to her eyes and saying, "not good." It just wasn't worth keeping the mirror up if it was only going to upset her. She still recognizes herself, which is a blessing. I have heard of caregivers who needed to cover the mirrors because the patients thought it was a stranger looking back at them.

♥

I wanted to make sure you saw that last paragraph about the mirror. Sometimes it is best to go ahead and put away a mirror or cover it up. If looking at her reflection is causing confusion or is upsetting, it's not worth keeping it out. Sometimes, a patient will think they are younger, and when they look in a mirror, they see an older person staring back at them. Can you imagine how scary that must be for them?

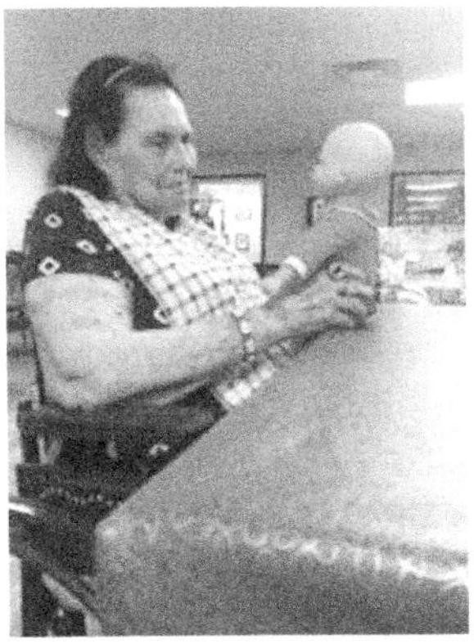

Mom Chronicles July 23, 2019
She's in a good mood so far!! While waiting for dinner to be served, she's pushing the button to have the baby doll talk to her.

Her roommate's hubby said she didn't fight the aides today. Hallelujah!

I also talked to two nurses to thank them for calling me Sunday to try and help her. One nurse said that Mom has taken to her for some reason and likes to come to sit in her office and "talk" to her. She said she sat in there for about 6 hours yesterday. When someone tried to take her out, she yelled, "no." The nurse said she didn't mind. She thinks Mom is a sweetheart. Fingers crossed that she doesn't panic when I try to leave today!!

Mom Chronicles July 23, 2019
*This one is not about Mom. I like to share things from friends who privately message me about their experiences or friends' experiences. Here is one from my friend Rhonda Youngblood, who permitted me to share! I hope this helps! I know I'm going to try it with Mom. I just need to think of some sight words to use. I may try photos or images too.

"I wanted to tell you something I learned from a friend last night. His pawpaw had dementia/Alzheimer's and got to where he couldn't speak much. They wrote words that were very important to him in large bright letters and placed them around his room—cows, Colita (that's where his ranch was), family, ranch, etc. He could see them easily, and they triggered his memory and comforted him. (It also gave unknown caretakers, therapists, etc., some conversation starters. They didn't use people's names, just "things" he loved. It was a comfort to him. Just a thought!"

Thank you, Rhonda!

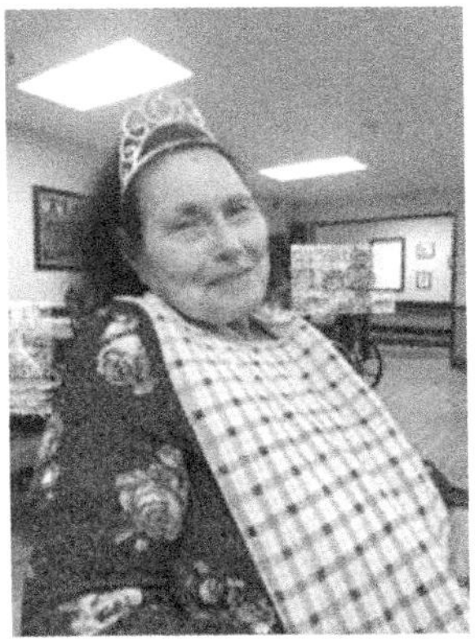

Mom Chronicles July 25, 2019
It's so stinkin' cute to see the aides curtsy in front of Mom and call her "my queen."

We also found a new drink that just puts her in "heaven" - Strawberry Nutrition Shake!

Last but not least, I signed off on two new meds for her. One is Celexa for depression. As I'm reading up on it, it says it's also good to reduce agitation in Alzheimer's patients. The second medication is another pain pill to see if we can get this pain under control. She's in a fantastic mood so far!!

Mom Chronicles July 26, 2019
Josh visited Mom with me this afternoon. I let him experience the joy of giving her one of the costume jewelry rings.

I also redid her nails with blue and silver today. You guys know I am a Houston Texans fan, so I had to look at the silver linings when putting these colors on her: 1) she has no clue these are Cowboy colors, and 2) Zeke didn't arrive at Oxnard today! I know, I know, I'm going to hear it from my Dallas peeps. 😊 (Bruce is still asleep, so I will definitely hear it from him in a few minutes.) These Color Street strips are truly the best things ever referred to me for Mom! I don't have to wait for polish to dry - she simply wouldn't understand the waiting process.

After that, I helped Mom play in their bi-weekly bingo game. She won one of the games!! She recognized a few of the numbers but not the majority. It was a great visit!

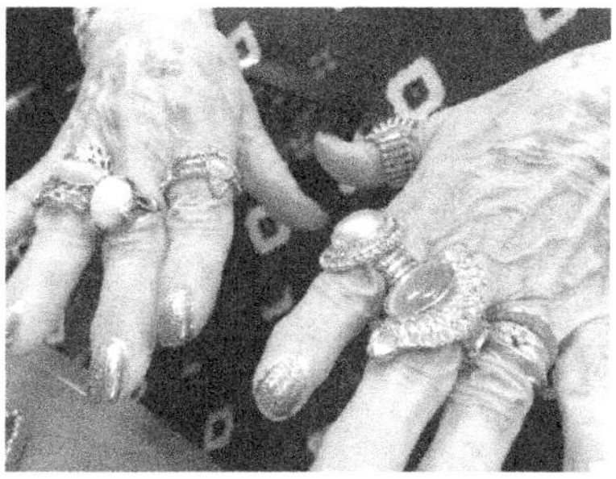
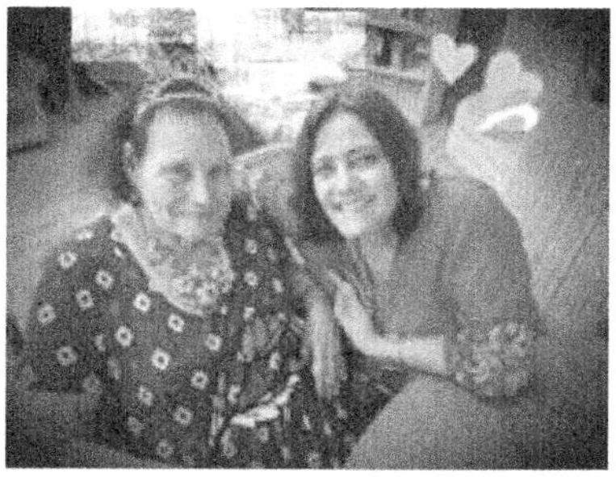
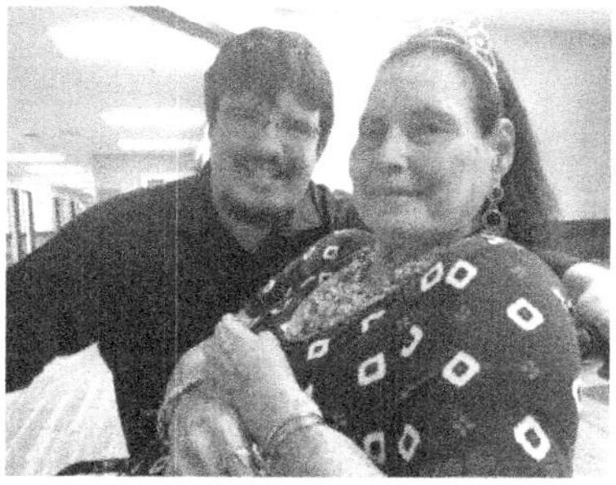

Mom Chronicles July 29, 2019
The diagnostician stopped by for a moment and said the aides reported coughing during some of her mechanical soft meals. Some of this visit spurred from a few days ago when they refused to give her strawberries because of the mechanical soft diet assigned to her. (Mechanical soft is food chopped up with no raw veggies or fruits allowed.) Canned is okay, though. I was a little upset with this because I think she can still be on regular food but just cut up since she doesn't know how to cut her food. She has, however, choked several times (or food going down the wrong pipe), so I'm probably wrong. (Yes, Bruce, I just admitted that I can be wrong sometimes.) 😊

They will do a swallow test on purées, mechanical soft, and regular food to test her swallowing. I know that difficulty swallowing is part of the last stage of Alzheimer's, so I'm probably fighting this by not believing she can't have regular food. She just still seems more alert than folks in the last stage, even though she has signs of everything else they experience.

They should be doing the test at the end of the week. I signed a consent form that allows me to be here during the test. That way, I can monitor it for myself. I need to believe they just want what's best for Mom, so we will see what the test says.

Right now, we are just waiting for dinner to be served. She's in a great mood so far. The greeting cards sent by several friends made her happy.

Mom Chronicles August 1, 2019
I got the call at 8:30 this morning that they would do the swallow test at 1:00 pm. Luckily, I was able to attend. She did fine. They said she could keep being served a regular diet. She can keep eating strawberries!!!!

I also worked with the director of nurses on another health issue. They have to do things slightly different from the memory care center because of state rules, so we will try other things to see what works. For example, we have been using a diaper AND an incontinence pad to line the diaper to help keep her dry. Apparently, the state frowns on this. So, she will need to go back to just using the diaper only. This just means they will need to keep an eye on her more closely and change her often to keep her dry.

I'm also going to try buying some dresses (muumuus) to see if that makes it easier to dress/change her. I need to try and find sparkly, flashy ones so that she accepts the wardrobe change and doesn't fight it.

Mom Chronicles August 2, 2019
It was a rough evening. At dinner, she did not have much of an appetite. She seems to be hurting, which may have caused the lack of appetite. When it was time for me to go home, I tried to leave several times over the course of 2 hours with the phrases that work every other time. She would cry. I tried redirecting with:

- 💗Photo album
- 💗Face Time with Bruce
- 💗Phone call when Josh
- 💗Skype with Sheila
- 💗Coloring - epic fail. She forgot how to color.

Redirection would work during that moment - she would smile and laugh - and then when I tried to leave again... waterworks and fear. I asked them to get her ready for bed early since she was more upset tonight, but they still hadn't come down to the room by 8 pm. I had to forgive myself and go ahead and leave. It broke my heart, though. I hated leaving her that way. I need to keep telling myself she was probably just fine 5 minutes after I left. On Monday, I'm going to ask them to start giving the pain pill and anxiety meds before dinner so that they have time to kick in when it's time for me to leave. In about another week or so, I will start going every other day to see if that helps her adjust a little more. She is doing well most days, though.

Rough evening. Alzheimer's sucks.

Mom Chronicles August 3, 2019
Thanks, Jennifer Hood, for telling me about a store called Austin's!! She loves the dresses, and I can't beat $5.99 per dress!! This will help the staff change her easier now.

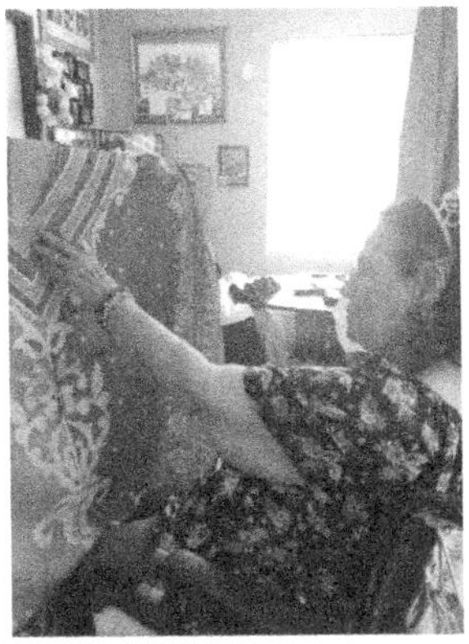
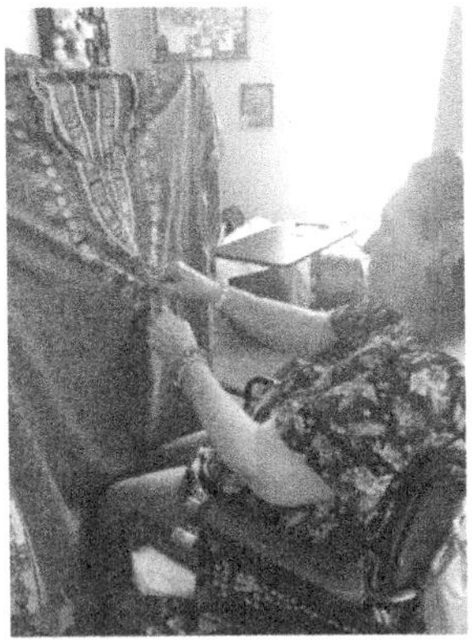
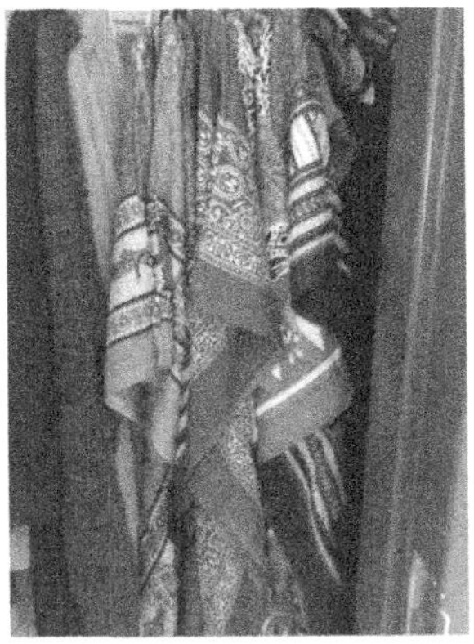

Mom Chronicles August 3, 2019
What a difference 24 hours makes! Mom was in a great mood today. She didn't seem to be hurting, and she enjoyed getting the new dresses. We also brought Simi to visit her, and not only did Mom enjoy seeing Simi, but so did all the other residents. We were able to leave after dinner with no drama, crying, or pouting. Alzheimer's was not so sucky today.

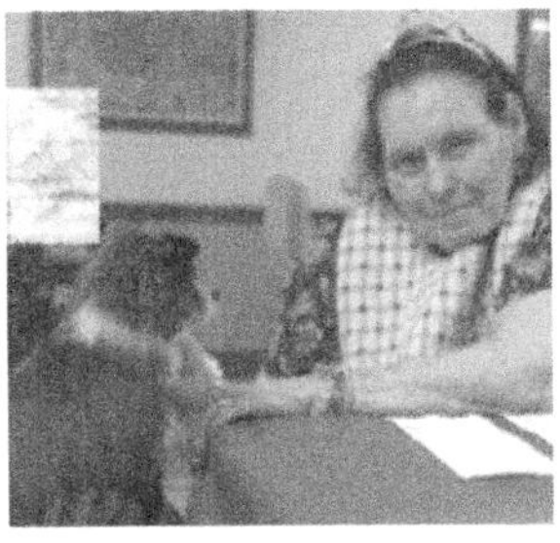

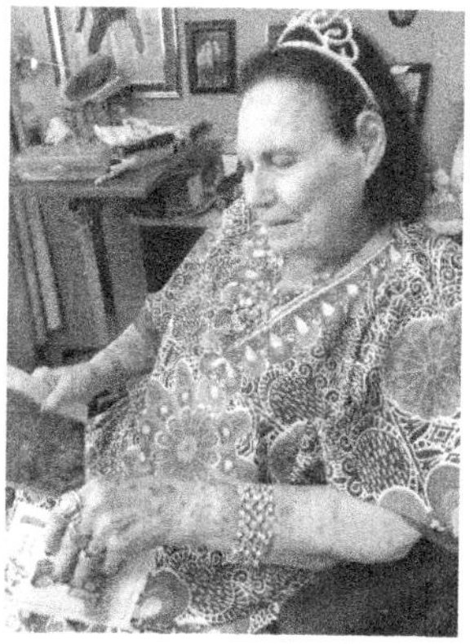

Mom Chronicles August 5, 2019

When I arrived, Mom was sitting near the nurse's station. I'm not sure why she was sitting down there, but she was happy to see me. I wheeled Mom to her room, then showed her some greeting cards from the memory care center. Shauna Sweetser had given them to me Friday when I went back to pick up some of Mom's things that had been found. Mom LOVED all the cards!! Thank you, Shauna, for having them made for her. It made her day! Mom was also in one of the dresses. She seemed to like it. She had a good appetite too. When I left, I took her to the TV room and nabbed the remote control (there was only one person there who wasn't watching the TV). I turned it off the SyFy channel, which freaks Mom out, and found a black and white old movie playing. She was mesmerized by it. With that holding her attention, I was able to leave without any tears or drama. Good visit!!

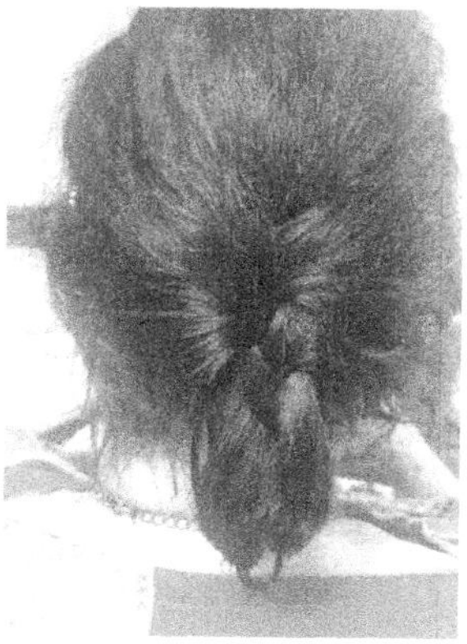

Mom Chronicles August 6, 2019

When I arrived today, she was sitting in the main hallway near the administrator's office. I noticed someone had taken the time to braid her hair in the back, which I thought was extremely sweet.

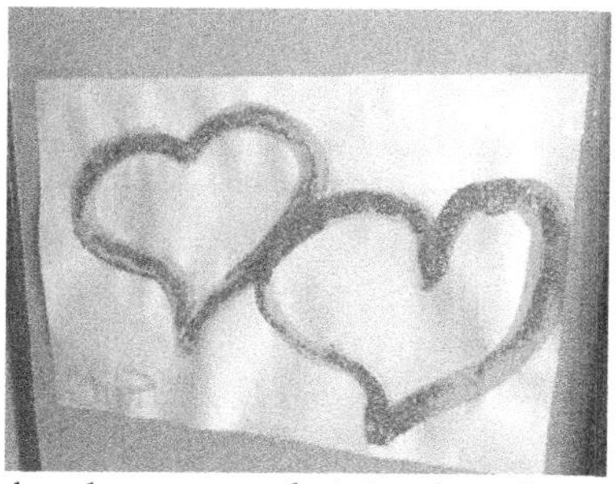

She was also right across the hall from the activity director's office. Miss T saw me with her and brought me a picture that they made together today of 2 hearts with glitter. That made me happy that she took the time to work with Mom on the picture.

I changed out her nail color, and we listened to music. She seemed a little more subdued and did seem to be hurting again. I'm not sure if they have started giving her the anxiety meds earlier as I asked or if it was just the pain. She wasn't excited as usual about her nails or a new ring that I gave her. She also only ate half of her meal.

After dinner, I wheeled her to her room. They had the news on in the main TV room, and it was freaking her out because it was more coverage of the shootings. So, we put the Hallmark channel on in her room. Much better. Love is always a better story!!

I was able to leave without any tears. I'm going to skip a day to try and help her adjust a little more. I did fib, though, and told her I would see her tomorrow. She won't remember, and it gives her hope, so I don't feel bad about that.

Mom Chronicles August 10, 2019

Thursday was a stressful visit. She was asleep when I got there, and while I watched her sleep, her body was jerking like crazy. It wasn't a restful nap at all. I learned from the daughter of Mom's roommate that they had tried to change her, but she refused, so they left. After hearing this, I shared with the DON the things to say to her that usually work. Some of the aides know; others just haven't learned yet. She said she would try to keep getting the word out to each shift. I also learned that her skin is breaking down from one thing we tried to keep her dry. Luckily, the DON monitored this and realized it wasn't working, so we are back to the original method of keeping her dry. I also had to get someone to help me get her up for dinner. I expressed my concern that if I wasn't there, would they have taken her to dinner, or if they brought her

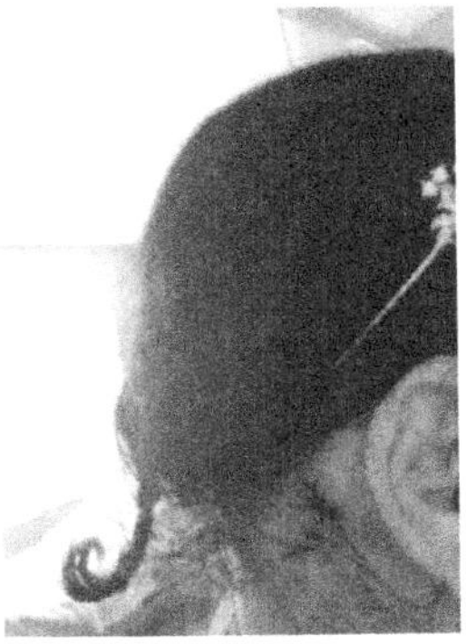

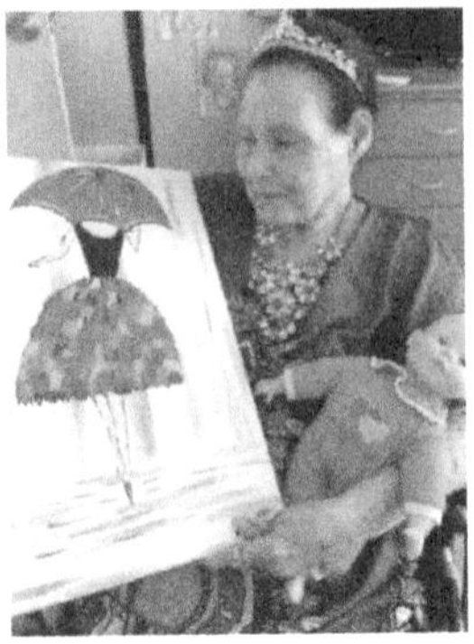

dinner to her, would they cue her. She needs help with using a fork or spoon to eat now. They assured me someone would help her on nights I'm not there. I'm just going to need to go in faith that they will (or get a camera for her room to ensure they will).

Yesterday, she was awake and up when I arrived. Someone had braided her hair again, and she was in a good mood. We put together a puzzle and played dominoes. I also gave her the painting I did Thursday night. She loved it. Sheila is here this weekend, so she will be the one visiting her and making sure she is okay.

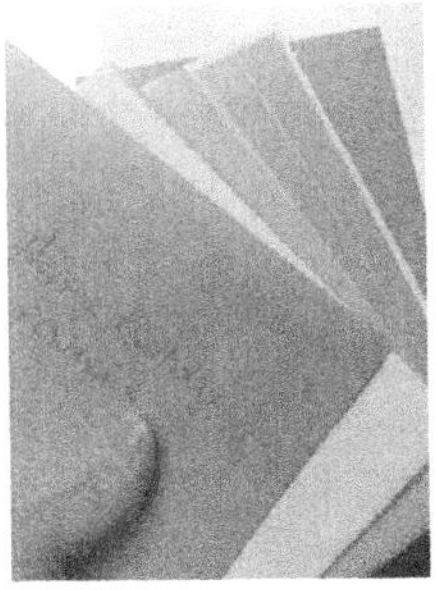

Mom Chronicles August 12, 2019
Mom's birthday next week is going to be great! Thank you to my amazing Region 10 friends who have contributed to "Operation Happy Birthday Mom"!! I have a ton of cards to surprise her with next week.

Mom Chronicles August 12, 2019
This is a long post tonight. Tonight, I am physically, mentally, and emotionally tired. When I arrived at the center, I couldn't find Mom. It turns out she was down in the physical therapy room. The therapist can get her to do all kinds of arms and hands exercises, but he can't get her to do any leg exercises. This is because her legs are so "frozen" - more on this in a moment.

I saw the DON, and she said she's keeping an eye on Mom's sores. She wanted to come down when they changed her before dinner. They finally got there, so she was called down and was able to see the skin breakdown on one side. She is trying a silicone bandage to see if Mom's skin can handle it. My sister, Mom, nor I can handle any adhesive on our skin. Well, the DON left, and the aide continued to change her. We noticed the other side is even worse than the side the DON just bandaged. So, I went right back down to her office to get her to come back and see them. She bandaged two more places and told the aides that Mom is to be checked every hour to an hour and a half and to keep her out of the wheelchair for a few days to relieve some of the pressure on these spots.

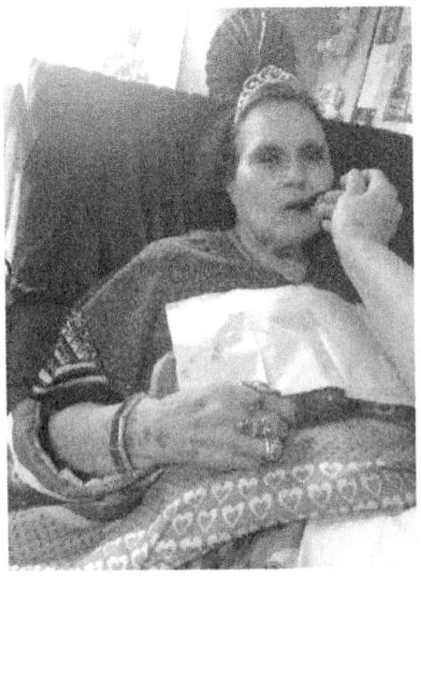

Without going too much into the TMI (too much information) zone, she wanted to keep Mom free from clothing in those areas. Well, as you all know now, anything out of the ordinary freaks Mom out. So, for the next hour, while we waited for dinner to arrive in her room, we looked through the photo albums, looked at the pictures on the wall, and watched Hallmark. Those things helped to stop her from crying.

The food finally arrived. We tried to sit her up on the side of the bed, but she couldn't support herself. [Remember one of the Stage 7 signs: they can't sit up on their own anymore.] She has relied on the wheelchair back for over a year and a half. So, we had to bring the bed up to a sitting position, which again was out of the ordinary and freaking her out. She also couldn't straighten her legs. They are permanently at a 90-degree angle. Because of this, the tray couldn't fit over her lap, so I had to feed her completely tonight. Every bite. I don't know why this affected me tonight, but I had to stop the tears from spilling out while feeding her. When I got in the car to leave later, the emotions just spilled over, and I had a good crying spell before leaving the parking lot. And when I met Bruce halfway on the way home before he went into work, they spilled over more. So much so that he said he was going to get his team started and then come home. I have a great guy. I tried to tell him I was fine, but he knows me. I was struggling tonight.

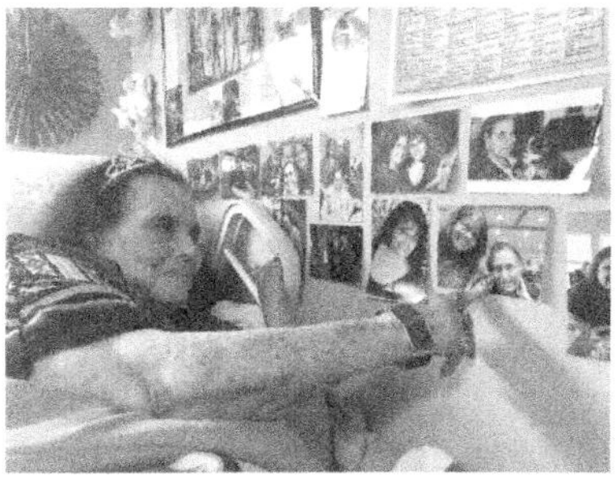

I know it was just a combination of:

- feeling sorry for her because of all the pain she's in,
- completely feeding her like she was a child,
- being "hangry" myself since I usually leave her place much earlier to get home at a decent time, and
- just being tired, period.

I'll be better tomorrow. Now I just need to decide if I'm going to stick with the plan of going every other day OR to go every day until they get her sores cleared up. I feel like I need to go every evening to make sure they follow through with the DON's orders. Have I mentioned lately that Alzheimer's sucks?

Mom Chronicles August 14, 2019

I am officially the founding member of the "Yes, I cry when I'm mad too" Club. And then I get MAD at the fact that I'm a member of the "Yes, I cry when I'm mad too" club. Ugh!!

When I arrived at the center, I asked the DON how Mom's skin was doing with the sores and the silicone bandages they were trying. She said her skin is looking better and that the silicone bandages aren't tearing her skin like regular bandages. She said the bandages wouldn't stay on, but they keep applying them to give her some protection. I was excited to hear the skin was getting better. I understand completely that she is reporting to me what the aides/nurses say to her and just physically hasn't had the opportunity to go down to Mom's room and see for herself. She needs to trust her nurses and aides to report things truthfully to her.

Well, something inside me whispered to stay until they changed Mom again so that I could see for myself. So I asked if they would change her right after dinner (6:00). Finally, around 7:30, the aides came down. I know they are busy, but I was right there when the DON asked them to change her now (because we both could smell a heavy aroma), and the aide said she would be right down after assisting two others.

Now here is where my "I cry when I'm mad too" club was formed. Mom's skin is way worse than Monday night. It's not a detrimental stage, according to my paramedic hubby, whose opinion I value deeply. But he and I both know how sensitive her skin is, and if they don't get a handle on this ASAP, it will get to that detrimental stage. So I talked to the nurse assigned to Mom's hall and expressed how upset I am that there are MORE sores and that the ones from Monday are worse. He said he would go down there and apply more silicone bandages.

I will come up here in the morning and ask to speak to both the administrator and the DON, show the pics I took of her skin from Monday and this evening, and tell her that these sores are worse, not better. I am also getting the camera paperwork set up and telling them that I will be monitoring now to ensure she is getting changed as much as she needs to be changed. Mama Bear is going to bat for her 77yr old cub. Now, who wants to join the "I cry when I'm mad too" Club? Membership forms are being created now!!

Mom Chronicles August 15, 2019

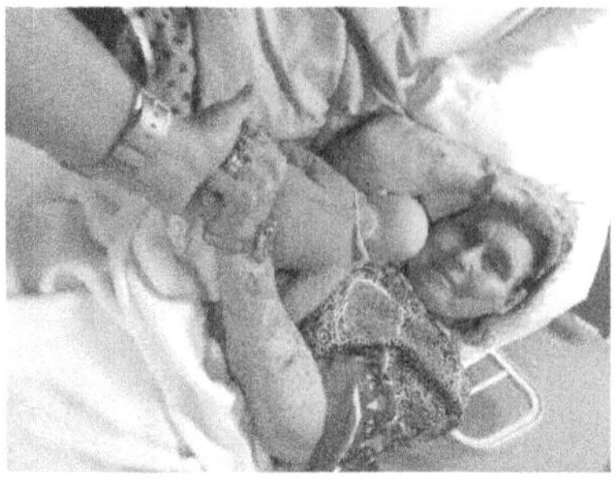

The staff was all in a meeting when I arrived about 30 minutes ago. The DON's assistant came out of the meeting, and I spoke to him about my concerns. I brought a list with all kinds of things that may help Mom - like phrases to use, straightening her up in the wheelchair, etc. So instead of being a helicopter parent, I am a helicopter daughter!

He mentioned they would order a heavy paste to put on her sores that will act as a barrier and a "bandage." It should be in today. They have her in bed, and right after our chat, he came down to turn her, so she's off her left side. It sounds like they will be keeping her in bed for a while and shifting her often.

I brought up Hospice for the second set of eyes and better pain control, so he said he would share this with the DON to have her address it with the doctor tomorrow. I printed off a list of Alzheimer's hospice "qualifications" and shared that she meets most everything on there. The primary doctor is supposed to be in tomorrow, so I will see if I can be here at the center when he's here.

She's resting now, so I'll head back to the office in a few minutes. I'm just waiting for the business office lady to get out of the meeting, too, so that I can get the camera permission slip. I need to get that installed ASAP.

Mom Chronicles August 16, 2019

Do you know the "terrible 2's"??? There is also a "terrible 77's". Oy!!! Lord grant me patience and seal my mouth shut!!!!!! I'm about to ground her!!!!

Mom Chronicles August 18, 2019

She loves her baby doll.

Mom Chronicles August 18, 2019

The fun thing about a captive audience is that I can pick on her. I do silly things to make her smile and laugh. And yes, I desperately need a pedicure. Don't diss the toes! 😉

Mom Chronicles August 19, 2019

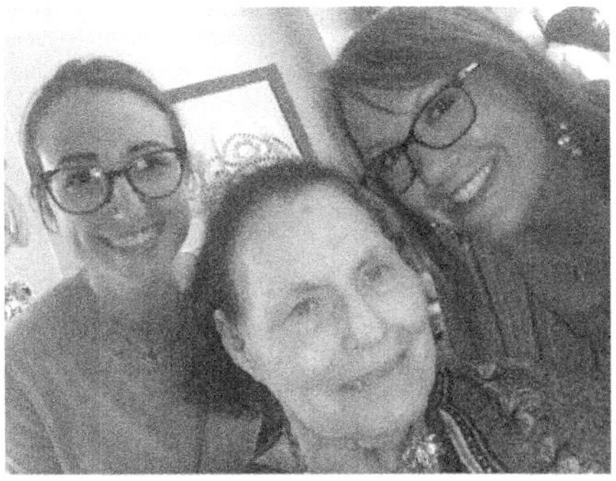

There are some negatives and some positives today. I'll get the icky stuff out of the way first so that I can end on a good note.

I took a personal day off to get the camera set up in her room. While there, the morning aide changed her at 11:30 - before lunch. He was very careful with her, and she only whimpered a little bit. I made sure he knew how much I appreciated him by thanking him several times. I stayed with her through lunch and then took her back to her room. We turned on the Hallmark channel. I left around 1:30.

Before I left, the aide who had changed her at 11:30 said the 2-10 shift aide should be by after 2 to recheck her.

Well, according to the camera, one stopped by to say hi to Mom about 3:30, but she was not changed until almost 5:00 - before dinner. Not acceptable! She went 5 1/2 hours without being changed. I will be having a chat with the DON tomorrow to let her know that the afternoon aides didn't follow her instructions.

Now for the positive. Leanne Holden and Madison Bowes from the memory care center stopped by at dinner time. They shared this picture with me and permitted me to share them. Mom was soooo happy to see them. It is such a blessing to have people who care about my Mom take time out of their day to visit her. Thank you both so much!

Mom Chronicles August 20, 2019
Today is my Mom's 78th birthday. I didn't think I would have her this long. I will be taking a cake, a few presents, and half of the cards we received (the other half will go with Sheila when she comes up this weekend so that she can celebrate with Mom too.)

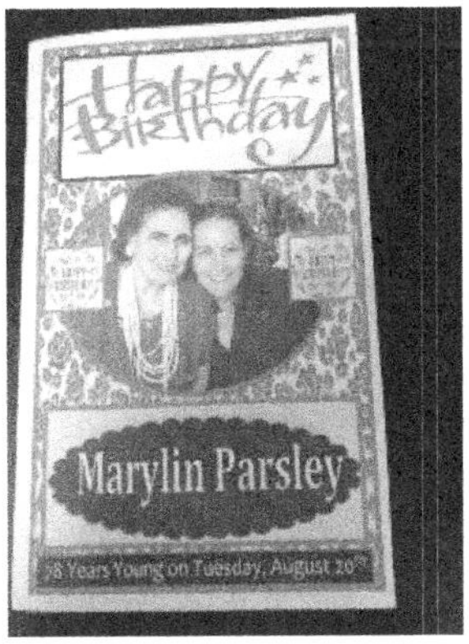

I came in to work this morning and found this beautiful homemade, multi-page card from my co-workers. This right here (along with ALL the other cards we received) means the world to me. I'm so grateful that you all would take a few moments out of your day to create something that will make a lady who most of you have never met smile. Thank you, thank you, thank you!

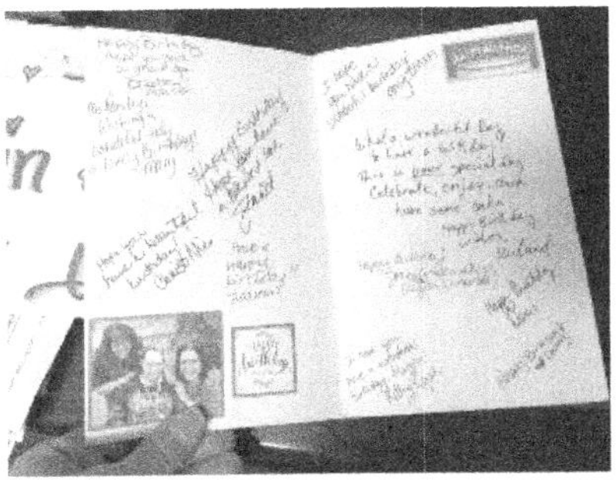
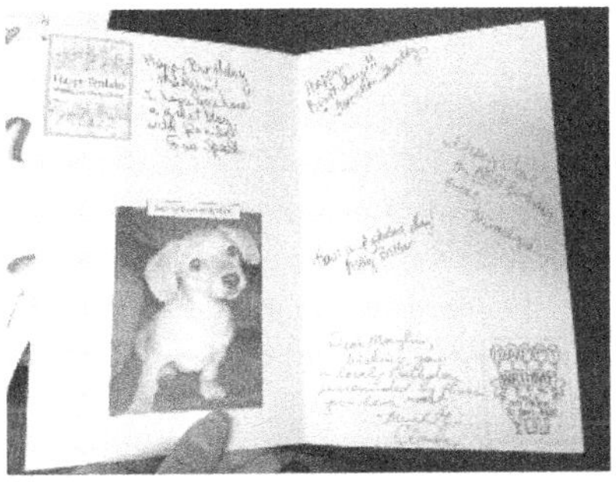
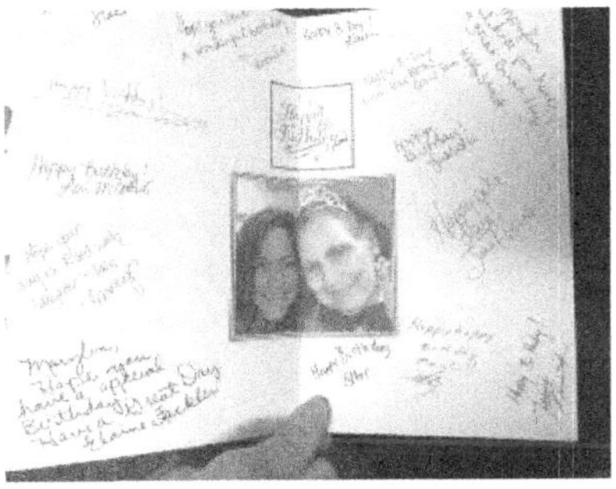
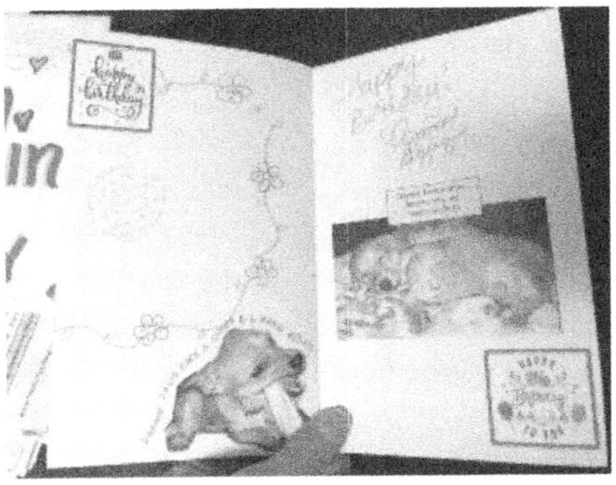
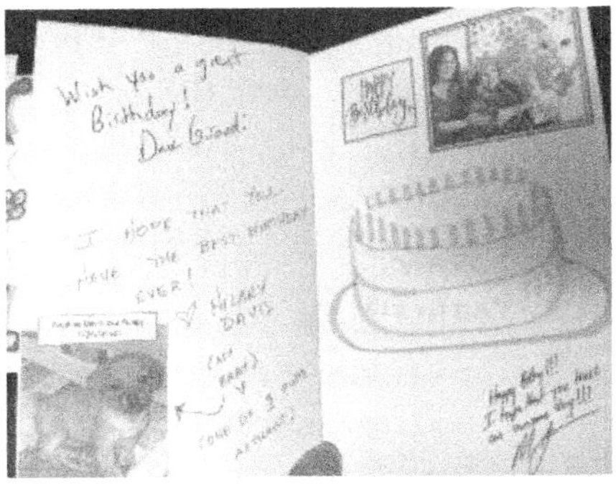
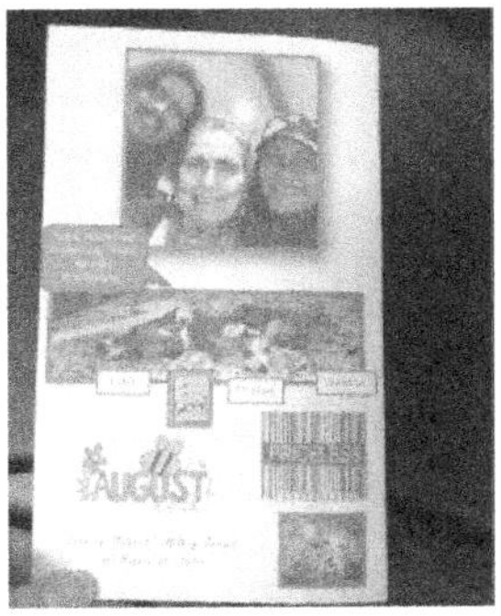

Mom Chronicles August 20, 2019

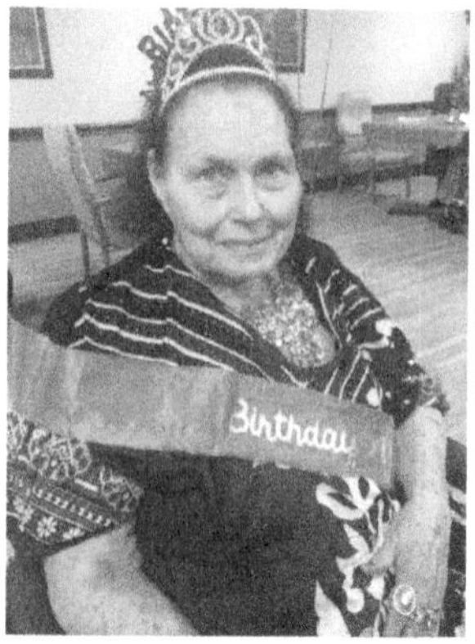

Happy 78th birthday to my Mom!

First - here is a real quick update. I had a chat with the DON about what I saw yesterday/last night through the camera. She agreed that 5 hours is too long between checks/changes. She was very nice and glad that I had the proof that some of her staff were not doing all they should be doing. She was also glad to see the 3rd shift CNA doing her job correctly and checking on Mom every 2 hours. She wasn't negative at all about us having the camera. So I think all is going to be well.

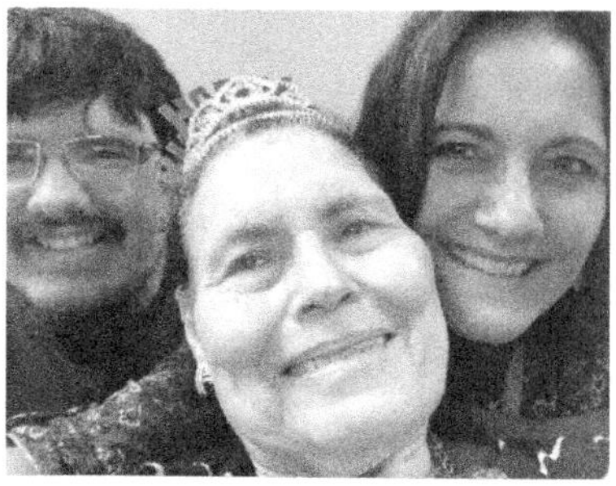

Now for the fun part - Mom's birthday!

She enjoyed all the cards, the gifts, the cake, and the decorations. Thank you all for making it special! I brought half the cards today. The other half will go with my sister this weekend when she celebrates with her. You all mean the world to my family for helping us celebrate with her!

♥

As hindsight is 20/20, we now know that August 20, 2019, was the last birthday she celebrated on earth. I'm so glad we were with her and that she seemed to enjoy the "party." We are truly grateful to all our friends who sent cards. I know not everyone was mentioned, but you all are blessings in our lives!

Mom Chronicles August 22, 2019

There were several things tonight that I wanted to share:

1) the baby was temporarily replaced by a puppy. I'm not sure how long that will last, but she kept petting him and brushing the hair out of his eyes.

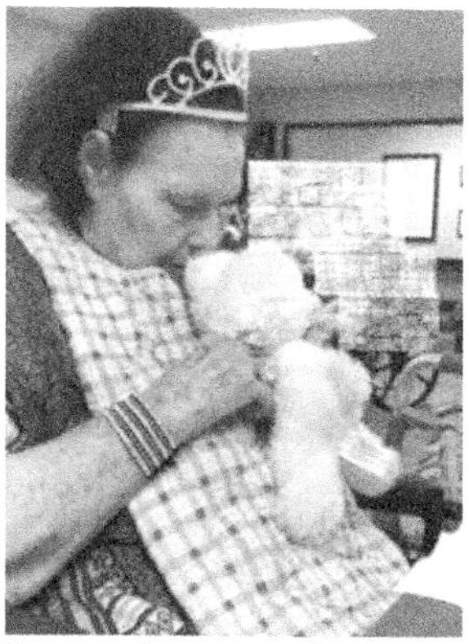

2) several of her nail polish strips needed replacing, so she picked the same color. While I was taking the polish off, she was glowering at me and was confused. I promised her they would look beautiful when I finished. Sure enough, she was fine once she saw the color back on her nails. But she was MAD while I took the old polish off!

3) while waiting for dinner, I had her open more birthday cards. She loved them all.

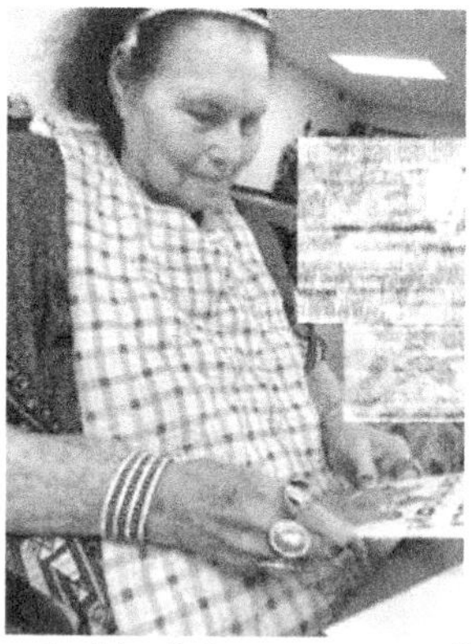

4) after our visit, I checked in through the camera several times, and I noticed she was trying to put herself into bed. Well, that would have been a disaster because she is not strong enough. She would have fallen. We couldn't get hold of the center, so I texted the DON. She had a special number for the center and was able to get hold of someone immediately. Whew! Crisis averted! We need to keep her in the TV room in the evenings instead of letting her watch TV in her room. That way, she can't try to do that again and will be safe until it's her time to go to bed.

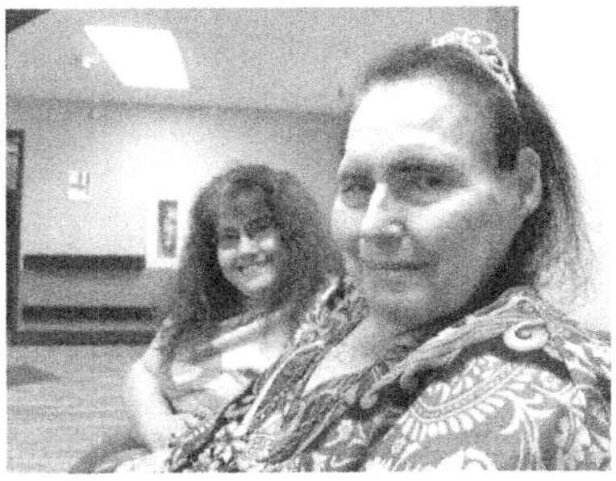

Mom Chronicles August 25, 2019

Sheila, Simi, and I spent a few minutes with Mom this evening before Sheila left Dallas to return home. Mom was in a good mood tonight.

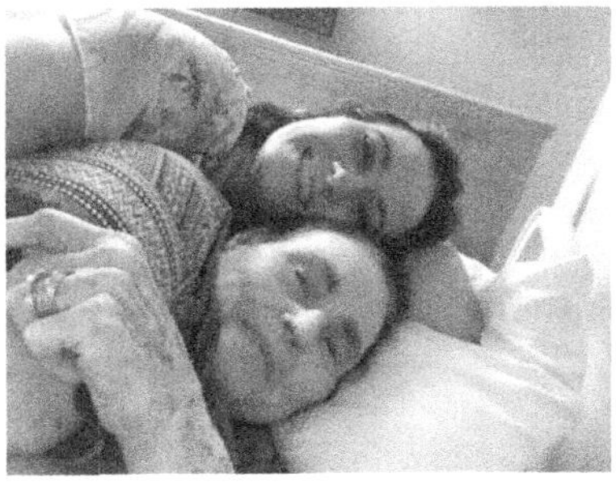

Mom Chronicles August 26, 2019

Concordia Lutheran's Children's Church Birthday Cards and Mom and Daughter Snuggles... just what the soul needs sometimes. Thank you, Gloria and John, for having the kiddos in Children's Church make cards for her. She LOVES them!

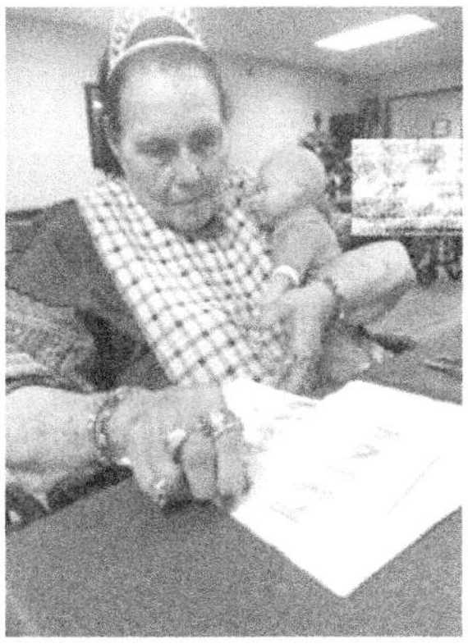

Mom Chronicles August 29, 2019

One financial strain is off our plate. Mom was officially approved for Medicaid, so our caregiving cost just went down significantly. We only have a small portion of the nursing home care cost we are responsible for each month. Hallelujah!!

The staff members are still caring for her very well. When I see an issue through the camera, I let the DON know, and she takes care of it immediately.

All is well with my Mom. Oh, a birthday card came in from my dear friend Lea who lives in California. Thanks, Lea Cates! She loves it!!

Mom Chronicles September 3, 2019

When I arrived at the center, Mom was lying down. She was upset because the unicorn stuffed animal that Sheila gave her for her birthday was not "talking" to her when she pushed the tummy. So I changed it out with the doll and showed her the doll talks. She was better after that.

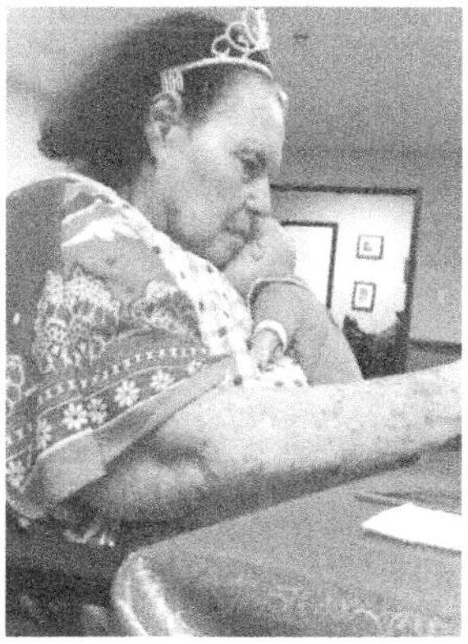

She was also upset that they had placed a pillow between her legs to try and relieve pressure. She acted like it was hurting - and it may have been because her legs are so "frozen" together. That's the best way I can explain it. She kept pointing to it and was about to start crying. I took the pillow out, and she was better after that too.

We got her up and took her to eat dinner. While waiting, she was hugging and kissing her doll on the forehead. I was able to grab a quick video of that before she stopped. The only phrase I could get out of her today was, "I love you." She said that over and over. That's not a bad phrase to get stuck on, so I'll take it.

Mom Chronicles September 5, 2019
The director of nurses just texted me to say that Mom gained 7.8 pounds this month. That's great news because that means she has a good appetite. They do feed them well there, too, from what I have witnessed. However, I will keep watching for water weight on her legs just to be safe. She struggled with that issue some at the other center.

Mom Chronicles September 7, 2019
Today we had a very special visit from Robin Nikula (Ted's daughter/my stepsister), her daughter Sarah Metcalf and Sarah's daughter Holly. When Mom lived in California with Ted, they had tons of photos of her grandkids. Holly was one of the great-grandkids I remember Mom talking about the most. I think most of the other great-grandkids were born after Mom and Ted moved away from California to live here in Texas. They brought her a beautiful card and necklace today. Robin also gave me a ton of necklaces and wall art that I can give to Mom at various times. Thank you, Robin, Sarah, and Holly. You brightened Mom's day today!

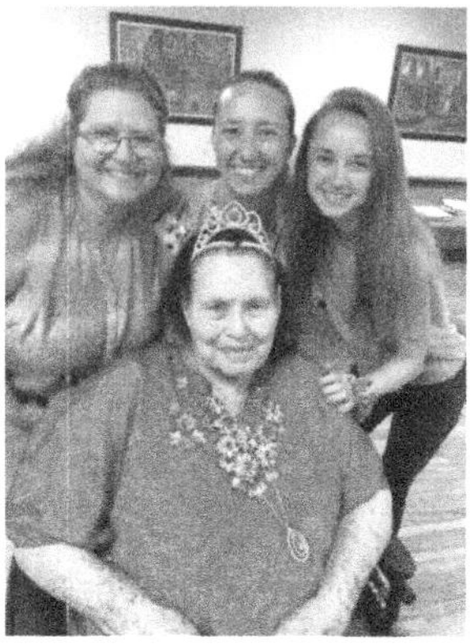

Mom Chronicles September 10, 2019
Mom had a mini-meltdown a little while ago. I checked in through the camera, and they brought her back to her room to lay her down. She was crying and crying. They just brought her lunch, and she has settled down some now and is eating. I'm not sure what she will be like when I get there tonight. It's times like these that I want to leave work and go to her, but I have too much to do. And I realize that I can't leave work over every little thing that upsets her. It's just hard.

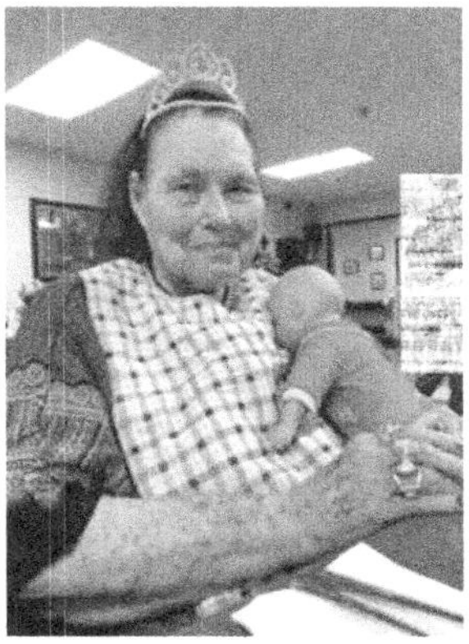

Mom Chronicles September 10, 2019
She is much better tonight. I learned from the DON that her meltdown was from her not wanting to do physical therapy. I asked her to talk to the doctor more about pain management. I just don't think it's under control yet. They had her resting all afternoon. When I arrived, I had to wait for them to freshen her up before going to the dining room. While waiting, we played with the balloon for a few minutes.

She's fine tonight. All is right in the world now.

Mom Chronicles September 11, 2019
I needed to come up here an extra day this week because the roommate's hubby accidentally unplugged the camera when he rearranged the table near Mom's bed.

I'm glad I came because Mom's face looks rubbed raw today. I know they showered her this morning, so I am afraid the aide scrubbed her face too hard. She has very sensitive skin. I had a bottle from my sensitive skin regimen in her drawer, so I applied it to her face. I'm hoping it will heal fast. She also decided she wanted to hold the other doll tonight. She is acting like she's never seen it before. It can be Christmas every day for her!! I also gave her several more birthday cards

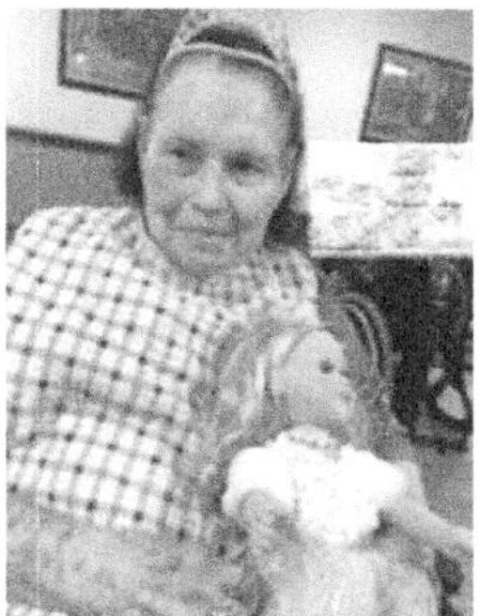

that came in over the past week or two. She enjoyed them all. Thank you, Sue Hill, Theresa Alexander, and Deborah Vick. Your cards were what we opened today.

Mom Chronicles September 11, 2019
Kindness goes a long way. I just looked in on Mom while they were getting her ready for bed. They talked to her and told her exactly what they would do each step of the way. She didn't fight them at all this time. She cooperated fully. And when one of the aides told her good night and that he would see her tomorrow, she put her fingers to her lips and "blew him a kiss" and said okay. It wasn't in a romantic way but in a "thank you for taking care of me way." I bet she sleeps well tonight since she didn't go to bed so agitated.

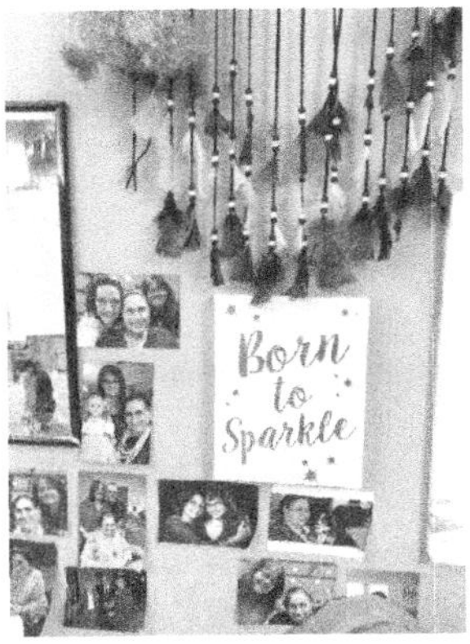

Mom Chronicles September 14, 2019
We stopped by to visit Mom after the RV show. She didn't like her dinner tonight, but I was able to get her to eat a little bit. I then fixed her fingernails. She is progressing so much in this disease that she doesn't understand why I'm taking off old polish to put on the new polish. When she keeps getting distressed with each nail I clean, I need to show her the new nail strips I'm going to put on her. After all ten nails were fixed, she was happy.

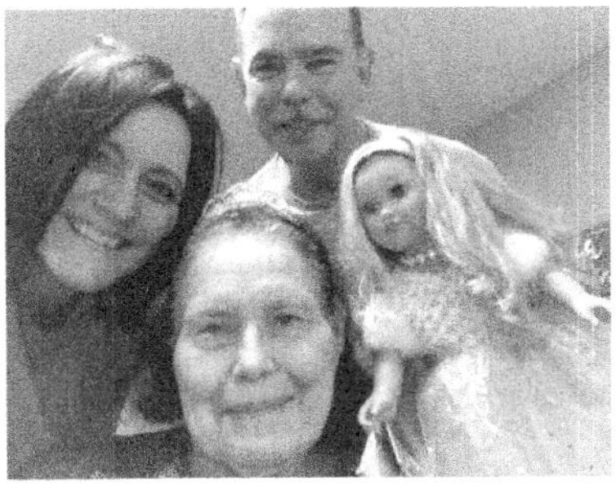

Bruce kept distracting her by making her doll dance to her playlist. That helped a ton! We were able to capture her "dancing" a little bit. We left her happy and content. Robin, here is a picture of one of the plaques you gave her. She was definitely "born to sparkle"! Thank you!

Mom Chronicles September 16, 2019
I had to do something today that I struggled to do because it might cost someone his job. One CNA (Certified Nursing Assistant) always talks a little rough with Mom - he's not very compassionate most of the time. When I'm checking up on Mom at the end of the day, I tend to focus on the recordings on the camera when he is on the screen. He worked an extra shift this past weekend and was very upset this morning. He will say phrases like "why do you have to act that way" to Mom. Ummmm... she has Alzheimer's. Yes, she's going to act that way. Well, he had already taken Mom to breakfast and came right back to straighten up her room. While there, he had a gripe-fest with the roommate's husband. He said some things that I'm not going to repeat here that caused both Bruce and me to be concerned that it could spill over into his care for Mom and the other residents. It wasn't about Mom but something in his life outside of work. I showed the video to the DON and the home's Director. After hearing it, they will show the video to someone higher in corporate headquarters to decide whether he gets reprimanded and trained or fired. I don't ever want to get anyone fired. However, I think this person could use some training to be a little more compassionate and learn the skills it takes to interact with an Alzheimer's patient. He also needs to reconsider practicing questionable activities outside of work that could potentially carry over to his job. Another positive thing that came out of the meeting is that they will do more in-service training with their staff on dealing with people who have Alzheimer's.

To end this on a positive note, I showed Mom 3 more cards from her birthday (I've been spreading them out.) One from Sue Hill, Sarah Metcalf, and a combined card from my co-workers (Beth Dolliver, Nikki Mickow, and Jala Hyde). Thanks, friends. She loved them!

Mom Chronicles September 18, 2019
I just watched a video from Teepa Snow called "**How Dementia Affects Language Skills**." It was eye-opening about dementia language skills. Are there folks who say bad words, mean words, racial slurs, inappropriate content in public places, and you just shrink because you are so embarrassed? Mom lost that "filter" a long time ago. Now I understand! What about conversation skills where they don't make sense? This video explains why!! It is worth the 30 minutes to watch! Go to YouTube and do a quick search for that video title.

Mom Chronicles September 21, 2019
Mom is in a good mood today. We haven't played "Mominoes" in a while. She wasn't dead set on playing the double five this time in every game. During one game, she decided to have all the dominoes face up. I need to play with her more often to keep the muscle memory going on playing the game.

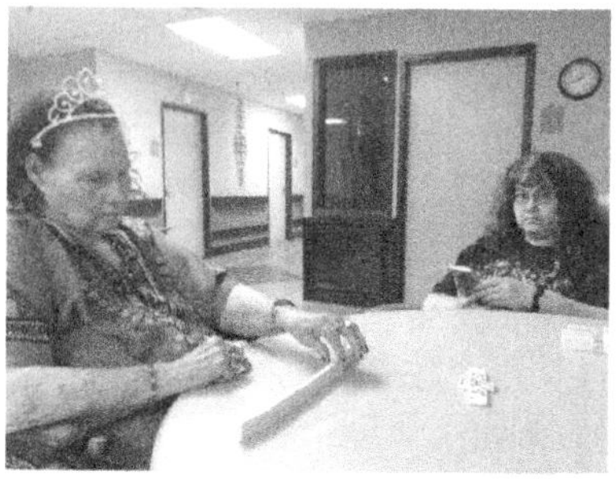

Mom Chronicles September 21, 2019
Here is one more fun video from today. Sheila and I do whatever we can to make her laugh.

Mom Chronicles September 22, 2019
Sheila found this unicorn with a recording device in it that Mom can press to hear our voices repeatedly. Pretty cool! We hope it helps her!

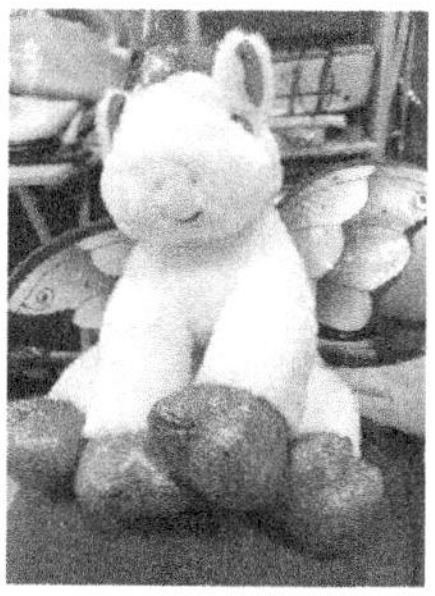

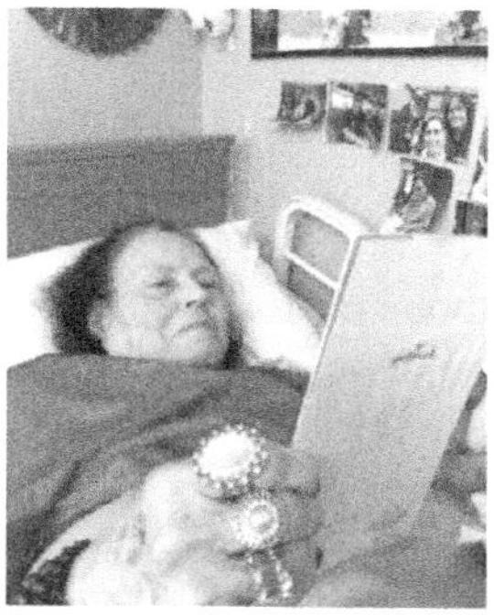

Mom Chronicles September 23, 2019
She is doing well today.

Laura Hodges, your cards came in, so I gave her one today. Thank you!!

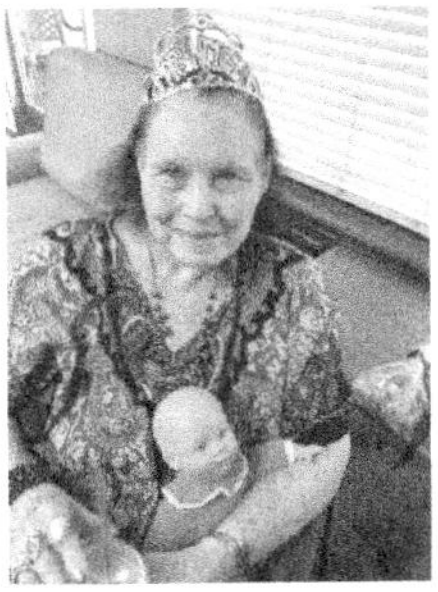

Mom Chronicles September 28, 2019

Strawberry shake. Check.

New princess crown. Check.

All smiles. Check!

Mom Chronicles October 2, 2019

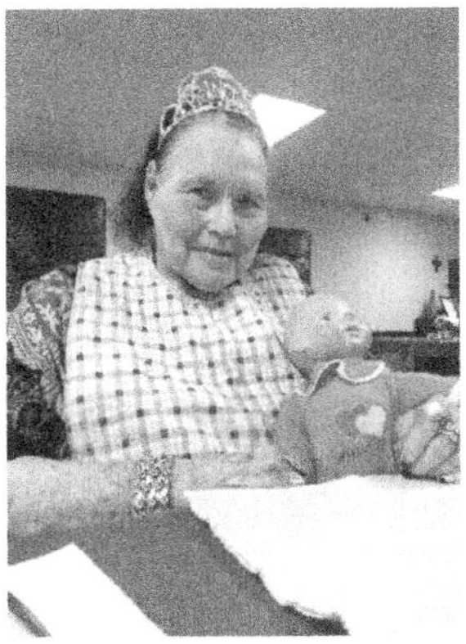

At dinner tonight, she snapped at me for a moment when she got frustrated with me trying to figure out what was wrong. She was frowning at dinner. She wasn't happy with the meal today. I asked simple questions like "are you full," "do you want a sandwich instead," etc., but it was too much. Finally, she snapped, "wait a minute." I could tell she was trying to process what was wrong, but she just wasn't able to tell me yet.

It turns out she had some ham stuck in her teeth. It was bothering her to the point that she didn't want to take another bite until she could clear that piece of meat. Well, what does the trusty daughter who always has at least three containers of dental floss in her purse do???? Right there in front of God, the CNAs, nurses, and other patients, I flossed her teeth in the cafeteria!!!

That was not the most pleasant experience because I was afraid she was going to bite me. But finally, I solved the problem, and she was able to continue eating. I wonder if I should switch careers to a dental hygienist.

The sad thing is that her teeth are in terrible shape. They don't get cleaned anymore (she couldn't handle it when I tried to have the traveling dentist clean her teeth last year at the other center - and the CNAs don't help her brush her teeth. I'm choosing my battles - the most important thing to me is to make sure she is changed regularly. The teeth will just have to go bad. I know I'm running the risk of bacteria getting in her bloodstream and causing infections. It's a catch-22.

Mom Chronicles October 4, 2019

During an important meeting this morning at work, I saw the nursing home calling me. My heart always skips a beat when I see them calling. I just don't want to hear bad news. I stepped out to take the call. This time, they just needed a little help with redirection. Mom wasn't cooperating with them. They put me on speakerphone, and I told her who I was and asked her to let the nurses help her. She said, ok. I had to repeat it a few times because she would come back and say she didn't know what to do.

When I was telling her bye and that I would see her later today, I said, "I love you." We do say this a lot in our family, and it's always comforting to hear it said back. Mom always does, but the words are usually slurred now. This time, she just said, "ok," I said it one more time just in case she didn't hear me. She said, "ok." I must admit that I had to stop the tears from spilling. I know that probably sounds dumb, but I love hearing her tell me she loves me. I know at some point those words will stop completely, but I'm not looking forward to it. I shared the story with my friend Beth at work, and she suggested I record her next time to get the words down permanently. Hopefully, she will say them this afternoon when I visit her.

Have I mentioned lately that Alzheimer's sucks? Well, it does!! Tears dried now. Back to work…

Mom Chronicles October 4, 2019

I recorded it (I love you) in 2 different ways!! This video captures one of the ways and is of both of us singing, "I love you a bushel and a peck and a hug around the neck."

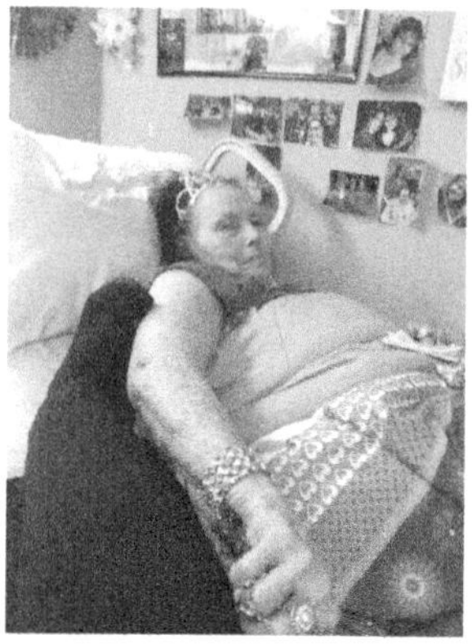

Mom Chronicles October 5, 2019

Momma Bear had to come out of hibernation last night. While I was visiting Mom, I was able to be there while they changed her. Well... I saw that she is very raw and blistered. I took photos and sent this to the DON and said I am NOT happy and very concerned. She replied, "Oh my!"

They haven't been able to get the cream she needs, so I had bought a diaper rash cream last week. She wondered if it could be the cream. I said no because she used it at the other center and then again during the first month she was here. She said the cream Mom needs is zinc oxide, so I went to the drug store next door to buy a regular strength and a maximum strength version.

No excuse. The nurses should be able to get the cream that she needs, and the CNAs should have reported her skin condition.

The DON (who has been great, by the way) has assured me this will be taken care of immediately. She wants Mom checked every 2 hours and that I can call her if I see it going past 2 hours through the camera.

I also had to report the aide last night because she had the mandate of checking Mom every 2 hours as well. She changed her at 10:45 pm and then peeped around the corner of the curtain at 2:30. She didn't walk in and physically check her. She didn't get changed again until 5:30. That's seven freaking hours of not being changed with broken-down skin. So yeah... Momma Bear is not happy.

I was so mad driving home yesterday I missed my turnoff. I don't want to move her because that's too traumatic for her. I still feel like we can get the problem resolved. I'm thankful for the camera!!

Mom Chronicles October 9, 2019

Today has been a little more eventful in this wonderful Alzheimer's journey.

I had just finished a training workshop for consultants this afternoon when I got a call from the nursing home. I was still in the training room, and luckily there were only a few people left. They needed me to talk to Mom to calm her down and convince her to let them give her a bed bath. I'm grateful for co-workers who understand what my family is going through because there was no way I could keep that conversation private. I was able to calm her down after a few minutes on the phone.

However, when I got to the center about an hour later, I learned that Mom has a new trick up her sleeves. She tried to bite them!! Luckily, they dodged it, and no skin was broken. I try to find humor in this journey as much as possible, so I asked if the state allows muzzles on patients. I said I could bedazzle it for her! They laughed and assured me they understand Mom's condition and they will just watch out for future potential bites.

At dinner, there is one table in the dining room with three women who are "challenging" because they constantly ask for things or a different meal. It's a constant, everyday deal with them. Well, today, two of them got into a tiff. They were shouting words that should not be repeated here. Mom was oblivious to it, but I was able to get dinner and an entertainment show (even though I wasn't eating)!!

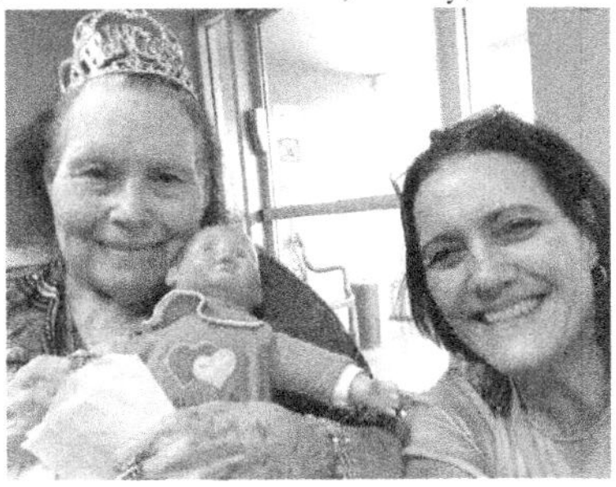

After dinner, I wheeled Mom to the TV room. We took a selfie, and she realized her baby doll was not facing outwards, so we had to retake the pic with the baby facing the camera. We had to make sure my baby sister was smiling for the camera too!!

Mom Chronicles October 10, 2019
A friend asked me a question about why Mom has learned to bite now. My gut feeling was that it was a defense mechanism, but I wanted to ask Jenni what she thought. As you may remember, Jenni Knutson is my friend and former director of the other center where Mom lived. She has a wealth of knowledge on Alzheimer's and dementia. Here is her response, and it makes perfect sense!!

"Yes, this is a very common defense mechanism when scared or agitated by Alzheimer's and dementia residents. Especially in the later stages. We all know how to bite, but we don't because we've been taught it's wrong. As Alzheimer's progresses, we lose our inhibitions or the ability to recall right from wrong. That's why often, women who were Sunday school teachers will begin swearing like sailors out of nowhere. Others will walk out of their room into the hallway of a community stark naked. They don't know they should be embarrassed or ashamed due to the lack of inhibition.

They try biting, hitting, scratching, punching, hair pulling, grabbing jewelry out of ears, or pulling necklaces until they break, but not everyone with the disease will do this. Caregivers often learn techniques to still get the shower done and not get hurt.

One technique is to sing a song as you're getting ready for the shower, such as "Old McDonald had a farm, E-I-E-I-? By stopping at the last letter, the resident will be focused on "what is that letter" and when they're focused on that, they are not thinking about a need to hit [or bite].

Not one thing works on all with this disease. Every person will need something different to feel safe or distracted."

Thank you, Jenni! By the way, Jenni is now the new director of a different memory care center opening in roughly six months or so. It will be a 3-point facility with retirement apartments for folks 55 years and older, assisted living, and a memory care center. I'm so happy for her!

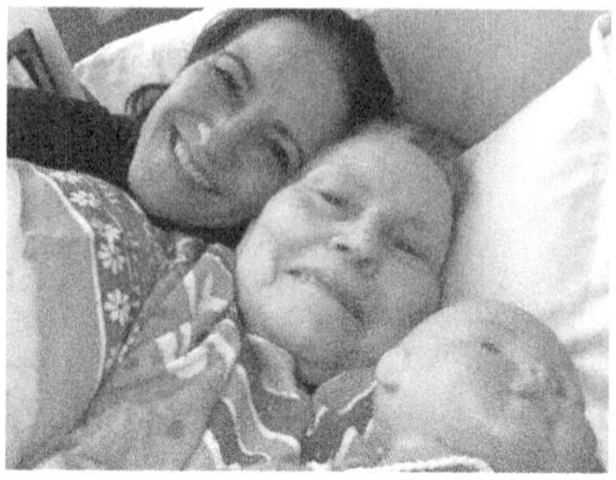

Mom Chronicles October 11, 2019
Mom was lying down when I got there, so I curled up next to her until the aides came to get her ready for dinner. Before that, I talked to the DON about a possible medication called Depakote Sprinkles that goes into food three times a day. Jenni learned about this medication from a friend who is an Alzheimer's Forensic Nurse. This medication might help with biting and hitting. She is going to talk to the doctor on Monday. The medication we are asking for should not leave her catatonic. Fingers crossed!

♥

As a reminder, these are ideas our family learned about and tried. None of what we share in this book should be considered medical or legal advice. We always recommend talking to doctors/professionals as there may be advances in medications and techniques to help in these situations.

Mom Chronicles October 13, 2019
Well... I had to eat a little crow today. Through the camera, I noticed that they still had not come to get Mom for dinner at 5:30 (they usually get her between 4:45 and 5:00). So I texted the DON to let her know. They finally got her at 6:00. I told the DON that it looks like they forgot her.

She said no, they didn't forget. They just had a patient actively dying on hospice, and they were trying to assist in that situation. Dinner ran late today. I apologized to her for my wrong assumption. I feel bad!! I will be a little more careful with what I think is going on when it looks like Mom is not being cared for properly.

Mom Chronicles October 14, 2019
Mom was in a great mood today. I gave her a new necklace that Sheila bought, and she had to put it on immediately. She loved it!

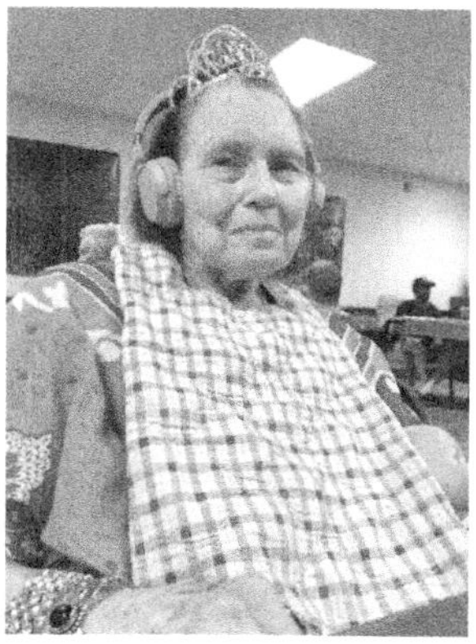

I also tested headphones with her today with her playlist to see how she handled having headphones on. The DON is curious to see if music therapy would help when she's combative. She be-bopped to the music, so the test went well. She would look sad when a song finished and then be startled when the next song came on. Since I could see the songs on the playlist, I chose her favorite Elvis songs. She just danced and danced with her head, shoulders, and arms!! My next step is figuring out what kind of device I can get that is not expensive and is easy to operate and charge for the aides. I don't want anything expensive since it might "walk away." Last but not least, a card came in from our friend Nena Sledge. She loved the card, Nena!! Thank you!

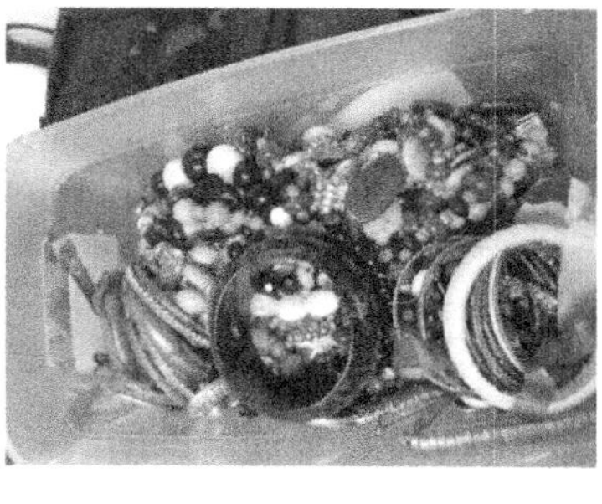

Mom Chronicles October 16, 2019
Connie Swiderski, you are amazing!!! Thank you, thank you, thank you! This jewelry will bring a huge smile to my Mom's face!!

Mom Chronicles October 16, 2019

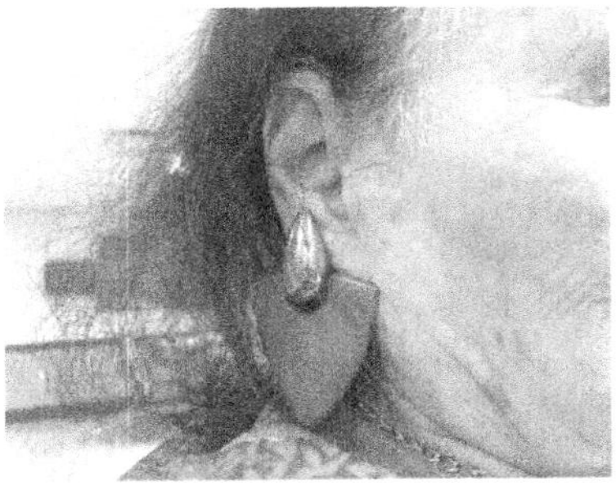

Mom was a little more tired than usual, but I changed out her nails today with a set from the new order of nail strips. She still doesn't like it when I'm removing the color first but is happy once she sees the new color. Her mind just can't comprehend the process anymore.

I also gave her the blue earrings that Connie sent in her box of jewelry. They matched her dress, and she loved them.

At dinner, I had to cue her a lot today. She needed guidance on how to eat today. She wanted to drink her cranberry juice like soup again. It's been months since I've seen her do this. So I'm just going to chalk it up to her seeming tired today.

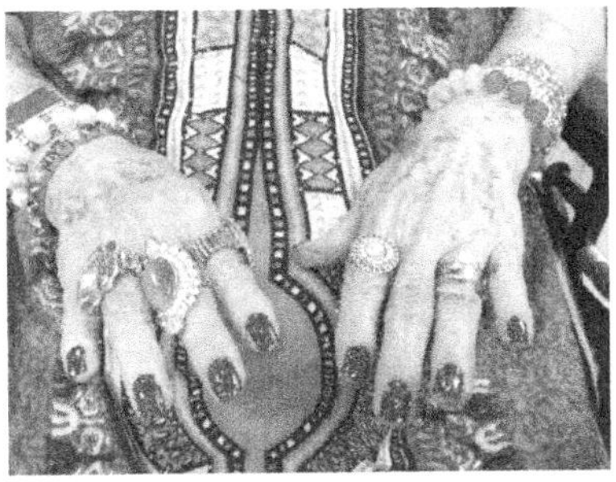

The head CNA stopped by and asked me if Mom likes having her bed against the wall. I said I don't know. I just know that she wants to see and touch all the photos on the wall. Apparently, the state looks at this as another form of restraint. I'm not sure I understand that, but I told them to do what they need to do to keep from getting in trouble with the state. Mom can't sit up on her own anymore, so I don't fear her falling out of bed. We will see what happens.

Mom Chronicles October 19, 2019

Several things today...

I added more photos to her wall. She didn't recognize many of them. At one point, she didn't even recognize Sheila and me in a photo even though I'm sitting right next to her. But then 10 minutes later she said she knew who I was. She mainly focuses on pictures of her. It makes me realize how appropriate the phrase she stated a few years ago is... "I remember me."

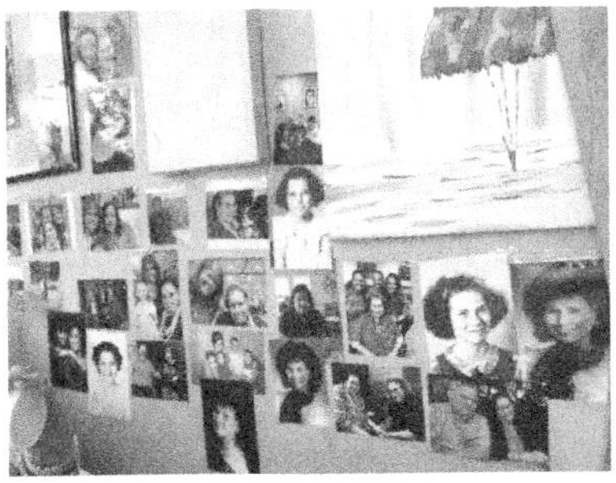

I also brought the new CD player, Elvis CD, and headphones. I wanted to do another test to see how she would react. She loves it! She's trying to sing. She can get the tune, but the words are very slurred, as you will hear. I heard "hound dog" at one point, and she does better with songs when there is a chorus repeated over and over.

Mom Chronicles October 21, 2019

I checked the camera last night in Mom's room during the tornado scare, and it was good to see that they took it seriously. The CNA spoke to me through the camera and said there was a tornado coming and that they had to get her up fast and get her into the hallway. She just didn't want me upset that they weren't "easing" her out of bed. I'm totally fine with that. I know Mom didn't understand a thing happening, but I'm glad she's safe. Also, the camera never went offline, so she didn't lose power there.

Mom Chronicles October 24, 2019
Here is a quick video from the Momster saying hi to everyone!!

Mom Chronicles October 25, 2019
Mom loves to look at the pics on her wall. With as much time as she spends in bed, I'm glad they provide her a little happiness.

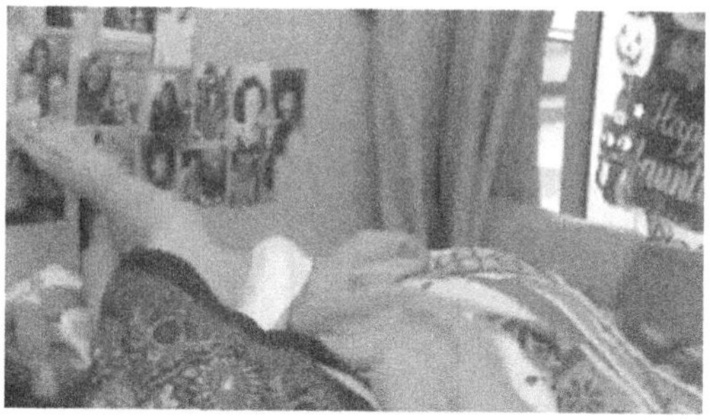

Mom Chronicles October 28, 2019
Mom was lying down when I arrived. She was doing her best to try and straighten/flatten out the hem of the sheet. She was fighting a losing battle, but it was keeping her busy. I noticed it was time to change out the polish on her nails, so I removed the old polish. As mentioned in previous posts, she does not understand the process of changing out polish anymore. She was giving me the evil eye the WHOLE time. I put the headphones on her to try and distract her. It took 3 Elvis songs before she started "singing." I was still getting the evil eye with a couple of smiles, but I powered through. I just kept smiling down at her and showing her the new polish strips so that she could hopefully make the connection. Once the new polish was on, she was happy.

Eating dinner was challenging too. I helped her eat part of it. (On Saturday, I had to help her eat the entire lunch.) After dinner, I took her to the TV room. I used my standard line that normally works, and she got mad at me. It was another "evil eye-madder than a hornet" look. I called in reinforcements - Bruce Face Timed in to get her laughing. I was able to leave after that.

I am starting to wonder if she knows me. It could be the new medicine she's on, but it just seems like she is looking at me differently now. Almost vacant, if that makes sense.

I'll take it day by day since I know things can change moment by moment with her. I know her and love her, and that's all that matters.

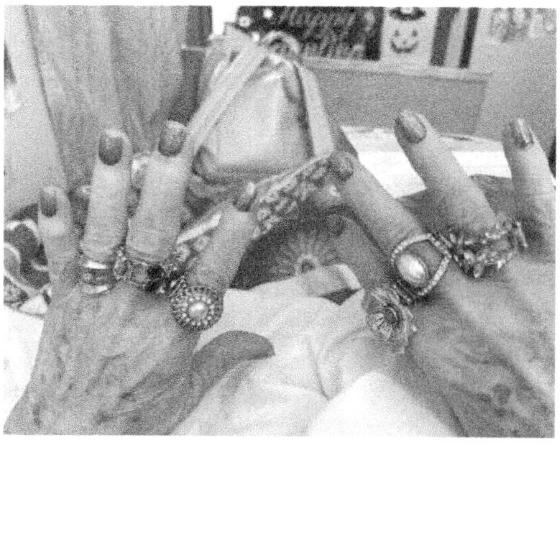

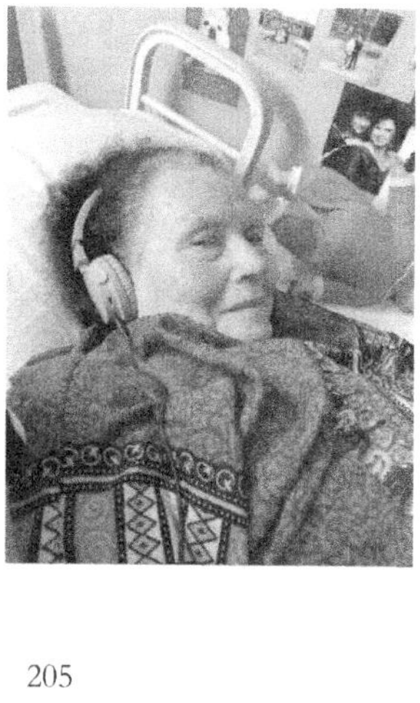

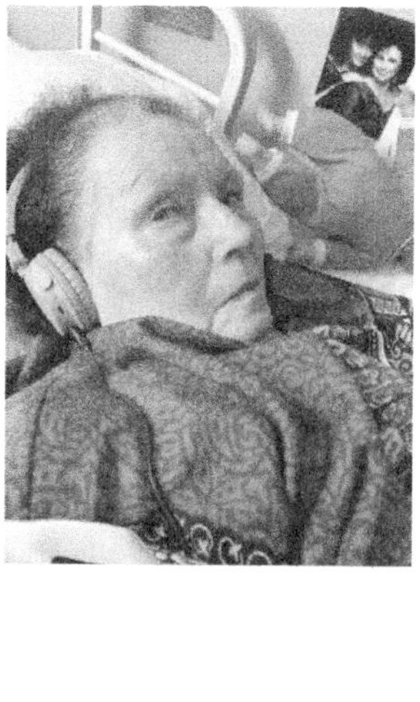

Mom Chronicles October 31, 2019
First of all, happy heavenly birthday to my Grandma Clark. She was my second mom, and I loved her dearly. Unfortunately, she also had Alzheimer's, and Mom took care of her for the last four years of her life.

Now... on to Mom. Mom was "out of it" tonight. I'm still going with the guess that it's the new meds. Bruce and I chatted about it. What is my preference? For her to be calm and not as agitated even if it seems like she doesn't know who we are or to have her know us and be more responsive but be highly upset with the aides to the point that she's screaming and biting? That's hard, but I think I want her to be calm and not scared.

Also, she got a marriage proposal and didn't even realize it at dinner. One of the residents was sitting at Mom's table at dinner time. He said to me, "her next husband is not going to be Indian... because that's me. I'm French." Now where in the world he pulled "Indian" out of the air, I don't know. I just smiled and went along with it. He has dementia too. Mom was clueless, but inside I laughed a little. Dude... if you only knew. She was married eight times. If she didn't have Alzheimer's, she probably would have married you too since Ted passed away last year. I do love my Momma, but she gave Elizabeth Taylor a run for the world record on marriages. Thank the good Lord above that Ted came into her life. She had never been happier than when she was with him. She found her true love at 60+ years old.

Back to this evening. Another thing about Mom tonight was that she had tears running down her face when I got there. She couldn't tell me what was wrong. She didn't seem to be hurting anywhere. Maybe allergies?? It was cold in there. Several other residents were wrapped in blankets. I asked her if she was cold, but she couldn't understand what I was asking her. She just kept looking at her nails to "answer" my question. Finally, about 15 minutes later, I noticed her rubbing her arms. That told me she was cold, so I went and picked out a sweater from her closet. I could tell she was happy when I put the sweater on her.

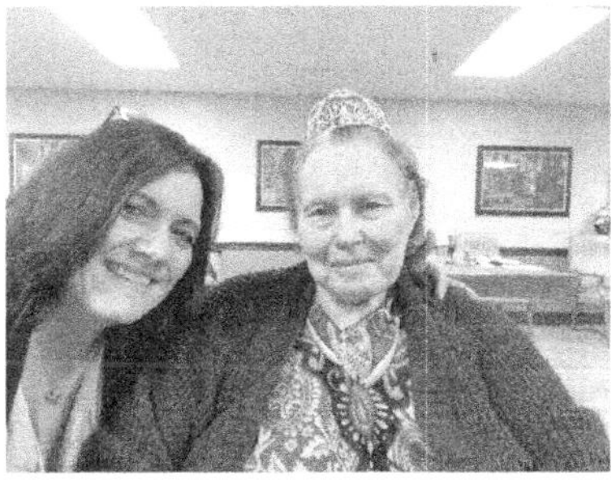

It's just so hard trying to figure what is wrong. She can't communicate with us anymore.

Finally, I Skyped Sheila in to try and see if that would brighten her up. Unfortunately, it didn't appear that she recognized her. After the call, though, she said she knew it was Sheila. I'm just not sure.

The days get more challenging with her, but that's okay. I'll take as many with her as I can, no matter how challenging.

♥

When a loved one with Alzheimer's can no longer communicate verbally with you, watch for nonverbal cues. Monitor for facial expressions, shifting, pacing, rubbing arms, clenching fists, and so on. You must become a detective. Remember all the "puzzle clues" I posted about earlier when she was more verbal? Puzzle-solving becomes more difficult at this stage because we have no context of what they are trying to communicate to us. They could be hurting, hungry, wet, or soiled, or any number of things. Like caring for a baby who cannot communicate, we must look for cues to determine what is wrong with our loved one.

Mom Chronicles November 2, 2019

My sissy is up this weekend and visiting Mom at the moment.

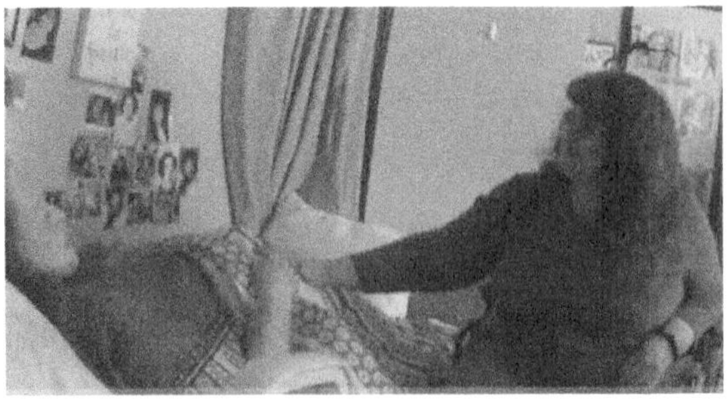

Mom Chronicles November 5, 2019

I haven't seen Mom since Thursday, and it's killing me. I want to see her so bad, but I've been sick (nothing serious – just a sore throat and non-stop coughing), and I don't want to get her sick. I thought I would be happy with taking a little break for several days, but it seriously is hard! I know I have limited time left with her, and I don't want to miss an opportunity. I'm hoping I can shake this soon so that I can get back over there ASAP. I'm afraid she will forget me if I'm not there.

Mom Chronicles November 7, 2019

Awww... the director of nurses just sent me this quick video clip. And she said that Mom smiled really big when she saw my video clip. I'm thankful I have a good working relationship with the staff there and that they show me they truly care about Mom. I'm hoping I get to see her tomorrow!

[This was the last time Mom ever spoke my name.]

Mom Chronicles November 8, 2019

I haven't seen her in a week, so it was fantastic seeing her today. She's very quiet but in a pleasant mood. They said she showered much easier for them today. The medicine seems to be working.

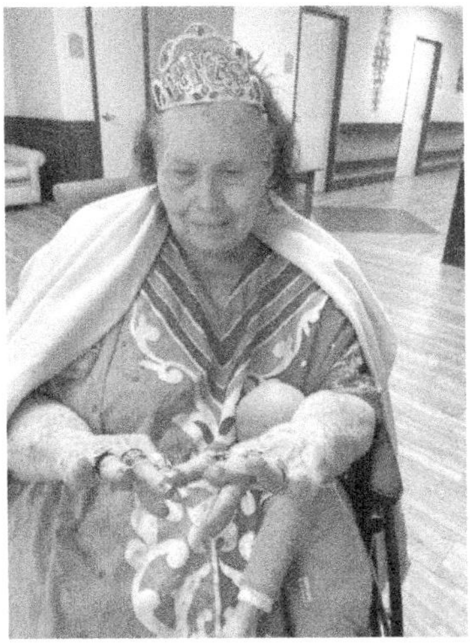

I spoiled her today with a strawberry shake, new bling rings, new fingernail strips, and a few new dresses. The beauty of the dashiki dresses is that they are beautiful, inexpensive, and comfortable. The not-so-beautiful part is that the seams come loose pretty easily. My sister will sew up a few of them next time she visits because she knows how to use a needle and thread. Me – not so much. I would rather pay someone or buy new dresses than deal with that. I'm grateful for a wonderful visit so far.

I love you, Mom.

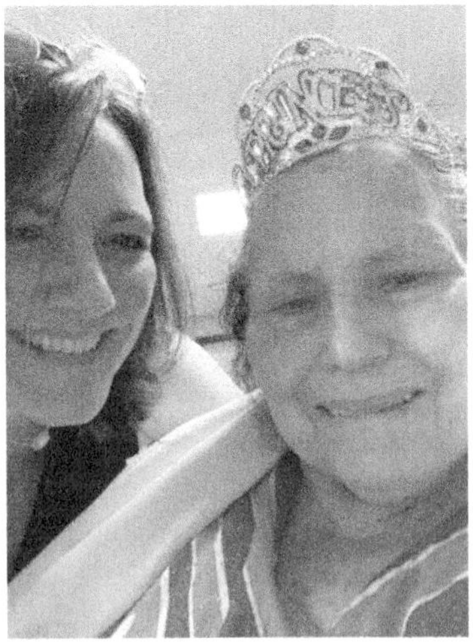

♥

My wonderful co-worker and friend Beth Dolliver was the one who sewed Mom's dress seams up since I saw her every day at work. She was a huge blessing for my Mom and me by helping with this task. If you need help with something for your loved one, ask around in your circle of friends and family. So many will be happy to help!

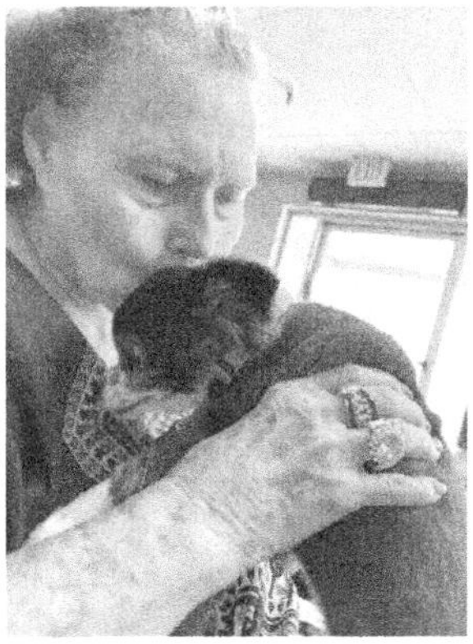

Mom Chronicles November 9, 2019
I had a short visit with Mom today. After getting Simi groomed, we stopped by the nursing home. She was sound asleep in her wheelchair in the TV room. The aide said she refused to let them lay her down after lunch. Like - the go to h-e-double-hockey sticks glare refusal.

I let her play with Simi for a few minutes, and then Uncle Quinton sent me a text about a Christmas memory he had of Mom and Grandma. They both played a mean trick on him when he was about seven years ago. They wrapped a huge box under the tree and kept telling him he had to wait until Christmas Eve to open it. You can imagine the torture this did to a 7-year-old. Well, on Christmas Eve, he was able to open the box. It was a clothes basket. He said he was soooo disappointed and heartbroken. They gave him his real gift afterward. He said it taught him not to get so wrapped up in what a gift could be. I'm glad Mom never did that to Sheila or me!!

Since he has an iPhone, we Face Timed for a minute. Mom kept stroking his beard through the phone glass. She didn't know what to think of the beard.

I have noticed some of Mom's dresses going missing. I saw one lady sitting by the nurse's station with one of them on while there. The sharpie is hard to see on these patterns, so the aide told me to get white cloth strips and sew them into the dresses so that the name can be seen better. I may need to beg Sheila or Beth to sew these in for me!!

When it was time to leave, I told the aides I would help them lay Mom down so that they could freshen her up. She looked like she was ready to fall asleep. She tucked the baby in by her shoulder and told me she loved me.

All is good in the world this afternoon!

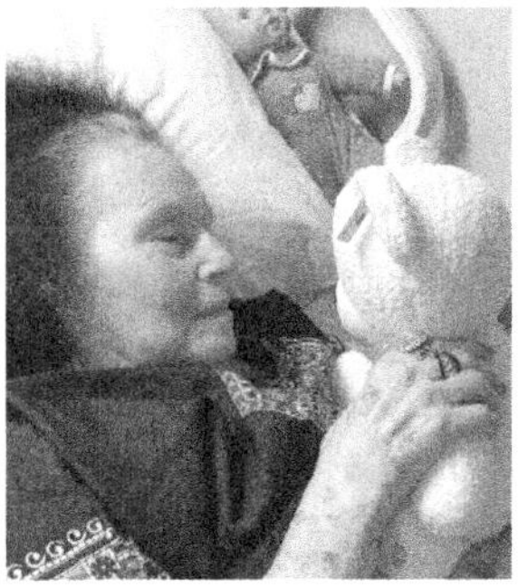

Mom Chronicles November 12, 2019
She doesn't know me today—Alzheimer's sucks. Maybe tomorrow will be better.

Mom Chronicles November 14, 2019
She was much better today. I'm still not quite sure she knew me, but I THINK she did. She laughed with me and told me a couple of times that she loved me. I wasn't getting the mean, confused stare like Tuesday.

I did have to feed her today, and the nurse told me they are putting her on weekly weigh-ins. She's gaining a little each week, and they just want to monitor it. I'm not seeing her legs swelling like at the other center, so I don't think it's water retention. She is eating well, so who knows. I'm glad they are keeping an eye on this.

Today was a great visit!

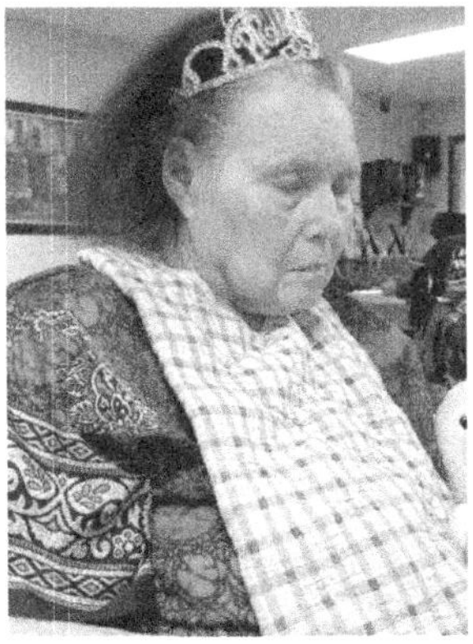

Mom Chronicles November 16, 2019
Are you sleepy?

"No."

And then she dozes off.

She is sleeping more and more throughout the days.

Mom Chronicles November 23, 2019
Sheila and I are visiting Mom after missing four days with her. She is alert and happy today. There is not much communication, which is the norm, but she is happy.

I redid her nails - she chose purple - and gave her a couple more rings. She is happy today! (And I think she knew who we were.)

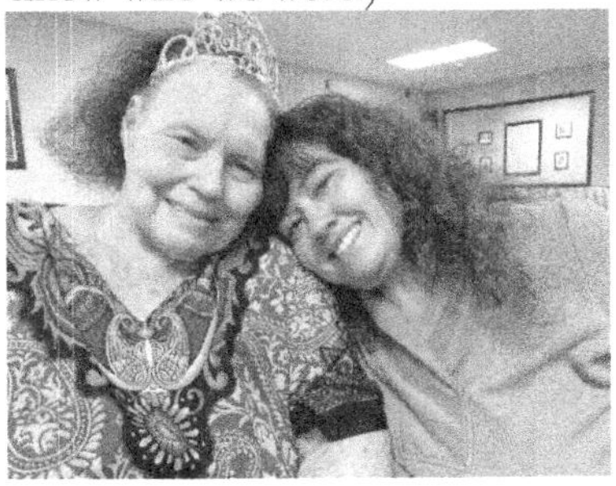

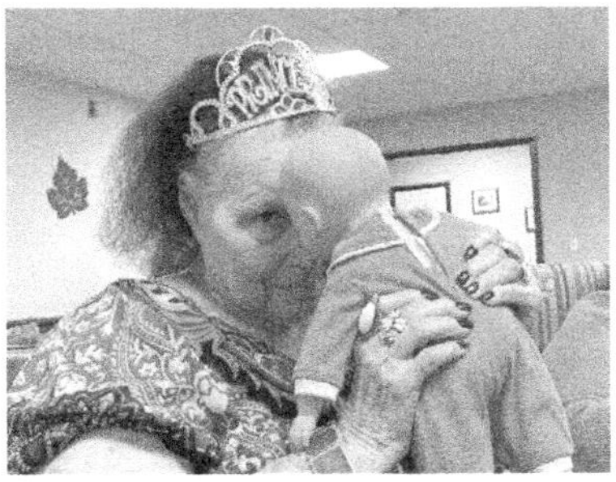

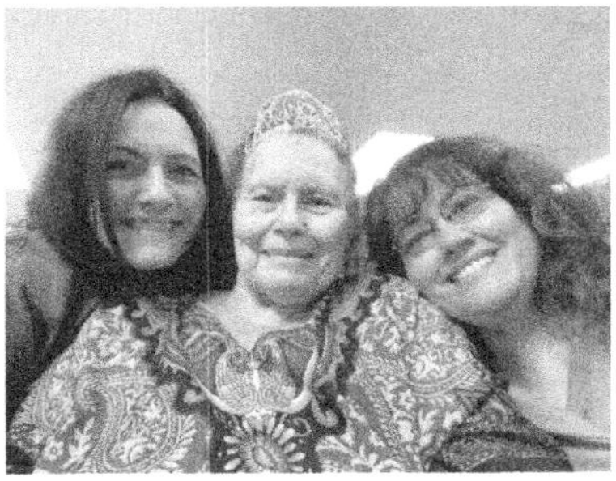

Mom Chronicles November 25, 2019
Today, she does not even recognize herself in the pictures on the wall. I'm telling her that the lady (or the young girl) in the photos is her. She is saying, "no, it's not." This is a first!! She's always at least recognized herself.

"I remember me" is not holding true today.

She's in a good mood, though, so I'll be happy with that.

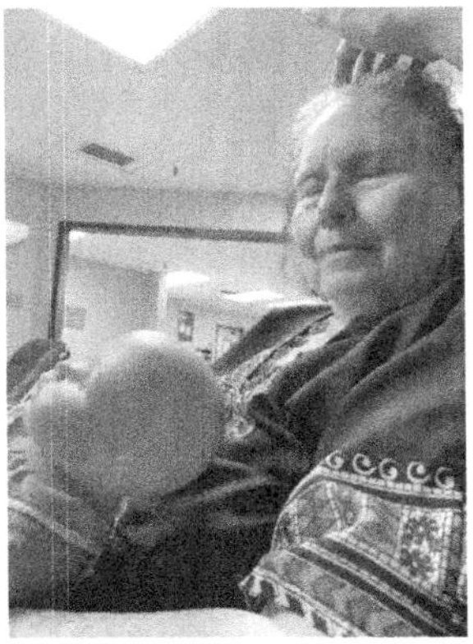

Mom Chronicles December 2, 2019
I had one of the best visits I've had with Mom in such a long time. She was smiling and alert. She only slightly dozed for a moment while waiting for dinner.

To me, she was "glowing." I had to help feed her. I also sent a message to the DON this morning asking if they could adjust her meds because she seemed too tired all the time and that she is at the stage where we need someone to help feed

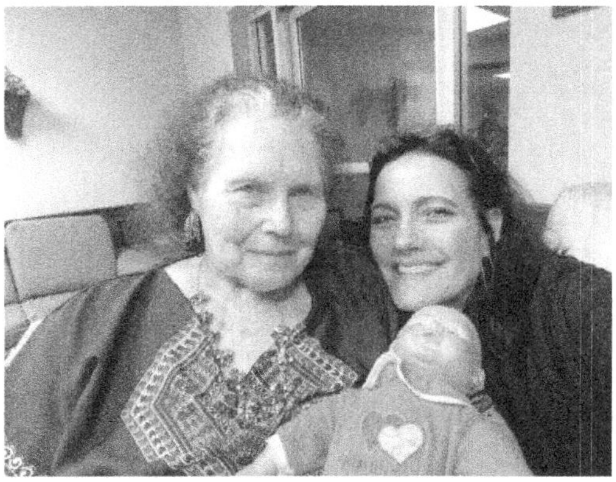

her when I'm not there. The DON said she would take care of it. After dinner, I rolled her to the TV room. I wanted Sheila to see her smile like this since Mom kept dozing during our visits, so we Skyped for a few minutes. I also finger-combed her hair because I remember reading that Alzheimer's patients need the sensory type of communication. I took a picture of her while I was doing that. She loved it! Look at that face!!

When I was about to leave, she told me she wanted to go home with me. The words were a little broken, but I knew what she was asking. She hasn't asked me this in a long time. It didn't make me sad. On the contrary, I was happy to hear her use several words together that made sense AND that she knew who I was!! I fibbed and said I needed to clean the guest bedroom out first, but I would take her home tomorrow. She laughed.

Tonight's visit was the absolute best one in a long time!!

Mom Chronicles December 4, 2019

She wasn't as alert tonight as she was on Monday. I tried to play a couple of rounds of "mominoes" with her, but tonight she couldn't remember how to set up her dominoes. In the first round, she tried standing them up "tall." In the second round, she placed them flat on the table. She missed a couple of matches as well. She was getting mad when I would tell her they didn't match, so I finally just had to let her play the way she wanted to. There was no sense in upsetting her.

Once dinner was served, I had to help feed her. The chicken was pretty dry tonight, so she kept getting meat stuck in her teeth. It bothered her too much to let me keep feeding her the rest of the meal, so I had to floss her teeth again. She tried to bite me this time - but not on purpose. I finally got those pesky meat slivers out and was able to finish feeding her. Oh, the things we do for our loved ones.

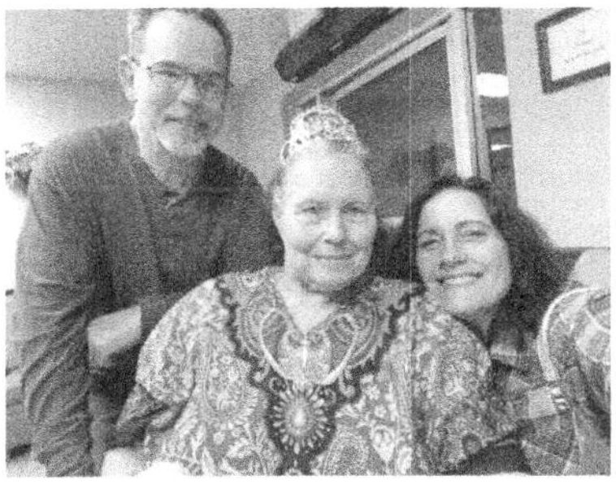

Mom Chronicles December 7, 2019

I didn't get to see Mom yesterday afternoon, so I monitored her through the camera at dinner time. They forgot her. I was not a happy camper. At 5:45, I sent a message to the DON letting her know that her roommate had already been fed by her family but that Mom was still in bed. Within 5 minutes, she had someone down there getting Mom up. I learned today from the roommate's husband that all they did was take her to the TV room and drop the tray off there with her. I have no idea if she ate or not. I will be having another conversation with the DON on Monday about this. I'm not happy at all!

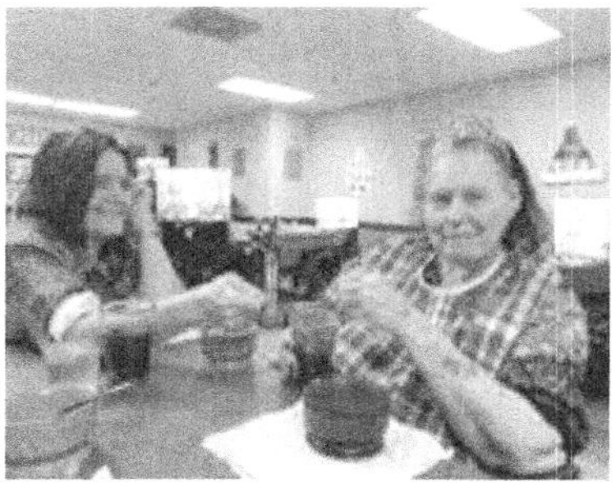

Bruce and I stopped by there this evening to visit and feed her before going out on a date night. He works so many Saturdays and Sundays that we don't get many of those. I think she recognized him, but we weren't sure at first. He helped feed her while I helped the aides get water and juice out to the residents in the dining hall, and then I took over. They were short-handed tonight. She was in a good mood tonight, and it wasn't difficult to tell her goodnight.

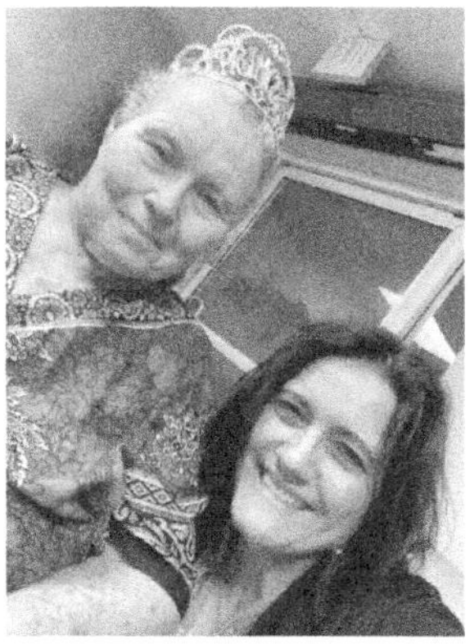

Mom Chronicles December 9, 2019

When I arrived there, she was lying down (as usual). I leaned down to give her a kiss, and she lit up when she saw me. She placed her hands on my face and just smiled and smiled. That made my day!

After getting her up, I took her to the dining room. I worked on her nails while waiting for dinner to be served. She picked the light blue glitter tonight. Again, her face lit up after she saw the finished nails. It was a nice visit.

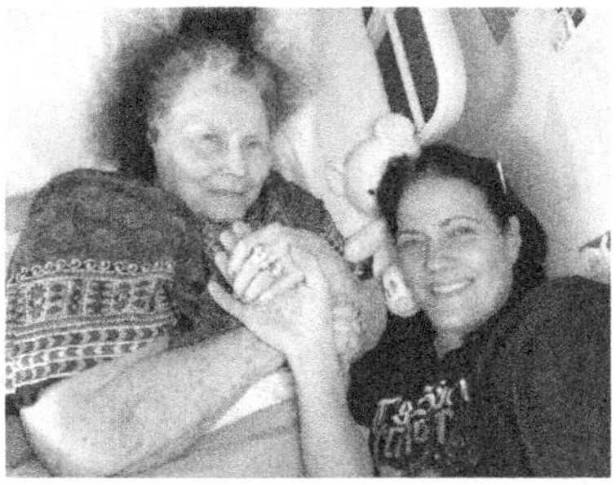

Mom Chronicles December 14, 2019

I got to the center early today. Since she was lying down, I simply curled up next to her until dinner time.

We are enjoying mommy/daughter snuggle time.

Mom Chronicles December 17, 2019

Two Christmas cards came in, and they made Mom smile! Thanks, Dani Gray and Darlene Hall!

Santa dropped by for a special visit to Mom. She (and all the other residents in the dining hall plus a few family members and nurses/aides) were all delighted! Thank you, John Sopko, for taking time out of your day to bring joy to my Mom. You are a wonderful blessing!

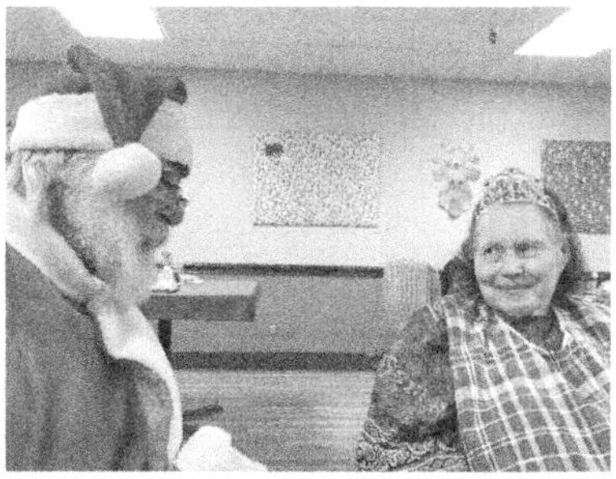

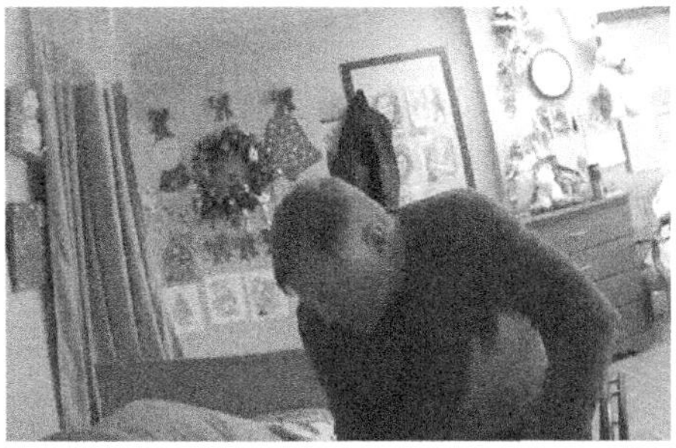

Mom Chronicles December 18, 2019

I just glanced back through the video today checking on Mom, and I saw this! Thank you, PK (Pastor Ken), for visiting Mom. I appreciate it so much!!!

Mom Chronicles December 21, 2019

- Visit from the three wise guys/gals
- New Christmas nail color
- Beautiful Christmas photos
- Alert and in a good mood
- Wonderful visit

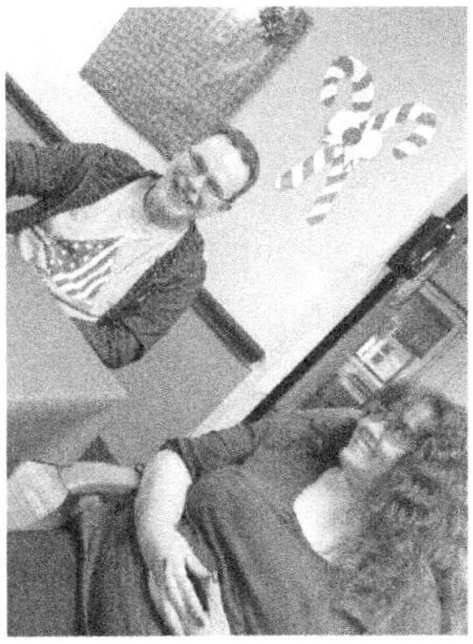
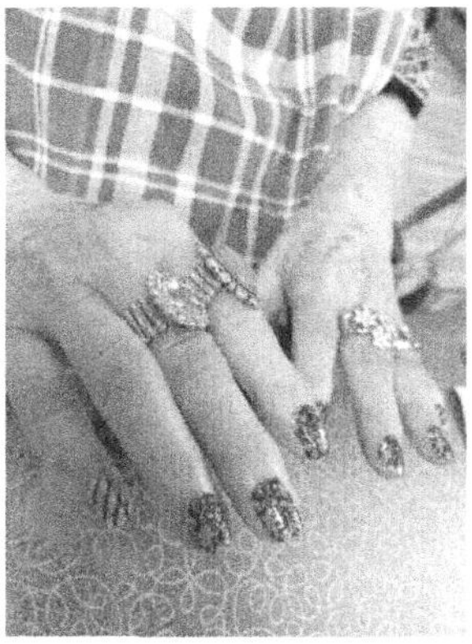
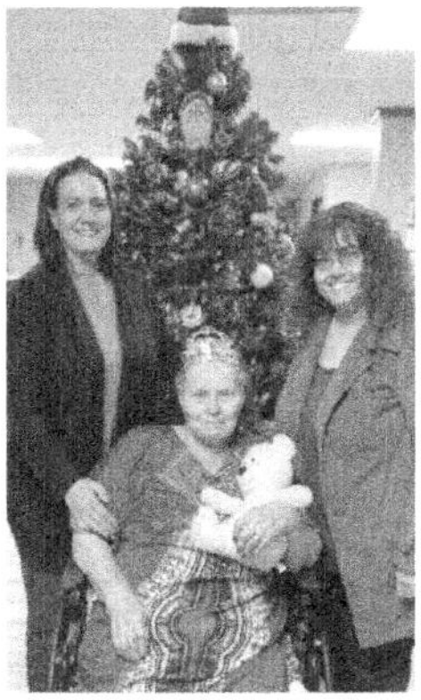
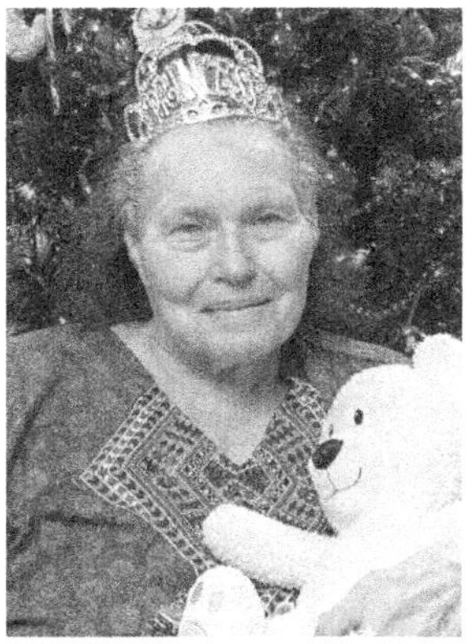

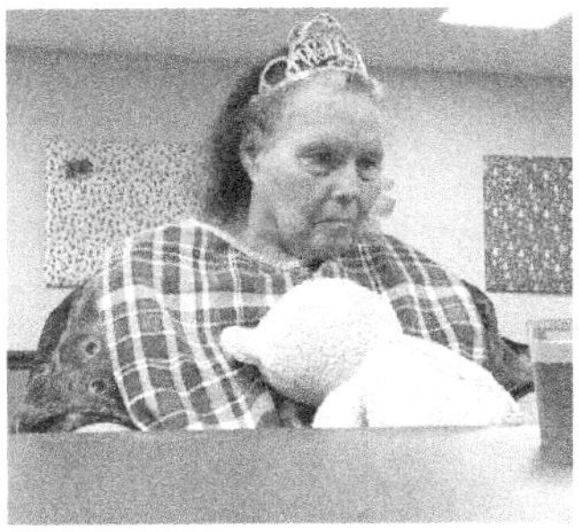

Mom Chronicles December 24, 2019
She's a little subdued tonight, but at least we got her to smile for a pic. We gave her a few bracelets and a ring for Christmas.

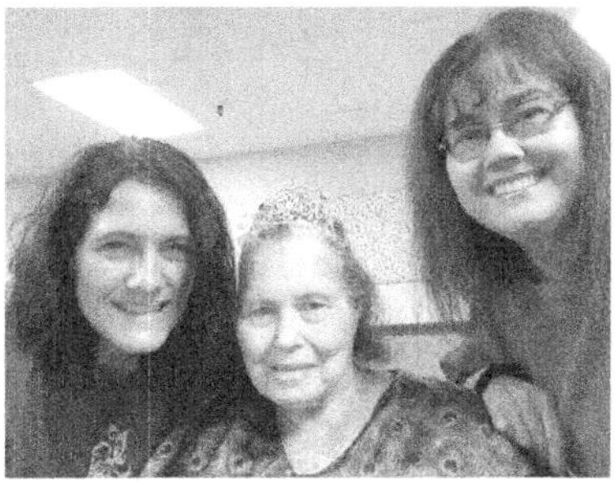

Mom Chronicles December 26, 2019
Sheila and I took Simi in for a visit. Mom was perky tonight and happy to see Simi, but she was not very hungry. I kept trying to get her to take one more bite, but she would turn her head and give me a resounding "no." She hasn't forgotten that word yet!!

This meal had many pepper specks (chicken fried steak and gravy), so she kept trying to pick out the pepper. We guess she thinks it's dirt or something. We kept trying to convince her they are spices to make her food taste better. She's didn't buy it. When we were leaving the nursing home, she pretended to cry to keep us from going. At least we left on a good laugh with her.

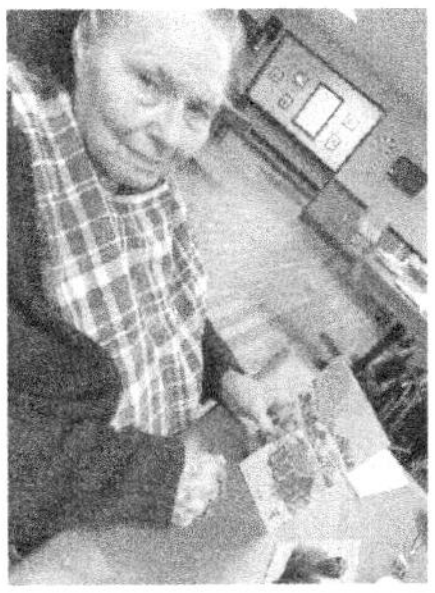

Mom Chronicles December 27, 2019
The Christmas card from Lea Cates came in (thank you!), and I gave a couple more cards from the stack that Sarah Metcalf and Robin Nikula dropped off a few months ago. She loved seeing the puppies and kittens. Thank you as well! They all made her smile. The other pic is of me trying to feed her dinner.

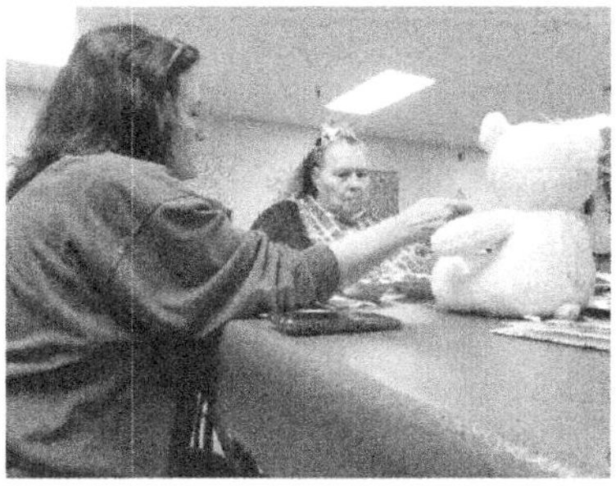

Mom Chronicles January 6, 2020
I haven't seen Mom in over a week. Sheila kept me updated while I was out of town. Last night she couldn't keep Mom awake to eat, and she reported that Mom has started having a cough. She finally got Mom to eat

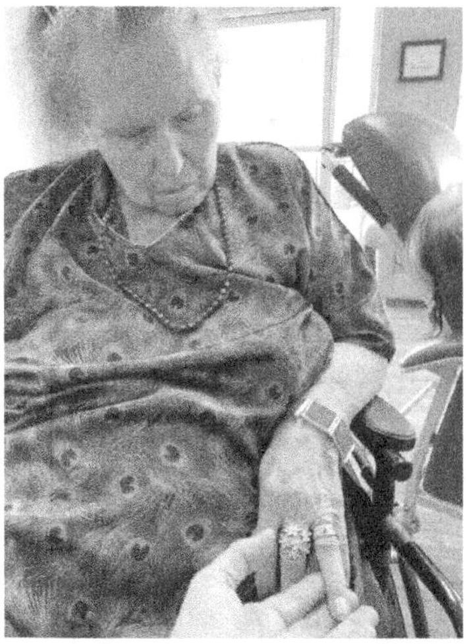

a little bit before she left for Huntsville. Today, I couldn't keep her awake while I fixed her nails with a red glitter shade. But, when she woke up, she LOVED the color.

During dinner, though, she was able to stay awake long enough to let me feed her. She tried to feed herself once, but she couldn't figure out how to hold the spoon. I'm supposed to try and let her feed herself as much as possible so that she doesn't forget the process. But, since she was so sleepy, I decided to feed her completely tonight to make sure she had some nutrition.

I also asked the DON to check her because of the cough and because I could hear the aide this morning through the camera say he could tell she's not feeling well. The DON listened to her lungs and said the right lung sounds diminished, so she has ordered an X-ray. The nurse on duty just told me they should be here shortly to take the X-ray. I don't know if they will update me tonight, so I will check in with the DON tomorrow morning to find out about the results. Also, I heard several residents coughing in the dining room, so it sounds like something is going around.

Finally, I gave her the two rings that Leigha Gaines bought her. She loved them. Thanks, Leigha

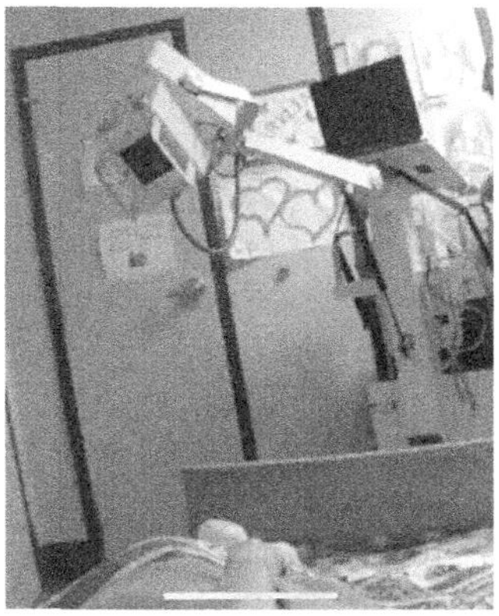

Mom Chronicles January 6, 2020
They just took the X-ray of her chest. It's pretty cool how they can do this in her room while she is in bed.

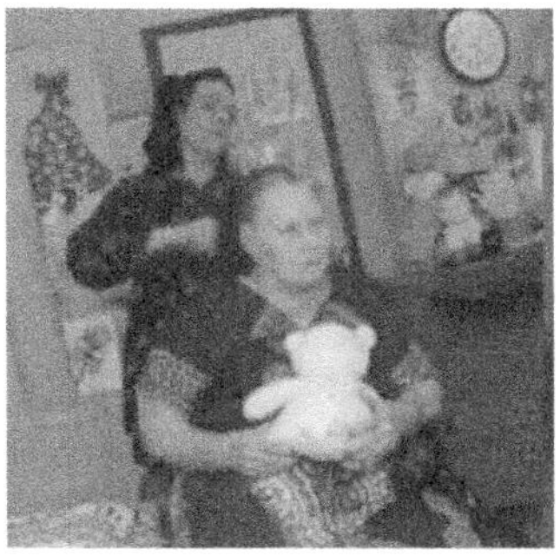

Mom Chronicles January 15, 2020
In this screenshot from the camera, I'm brushing Mom's hair and then placing her crown back on after her afternoon nap before heading to dinner. She loves to have her hair brushed.

Mom Chronicles January 17, 2020
I arrived about an hour earlier than usual today. When she saw me, she gave me a huge smile and was perky and giggling. I sat on the bed with her and just tried a little small talk, knowing that she couldn't understand

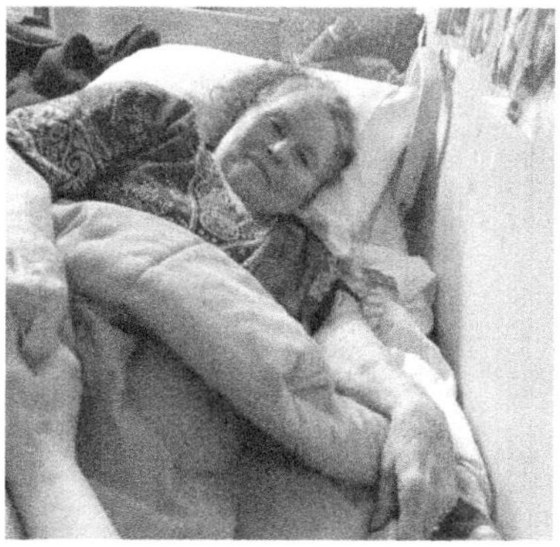

me. I just wanted her to hear my voice. I held her hand too. About 20 minutes into the visit, her whole demeanor changed. She looked at me like I was an alien, and I could no longer get any responses or sounds at all.

At dinner, they served her a sandwich and some crackers (and some other items). I started opening one package of the crackers. She took the other one and put it in her mouth, wrapper and all, trying to eat it. I took it away from her and showed her that I needed to open the package first before she could start eating.

I'm still getting the alien looks from her, so I'm not sure she knows me right now. That's okay. She knew me when I first got here, and that's what's important to me. So I'll take what I can get.

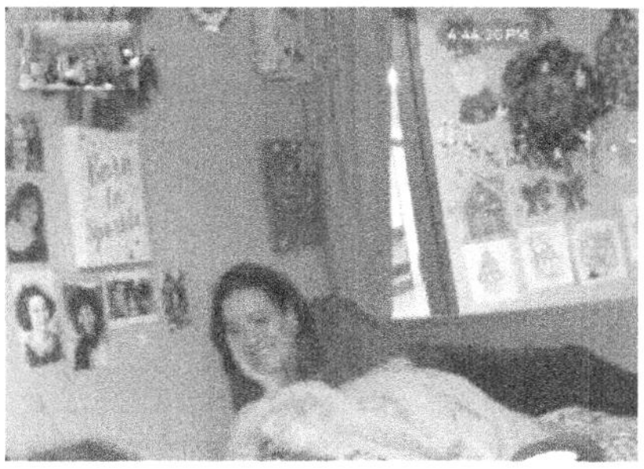

Mom Chronicles January 17, 2020
When I got home, I checked the camera for today's happenings. I now know why I was an alien about 20 minutes into our visit. The nurse had just given her meds 10 minutes before I walked in. So that makes it a perfect 30 minutes before the meds started kicking in to relax her.

The "Area 51 Alien" mystery is solved for the day.

Mom Chronicles January 21, 2020
I'm a stranger today. And I'm okay with it. I think I am getting used to it. I looked back at the video feed to see if they had given her medicine recently, but they hadn't. So, today is just a day she doesn't recognize me. But, tomorrow may be different with this stupid disease.

Seriously - I'm okay. It's not bothering me today.

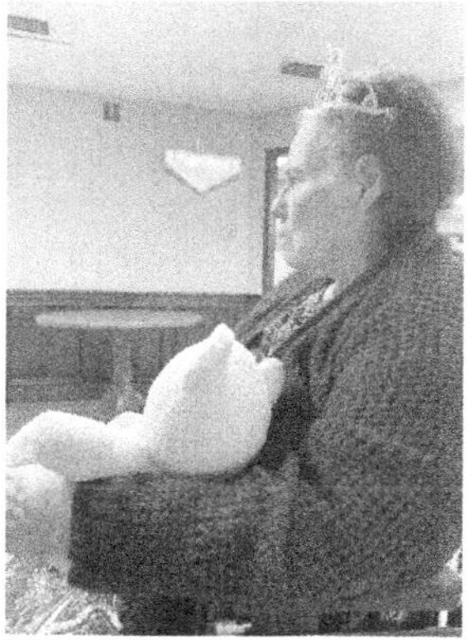

Mom Chronicles January 22, 2020
When I got there, she gave me a huge smile. (Yay!)

Then from that point on, there were no smiles and no communication. I just helped feed her in silence, other than having a small conversation with another lady at Mom's table.

As I was leaving, I pulled my phone out and asked her to take a pic with me. When she saw the camera, she smiled so big. She loves photos!!

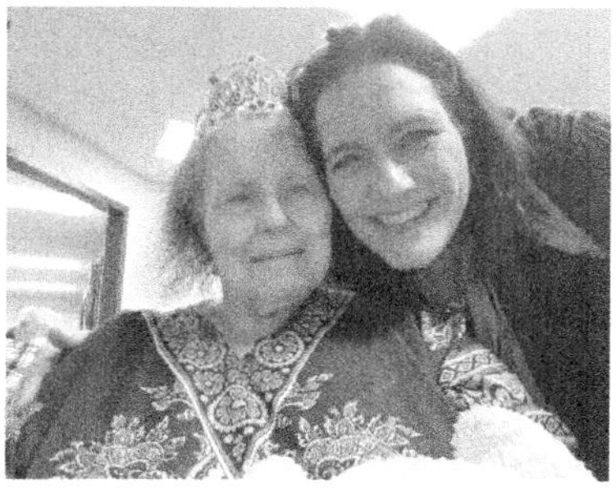

Mom Chronicles January 23, 2020
She lit up and said she loved me when I walked in!

We are listening to music. She could even mimic a sad facial expression on a "sad" part of the song. She has a look of pure joy on her face listening to Elvis.

She wanted the headphones back on when "Love Me Tender" came on. She's trying to sing it, bless her heart!

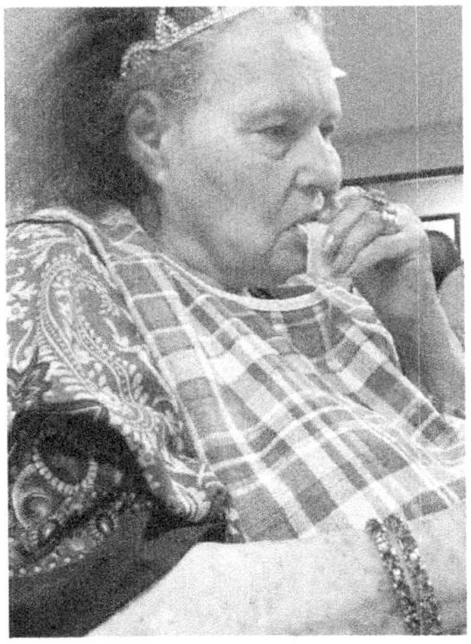

Mom Chronicles January 23, 2020

Stop the presses... she's eating cheese today! This woman has not eaten cheese since I was little. She's forgotten that she doesn't like cheese!! I just need to laugh when something unusual like this happens during this journey.

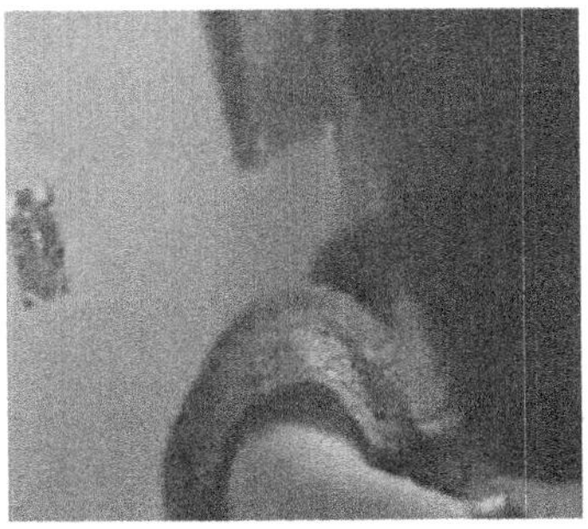

Mom Chronicles January 27, 2020
Bless her heart... Mom has no strength to hold herself up at all on the bed. A new aide was helping to get her back on the bed a little while ago and let go of Mom for just a second. Mom immediately started falling to the side. The aide caught her quickly.

Mom Chronicles January 29, 2020
She's in a great mood today. Her vocabulary is very small, but she's happy.

Quick update... The other lady who sits at Mom's table just came into the dining room and looked at me and said, "I'm hungry, momma!" So I told her dinner would be served in a few minutes.

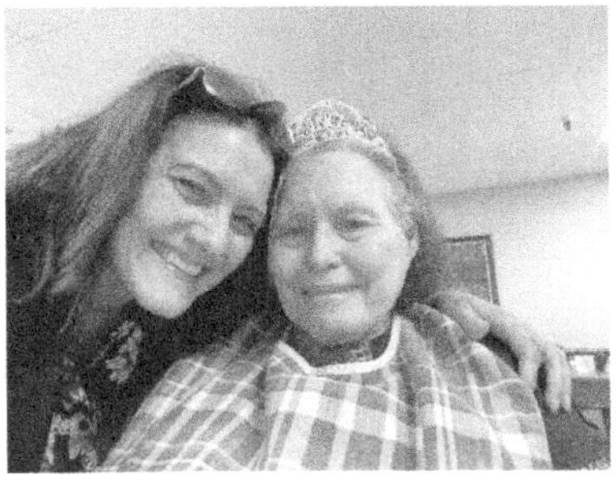

Mom Chronicles January 31, 2020
Yesterday's visit was another "first" in this Alzheimer's journey with Mom. During the whole visit, I was not able to get a single word out of her. No "hi," no "I love you," no answer of "yes" or "no" to the question of "are you feeling okay?" No words. I was able to get some grins, especially when I gave her the card from

Theresa Alexander. Sheila and I even tried Skyping. Mom grinned and blew a kiss to Sheila - but no spoken words.

I could tell she wasn't feeling well - she had a runny nose and is still coughing, which may have been a contributing factor.

I'm hoping to get a word or two during the next visit. Also, Sheila will be visiting this weekend, so she may be able to coax some words out.

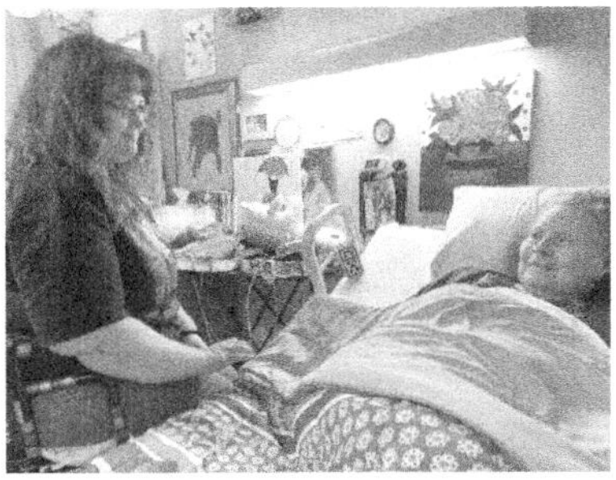

Mom Chronicles February 1, 2020
We are getting some words out of her today!! Yay! "Hi," "yes," "good."

Mom Chronicles February 1, 2020
Joshua... I have a special happy birthday wish for you!!

Mom Chronicles February 1, 2020
Feeding her dinner tonight was fun! She was so sleepy that she would chew her food with her eyes closed, and then I would have to get her attention to wake her up to take the next bite. But I did get her to eat the whole meal - it just took a while.

Now we are in the TV room, and she is nodding off again.

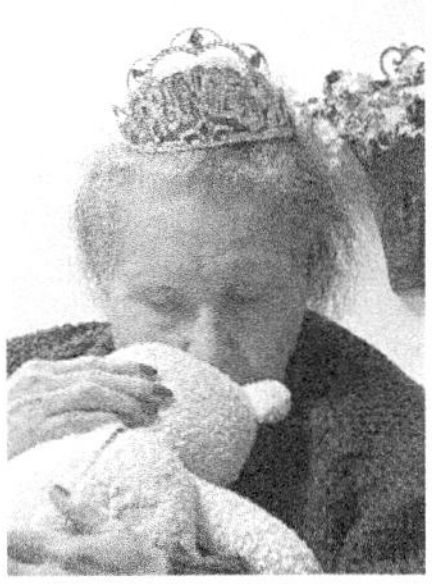

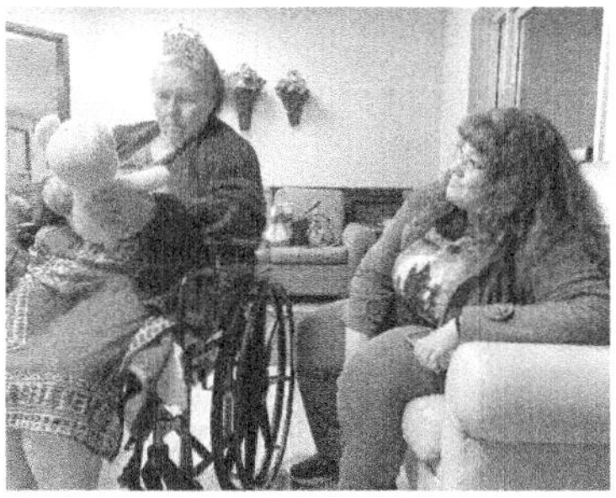

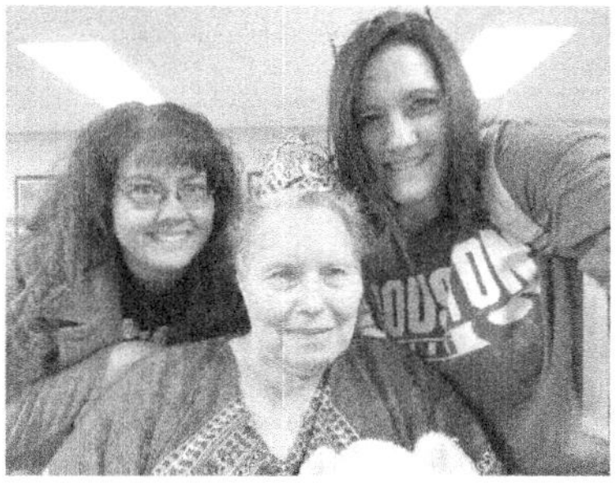

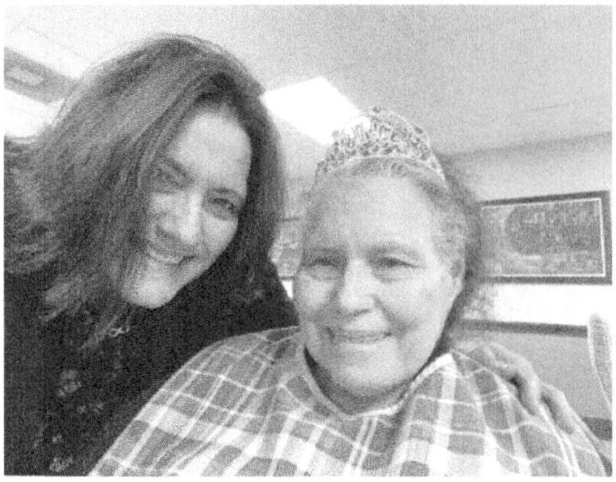

Mom Chronicles February 5, 2020
I'm with my sweet mom waiting for dinner: silent communication - lots of smiles. I ask simple questions (Are you okay? Did you have a good day?), but she isn't understanding. Instead, she just laughs, which is her sign that she doesn't understand what I asked.

She showed me her rings and nails, so they still bring her happiness.

Mom Chronicles February 6, 2020
I bought Mom a strawberry shake with a gift card that Theresa Alexander sent me for Mom. I haven't bought many for her lately because they are watching her weight. I felt it was time to give her a treat, especially since she hasn't been eating well lately.

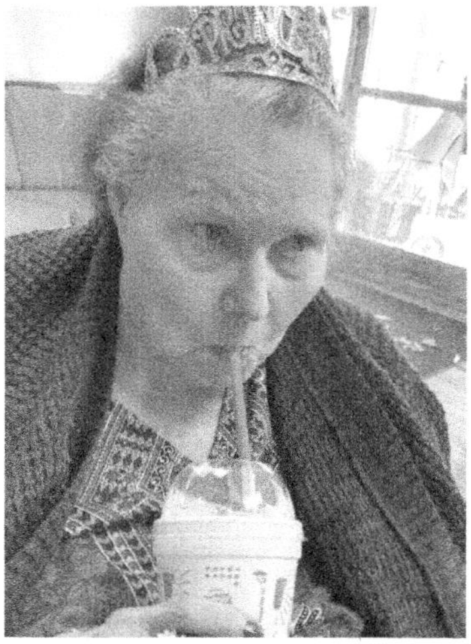

I also talked to one of the administrators. They are finally ordering her a larger wheelchair. I've been asking for this for months. It took my sister to ask to get it done finally. She is a little more "persuasive" than me sometimes. The administrator said she ordered a purple one because she knows Mom loves purple. Hopefully, it will be in soon.

Now we are just waiting for dinner to be served. I probably just spoiled her appetite, but I don't care. She's enjoying the shake.

One of the residents just wheeled up to me and asked if I lived here because I'm here all the time. I just laughed and said it feels like it sometimes. I don't want to miss too many moments with Mom, and she needs the most assistance at mealtimes.

Mom Chronicles February 10, 2020
I gave her Uncle Quinton's card when we first got to the dining room. She stared at it while we waited to be served. After she finished eating, she noticed it again and opened it. To her, she is seeing it for the first time again. Another smile. Thank you, Uncle Quinton! You made her smile today!

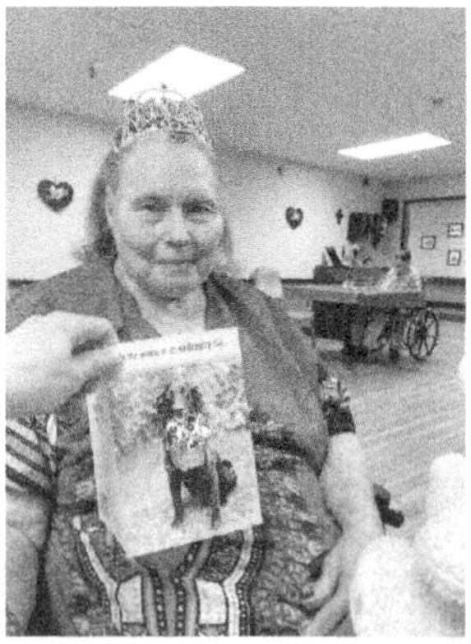

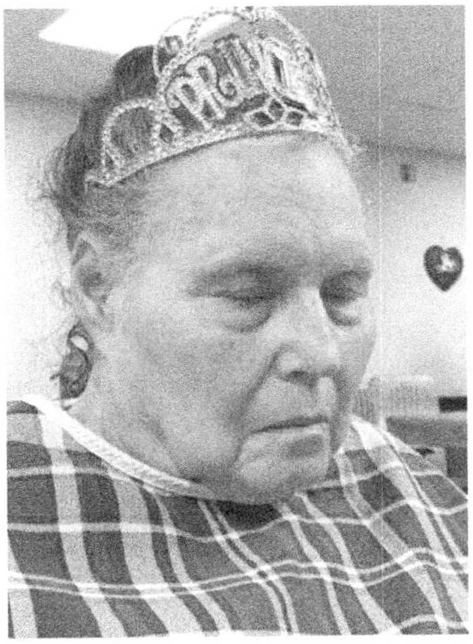

Mom Chronicles February 11, 2020
She is sleepy today. I'm hoping I can wake her up enough to eat when dinner is served.

On another note, someone fixed her hair into a little bun. It's so cute!

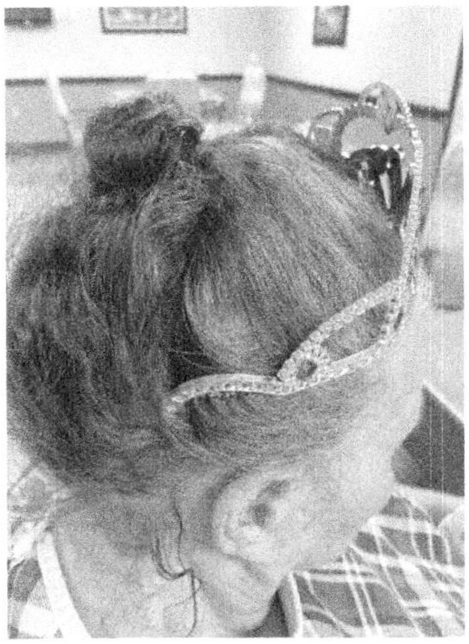

Mom Chronicles February 11, 2020
There was at least one occasion when an aide asked me if Mom had epilepsy. No, she doesn't. I noticed her hands shaking when she lived at the memory care center. It has progressed more to a jerking motion. Upon researching this, I learned that another symptom of Alzheimer's is body jerking, otherwise known as myoclonus. Mom tends to jerk the most when she's sleeping. Here is a short 30-second video of her jerking motions while we are waiting for dinner.

Here is more info about myoclonus: www.healthline.com/health/myoclonus#causes

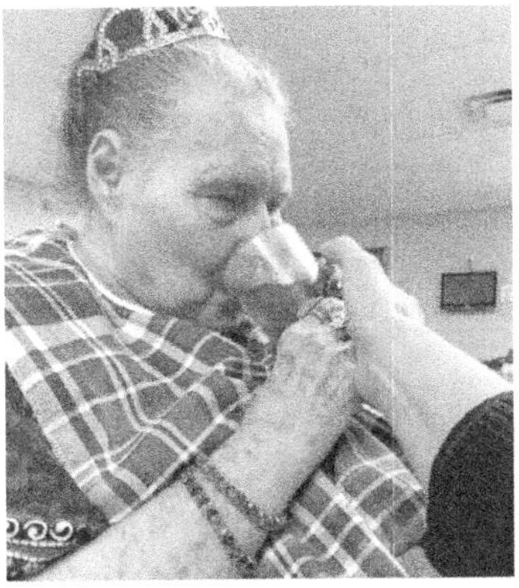

Mom Chronicles February 12, 2020
It took 3 of us to wake Mom up for dinner. My heart always skips a beat when it's hard to wake her up.

I was able to get her to eat half of her dinner. She didn't even want her dessert, which is very unusual.

When I wanted her to drink, she didn't want to hold her cup. So I had to place both of her hands around the cup and guide her to take a drink.

I'm sure tomorrow will be fine. Every day is a new day.

Mom Chronicles February 13, 2020
Mom was sound asleep at the table when I arrived. So I woke her up and tried to get her to say hi or anything to me! Nope. Nada. Nothing.

The aide comes by and asks, "Princess, are you okay?" Mom smiled and replied yes.

I tried again to get her to talk to me or smile. Nope. Nada. Nothing.

Bruce texted me and asked if he could FaceTime and say hi to her. I said sure but not to expect anything. We FaceTimed. She smiled at Bruce, said hi, and replied, "I love you," when he told her he loved her. Bruce hung up. I tried again to get her to talk to me or smile. Nope. Nada. Nothing. I bought a candy bar for her and brought it out to give to her. By golly, I'm gonna bribe a smile out of her.

But nope. Nada. Nothing. She ate the candy bar and just looked at me as if I'm chopped liver. All I can do is laugh. Alzheimer's life is an adventure!!

Mom Chronicles February 16, 2020
She was in a great mood, and I was no longer chopped liver to her today! Sheila has a great video of her and Bruce singing to each other. She should be posting it soon. Elvis made everyone happy in the dining hall yesterday.

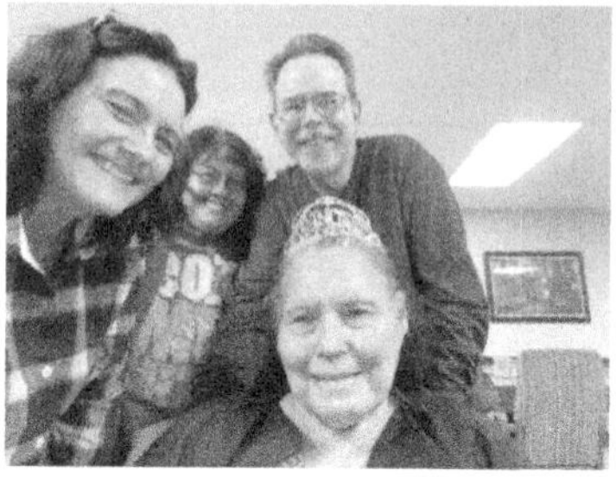

Mom Chronicles February 17, 2020
There was new staff assigned to Mom's hallway today.

- 😖 The camera showed no care at all since 7 am.
- 😖 They don't know the level of care for Mom yet (but they will very quickly!)
- 😖 Mama Bear had to come out when I got to the center this evening.

I'm not an intolerable family member - I try very hard to thank them often, be nice to them and let them know I know they are overworked and underpaid for what they do. But I do expect a minimal level of care, and I won't accept less than that. There are some things I pick my battles on and let slide. Others are non-negotiable. The good thing is she is in a fantastic mood today! She is smiling and laughing, and I'm getting more words out of her today than I have in a long time.

Mom Chronicles February 18, 2020
I just walked into her room and found a new crown for her. I can't tell through the camera who gave it to her. Someone is very kind for thinking of Mom. Sheila, did you bring this one?

Update: Mystery solved - one of the nurses gave Mom this crown with mardi gras colors. None of the other residents got one—just Mom.

Mom Chronicles February 20, 2020
I decided to do something I haven't done in about a year or so. I brought her a sandwich [from a popular sub sandwich food chain], chips, and a diet soda. She used to LOVE this meal. I wasn't sure if she would like it since her tastes have changed so much, but she loves it so far. Score!!

Update: The diet soda was NOT a hit. I got a scowl when she took a drink of that, so we are back to cranberry juice.

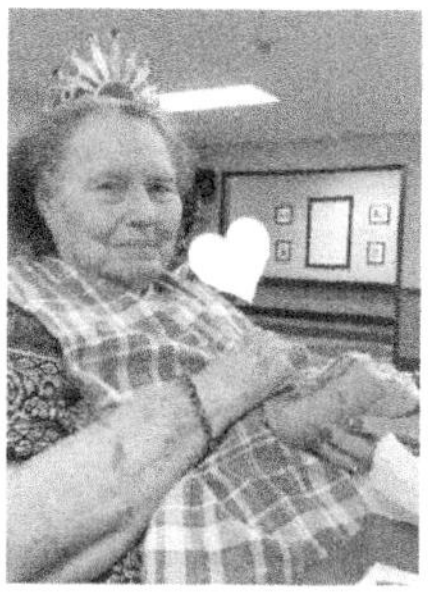

Mom Chronicles February 25, 2020
Mom "danced" with her shoulders and head bops when I played her 50s music playlist at dinner today. Even other residents in the dining hall who could hear my phone's music were singing and "dancing" in their chairs. I love making these precious people smile!

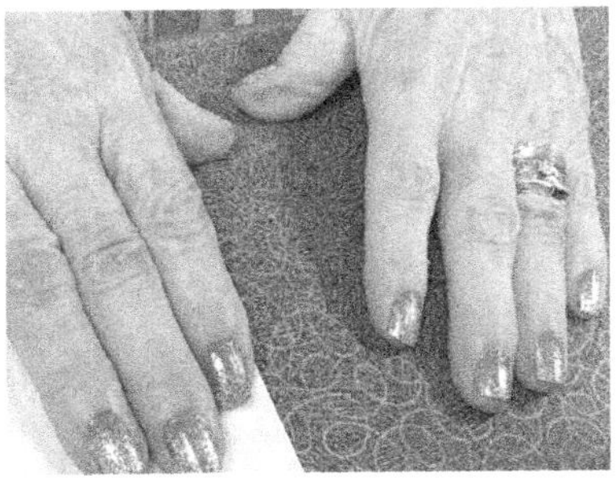

Mom Chronicles February 26, 2020
Oh, I could be so, so evil to my mom!!! They are serving boiled okra tonight. She does not want it (I can't blame her). She used to FORCE Sheila and me to eat this as kids. FORCE. The little mean streak in me wants to force her to eat it tonight, but I won't.

I did change out her nail polish today. And she's in a good mood.

Mom Chronicles February 27, 2020
A few days ago (may have been last week actually - time melds together for me), one of the nurses stopped by the dining room table where Mom and I were sitting and asked Mom if she remembered her. Mom smiled and then cupped the nurse's cheek. That was her way of saying either "yes, I remember you" or "yes, you are a sweet person." There is no way to know for sure.

Yesterday and today, Mom smiled and cupped my cheek too when I told her I loved her. So I choose to believe that is her way of saying she loves me, even though the words are difficult to come by.

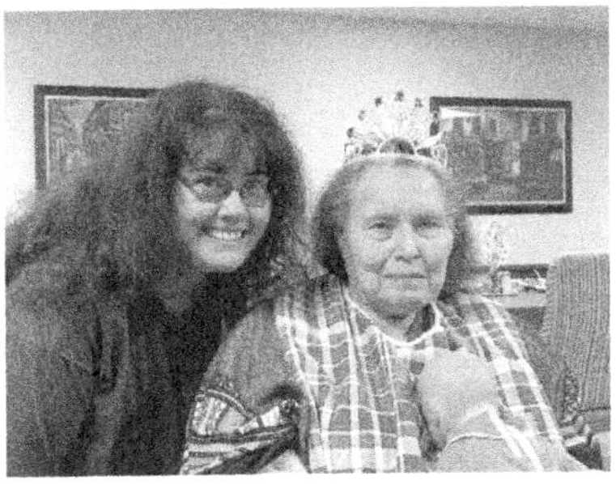

Mom Chronicles March 1, 2020
Sheila had dinner duty tonight. It took a while, but we finally got Mom to smile.

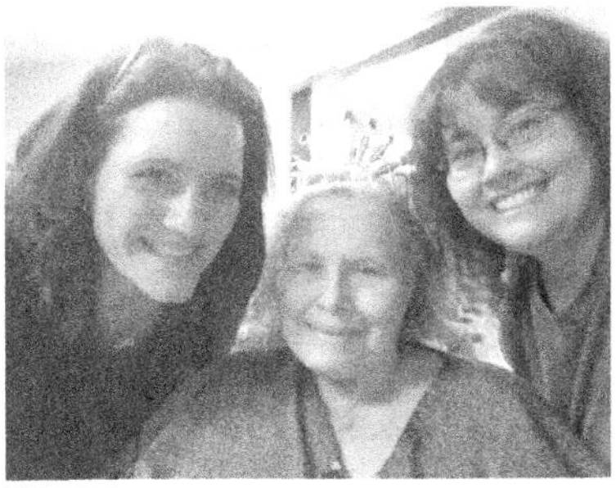

♥

Hindsight is 20/20. The world (and nursing home) was about to close down due to the COVID-19 pandemic a few weeks from this date. This photo is the one that Sheila, Mom, and I took together before she passed away. I will treasure this photo forever.

Mom Chronicles March 2, 2020
Mama bear had to come out again today. The condition of her skin is BAD. I showed the photos to the new DON, head CNA, and the director. Thank the good Lord I was able to be here on time to see it. I'm not happy! No excuse. Period.

Mom Chronicles March 3, 2020
She was trying to tell me something tonight, but I couldn't figure out what she wanted to say, so she got frustrated and mad. I tried reassuring her that I knew she was trying hard. I just kept feeding her, and she forgot she was mad at me. Redirection at its best!!

Mom Chronicles March 4, 2020
Mom was giving me a silly face tonight!!

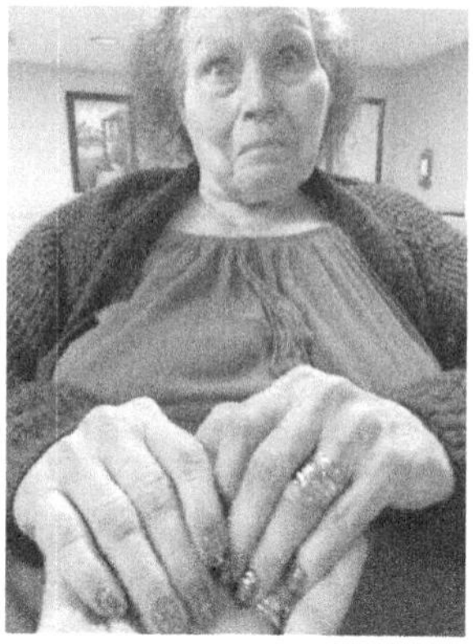

Mom Chronicles March 4, 2020
Where have these clips been all my life??!! I tried them for the first time on Mom tonight to remove her old nail polish. I left them on with the polish remover for about 5 minutes, and the old glitter strips just melted off. No more scrubbing! (The glitter strips are more difficult to remove than the plain polish strips.)

Full disclosure - I kept forgetting them in my car and finally remembered them tonight. Samantha Bradbury, thank you for giving me a set!! It made nail color change super easy for Mom!!

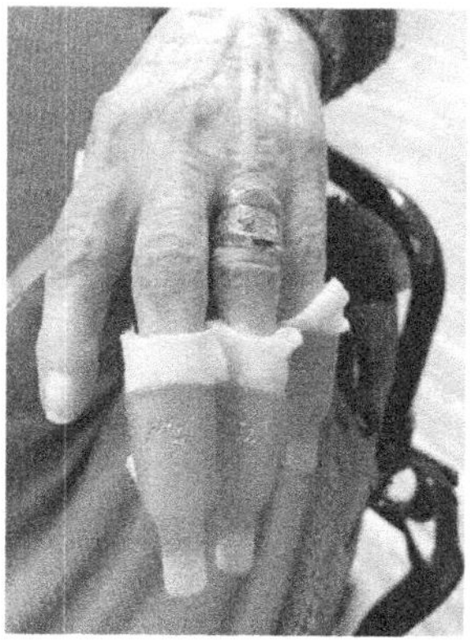

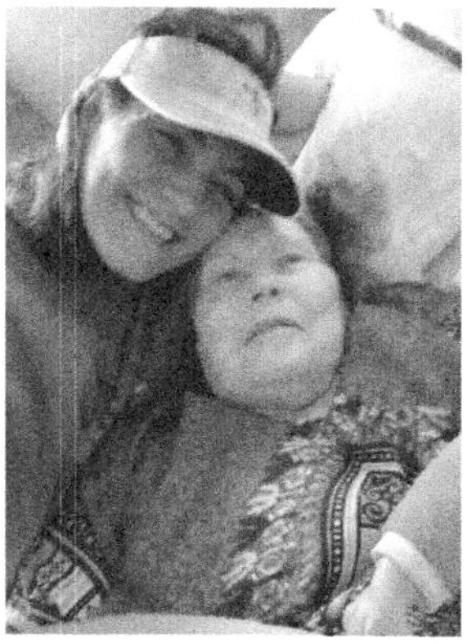

Mom Chronicles March 9, 2020
I got here early tonight so that I can see the condition of her skin. While waiting, she was trying to talk to me, so I started the video. It was all gibberish. The only clear word I could get from her was "no." I miss hearing her talk to me - even if it was the same story over and over—Alzheimer's sucks. You will probably hear me say that a few more times before this journey is over. I know it's not a nice word, but it's the only word that fits right now.

Disregard my hair. It's spring break, and I just don't care to go to all the trouble of fixing it.

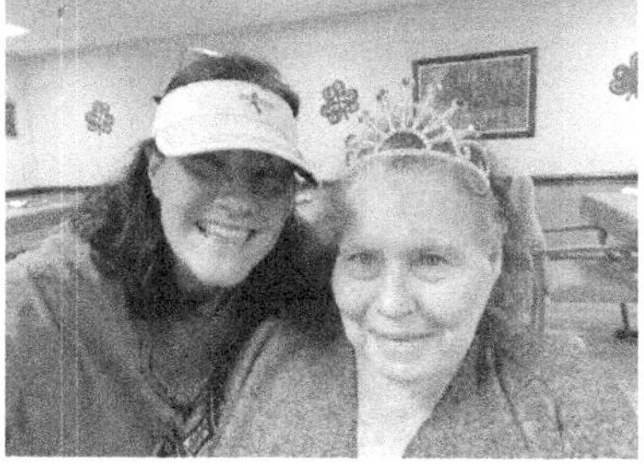

Mom Chronicles March 9, 2020
We are in our 5th year of this awful disease. Mom is now in the last stage. Communication is nil. I'm lucky if I can get a clear "I love you" out of her now. Most words are "gibberish. I recorded it today. One of the staff members (Shauna) at the memory care center she used to live at said to encourage her and let her know that we know how hard she's trying. Most of the time, I just pretend to know what she's saying. I miss our conversations, even if they were repeated over and over.

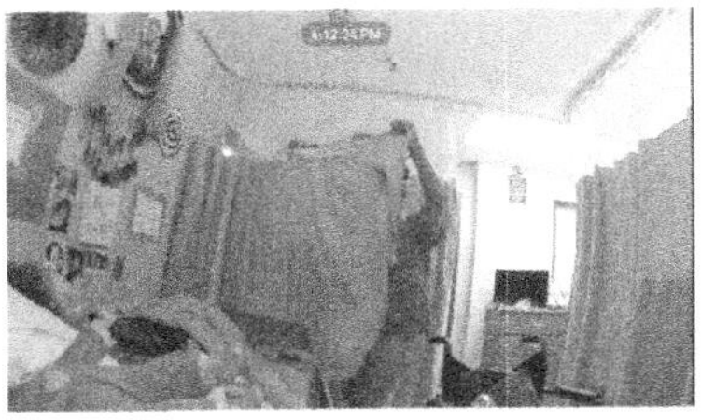

Mom Chronicles March 10, 2020
I couldn't stop by there today, but I just checked on her through the camera. The activities director stopped by and told Mom and her roommate that a group of ladies bought everyone at the center some new pajamas. How sweet!!

♥

At this point in our journey, the bottom fell out in the world with the COVID-19 pandemic. Little did I know that the visit I had with Mom on the 9th was my last real visit - other than the end-of-life visits we had in July. This photo was the last selfie with her sitting right next to me and not through a glass door or window. I'm so incredibly grateful we had the camera in her room because it helped me stay connected to her in some small way during the lockdown, and it allowed me to make sure she was being cared for as well as possible.

Mom Chronicles March 12, 2020
Well... I just got the call that they are locking down the nursing home to visitors. The director gave me her cell phone number, though, so that we can FaceTime with Mom. I'm grateful for that.

I understand why they are doing this, but it's going to be so hard. I'm on limited time with Mom because of her advanced stage with Alzheimer's. I don't want to miss moments with her. I don't want her to forget me entirely. Hopefully, this stupid virus stuff settles down quickly.

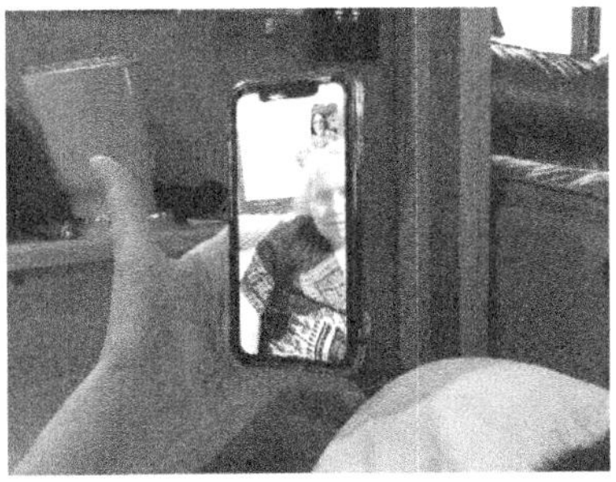

Mom Chronicles March 13, 2020
The director just let me FaceTime with Mom. She is in a good mood and seemed happy. I'm so grateful for technology and an understanding and kind director!

Mom Chronicles March 14, 2020
Through the camera, I could see they are following CDC's guidelines for no more communal meals. Instead, all residents are staying in their rooms for meals.

So far, they are dropping off the tray and showing Mom how to take the first bite. For breakfast, she didn't eat. They tried to coax her to take a bite when they returned to get the tray, but she refused. At lunch, it was the same process, but I can't tell if she's eating. They haven't come back to pick up the tray yet, so I won't know until then. I did hear the aide try to tell her and show her how to use her fork to take a bite before she walked out to help the next resident.

I sent a message to the director and asked if they could make sure she is served finger foods for as long as she will be feeding herself. She took care of it right away, so hopefully, dinner time will be easier for her.

**Update: In the time it took me to type the post, an aide came in and started helping Mom eat. Thank the good Lord. I know they are doing their best in a difficult situation.

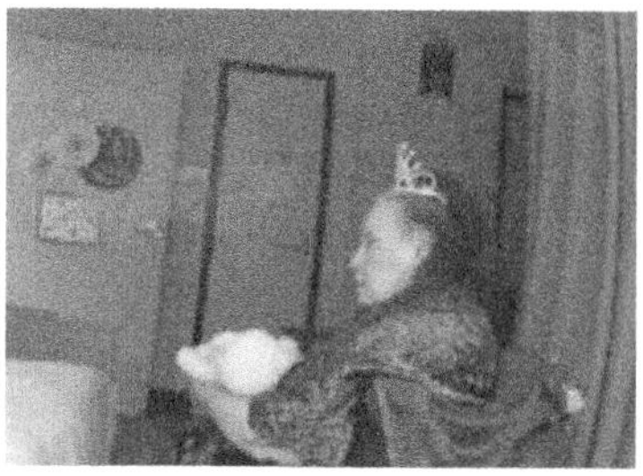

Mom Chronicles March 16, 2020
They have her up out of bed this morning. I miss her so much!

Mom Chronicles March 16, 2020
I had to laugh while doing a quick check-in on my mom. I could hear the activities' director, Miss T, in the hallway yelling - "can you all hear me?" They are about to play a round of Bingo. (Everyone is isolated in their rooms, and those playing Bingo are sitting in their doorways.) Of course, mom can't play (she doesn't understand how to play anymore), but nothing (even this stinky ole virus) gets in the way of the other residents playing Bingo! I love Miss T's ingenuity and on-the-spot problem-solving!!

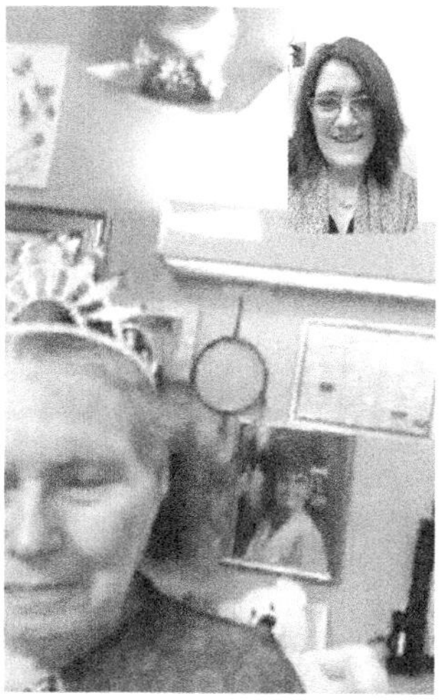

Mom Chronicles March 17, 2020
One of the sweet nursing aides just let me video chat with Mom. Thank you, Tammy Hernandez!

Mom Chronicles March 18, 2020
I'm not a happy camper at the moment and will be getting in touch with the director tomorrow morning. This is the first day in a while that Mom didn't get the level of care expected. I did call the nurse at 10:30 pm when I checked the camera, and luckily, she answered. She said she would be down there to help Mom shortly. Unfortunately, they are in a shift change, so it's going to be a little bit.

I don't know if they were short-staffed today or not, so I will just let her know what I saw through the camera so that she can address it ASAP. She is great, so I know she will take care of it. I feel so helpless with not being able to be there to help her. I have to be open-minded because I don't know what the situation was/is. I remember one time she didn't get the expected care, and it turns out a resident was in the process of passing away, so they were overwhelmed with that. I felt like poo after learning that.

I imagine things are going to be challenging for a while.

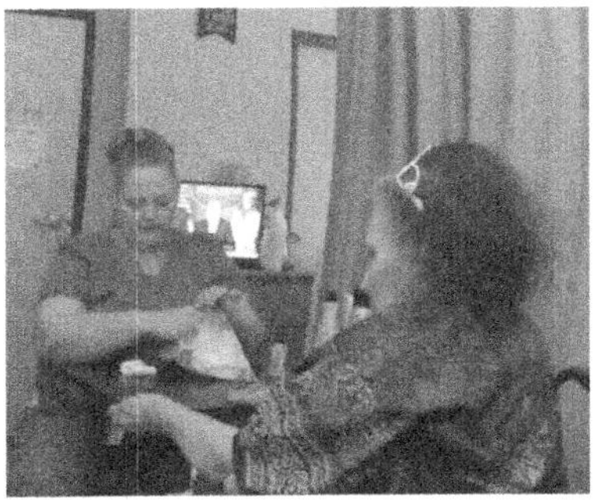

Mom Chronicles March 19, 2020

I was able to talk to the lead CNA this morning about my concern from yesterday. She resolved it immediately and understood my concern.

While talking to her, I also asked if any of the staff who knows how to apply Color Street nail strips would be willing to change the polish out on Mom. I usually change them out once a week. Tammy removed the old polish, and then another staff member applied the new strips. These staff members are truly going above and beyond for my mom and the residents. Thank you, Tammy!

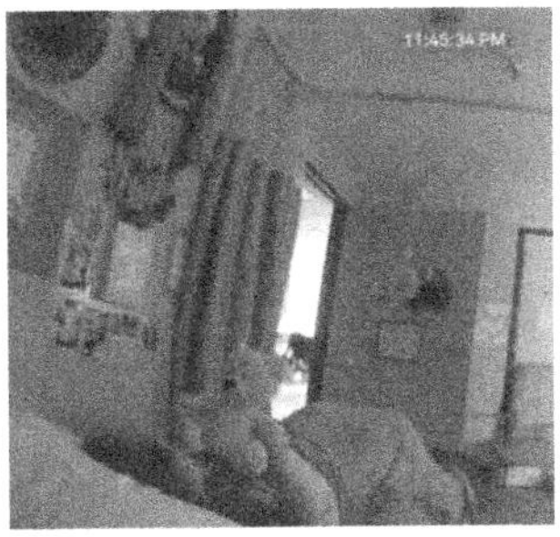

Mom Chronicles March 20, 2020

Mom and I both are wide awake at midnight. She's staying entertained with her bear. I am staying entertained with my phone. I think she's got the better deal. Joshua - I may need to snag Scraggly back!!

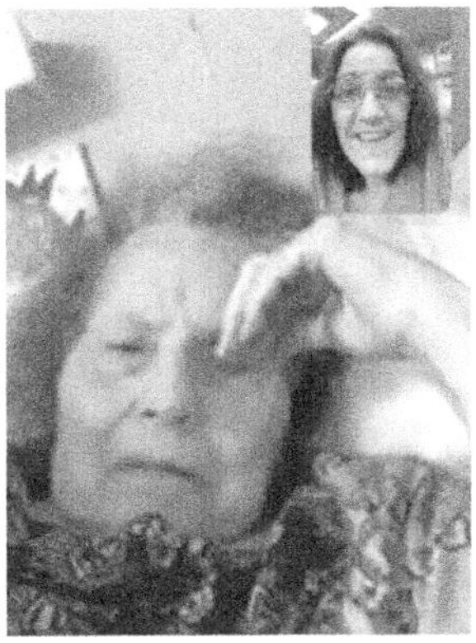

Mom Chronicles March 23, 2020

I had a quick video chat with Mom. She was able to say hi and yes to a couple of questions. She also tried to sing the "bushel and a peck" song. Then she kept nodding off, so we kept it short.

I'm thankful, thankful, thankful for technology and nurses/CNAs who care. I look dorky in the pic, but I don't care. I was able to say hi to my mommy.

Mom Chronicles March 25, 2020

Some of the aides forget just how important Mom's bear or baby doll is to keep her engaged. The aide brought a blanket to cover her legs but unfortunately put the bear on the bed out of her reach. Mom can't maneuver in the wheelchair by herself anymore, so all she can do is stare at the bear and not play with it.

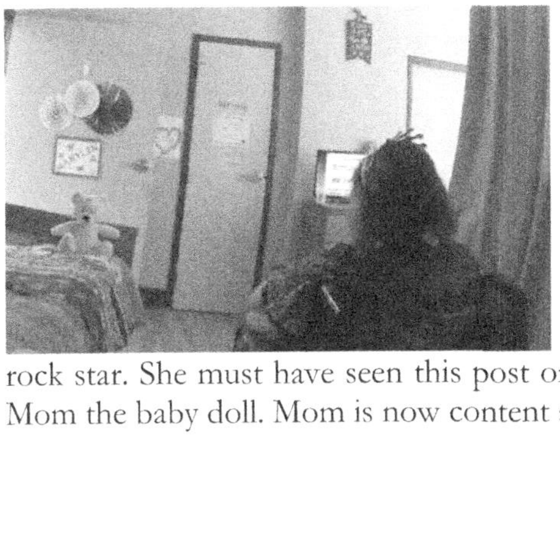

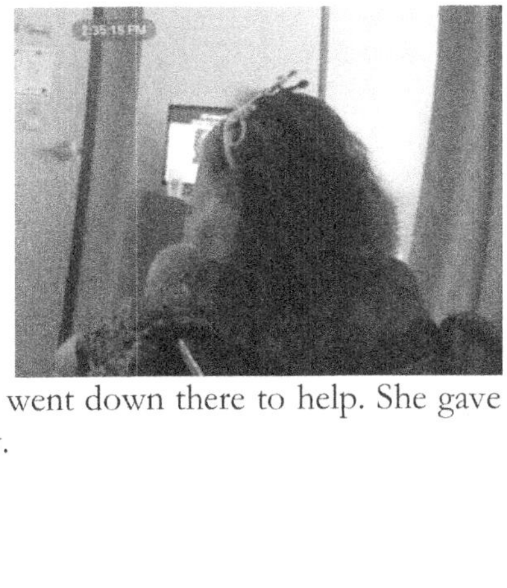

I am not going to call up there and ask them to bring it to her. I would rather reserve my phone calls for the important stuff. I just feel sad for her right now. Hopefully, an aide at the next check-in will give it to her. Update: Tammy is a rock star. She must have seen this post on Facebook and immediately went down there to help. She gave Mom the baby doll. Mom is now content and hugging/kissing her baby.

Mom Chronicles March 25, 2020
Mom doesn't have an appetite tonight. The aide is going to get a nutrition shake from the kitchen and see if Mom will drink it. I so wish I was there to try and help encourage her to eat.

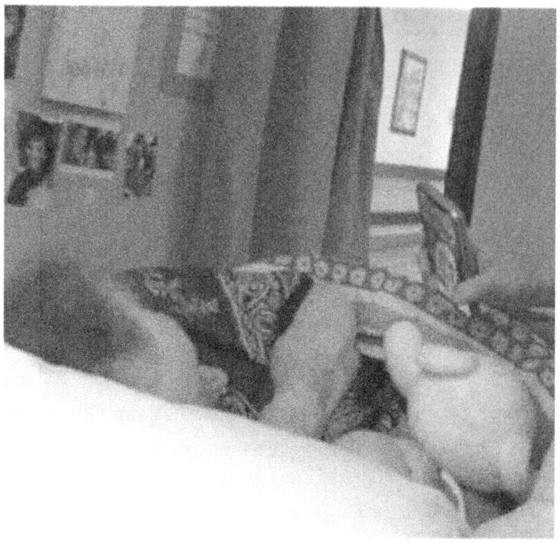

Mom Chronicles March 28, 2020
I just had a video chat with Mom. It was short and sweet. I got a "love you" from her. I'm so glad to hear those words when she can say them.

I had to put a sticker over my face in the pic before sharing. I am a hot mess right now. I'm still in my pajamas, and nothing is done so far to look presentable to the public. Thank you, Tammy, for the video chat this morning.

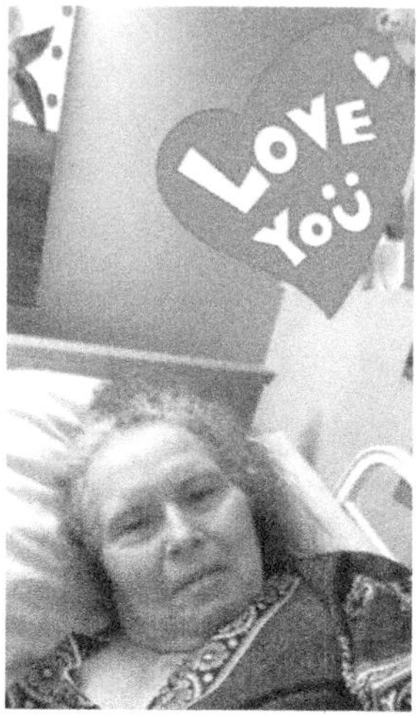

Mom Chronicles March 28, 2020
I love it when the aides take that extra few seconds to interact with Mom. The baby doll says words like "mama," "hello," etc. This aide, who is one of the best aides there at the center, pressed the tummy to let the baby talk to Mom before laying the baby down with her. I'm so thankful for nurses, aides, and staff who care so deeply for their patients.

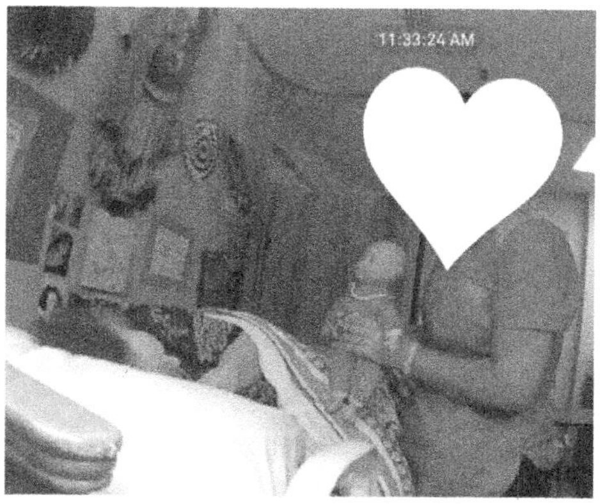

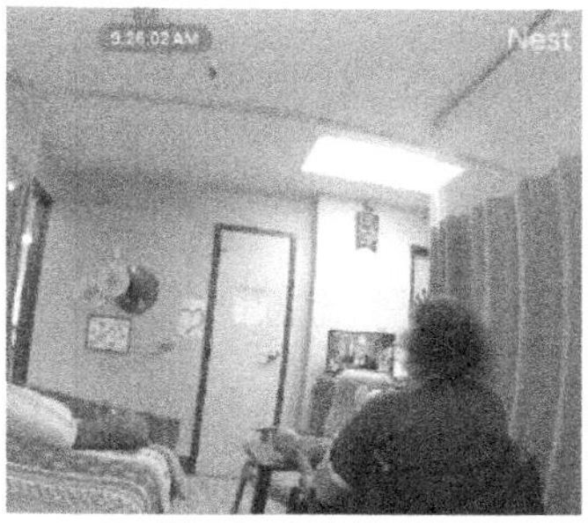

Mom Chronicles March 29, 2020
Mom is refusing her medications this morning. And by listening to the nurse, I learned Mom had a hard time yesterday swallowing the "whole" pills, so she crushed them up last night and this morning and put them in something easy for her to swallow. I'm guessing it is something to cover the bitter taste. She is still refusing.

She was pleading with her to take her meds. At one point, she even said, "I love you. Don't you want to live?" She was saying this in a nice way - not an ugly way at all. I know Mom didn't understand what she was saying - she doesn't understand anything except simple, familiar phrases. Maybe she will do better later and take her meds then.

♥

You can crush medicine up and put it into applesauce, pudding, milk, or fruit juice to cover the bitter taste. Check with a physician for ideas on the specific medicines your loved one needs to take that may need to be crushed at this stage.

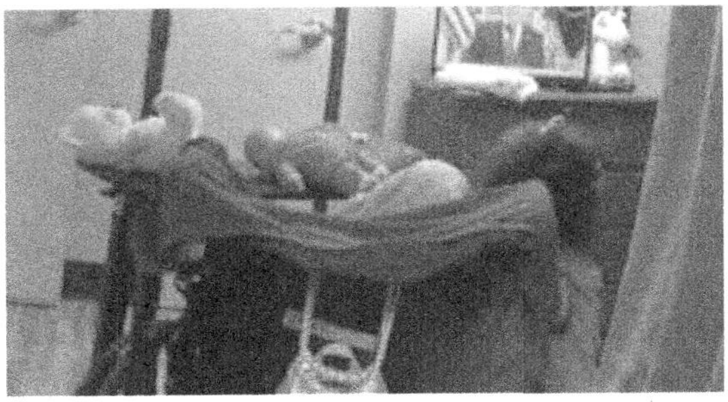

Mom Chronicles March 30, 2020

Mom fell out of her wheelchair at 4:30 pm. It looks like she must have fallen asleep and kept leaning over more and more to the right. To me, it sounded like she hit the ground hard, but they assessed her and didn't see any injuries. They said she slid out of her chair. That didn't sound or look like a "slide-out." They just called me a minute ago to report it to me. I think she is getting weaker and weaker—stupid virus. I want to see my Mom!! [It's hard to watch the video of her falling, so I didn't include it in the book.]

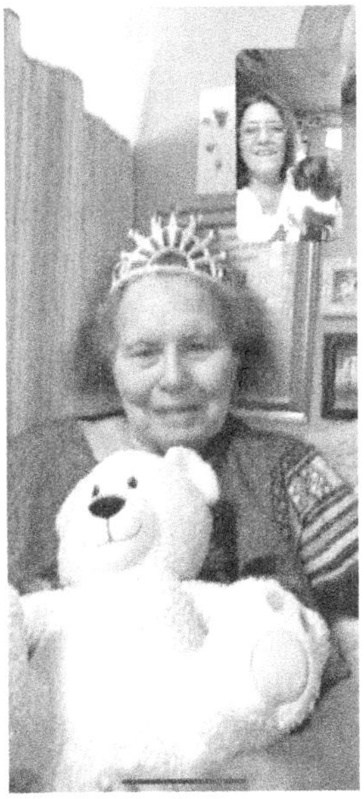

Mom Chronicles March 31, 2020

Mom is doing okay. She doesn't seem to be in pain from the fall. Tammy just video chatted with me so that I could talk to Mom. She was in a good mood and laughing. She was trying to talk, which is always a good sign. I feel better today, knowing she is not in pain.

Mom Chronicles April 1, 2020

Many of the folks at this nursing home go above and beyond for their patients. Mom's baby doll had fallen behind the bed. Miss T noticed that Mom's doll was missing, so she looked for it. She found it under/behind the bed. At first, she was going to have someone get it out for her, but she changed her mind and did it herself. What a beautiful lady who cares!! Tammy, please share my love and admiration for Miss T!

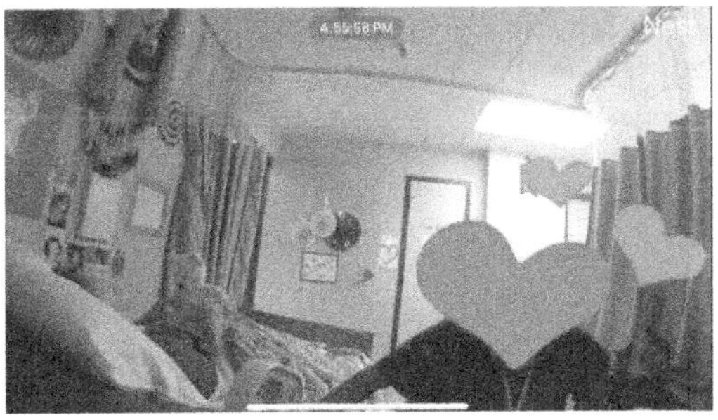

Mom Chronicles April 4, 2020

I've been noticing through the camera that Mom is refusing to eat a lot more lately - or only taking a few bites here and there. I listened to the nursing aide try to encourage her at dinner time tonight by saying her daughter was coming soon to visit. This fib doesn't bother me because, for someone with Alzheimer's, they will forget the conversation within 5 minutes anyway. With any luck, it will give her "hope" for that moment and encourage her to eat. It didn't work this time, though. I only saw her take a few bites. I know we are getting closer to the end of this Alzheimer's journey. I found this article that explains whether or not our loved one is "suffering" by feeling starved. According to the site, the loved one is not suffering. The part of her brain that controls hunger and thirst is shutting down. The body is adjusting to reduced food and fluids.

That brought a little comfort to me. I don't want her starving. It sounds like this is just the normal process. I just pray Sheila and I get to see her face to face again on this side of heaven.

www.scie.org.uk/dementia/advanced-dementia-and-end-of-life-care/end-of-life-care/eating-drinking.asp
(Dementia: Eating and drinking at the end of life, n.d.)

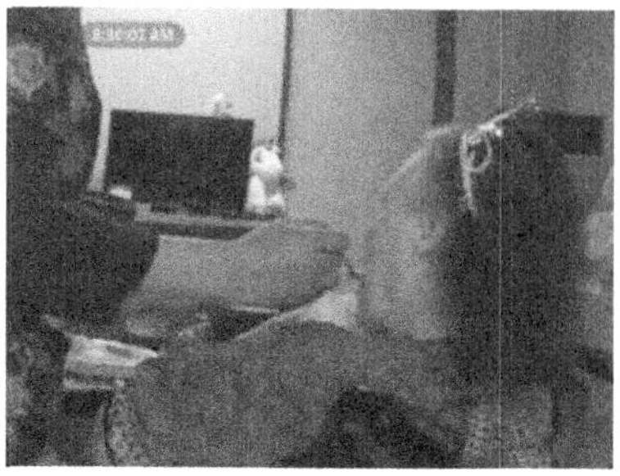

Mom Chronicles April 5, 2020
She's eating this morning. Hallelujah!

Mom Chronicles April 13, 2020
I haven't been able to talk to Mom via video for over a week. The staff are so busy - it's hard to catch them for a video chat. I can only imagine how hectic things are. I'm so thankful for the camera so that I can at least "see" her. She loves her baby doll.

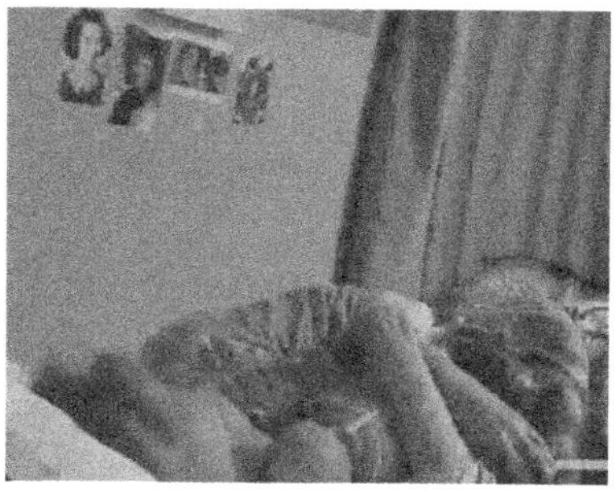

Mom Chronicles April 14, 2020
It looks like they tried a new wheelchair out on Mom. I'm not sure if this is the same one that was ordered several months ago. It has a different configuration that allows her to lay back and to support her legs more. They were having a hard time with her legs, though, because they are so "frozen" and permanently bent 90 degrees. I'm not sure if this will be her permanent new chair or not. They wheeled it back out after putting her back into bed.

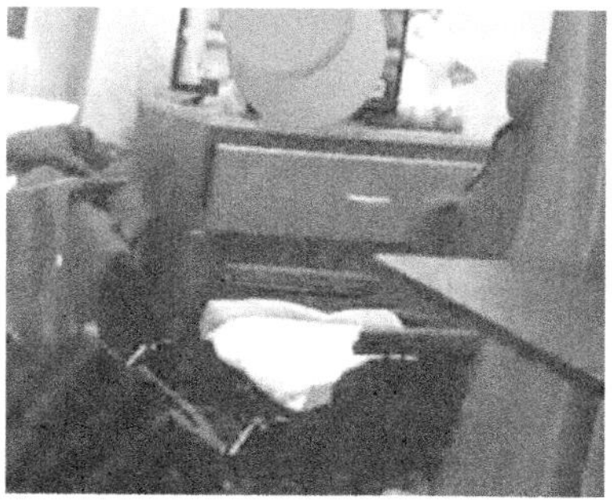

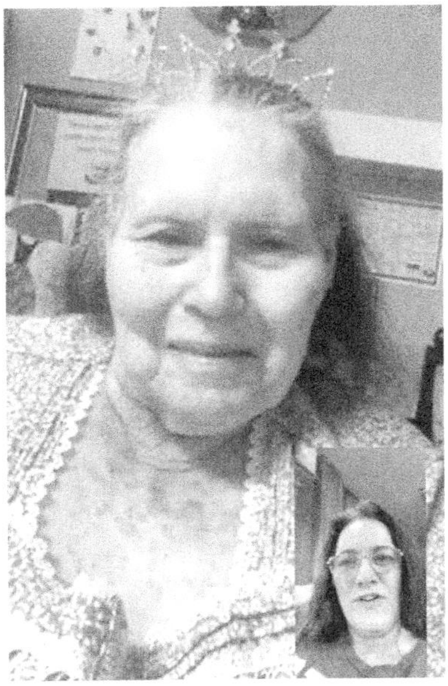

Mom Chronicles April 15, 2020
I was able to have a video call with Mom!! She was more awake and alert than the last several times. She didn't know my name, but she knew I was her daughter. They are also going to change out her nail polish today. Talking to her is just what I needed today! Thank you, Tammy!

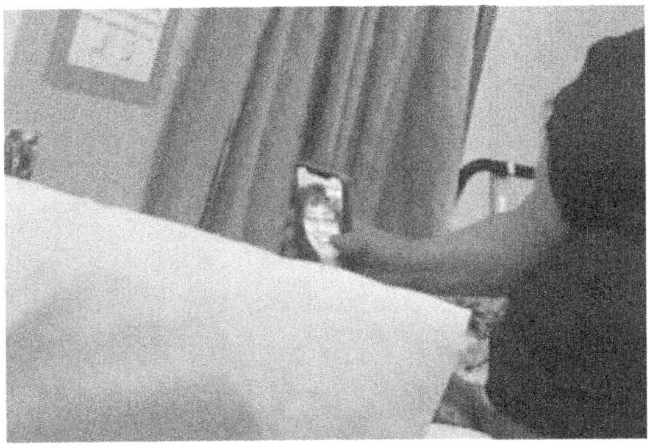

Mom Chronicles April 17, 2020
Sheila was able to video chat with Mom a little while ago. Yay!

Mom Chronicles April 17, 2020
The speech therapist came in a few minutes ago and tried several types of food out with Mom to see what consistency of food she needs. It takes her a long time to chew, and an aide reported that Mom had a hard time swallowing bites of food today. Mom kept refusing to try the pudding in the test. At the end of the test, she told Mom she would put her on some softer food and then check in on Monday to see how she's doing.

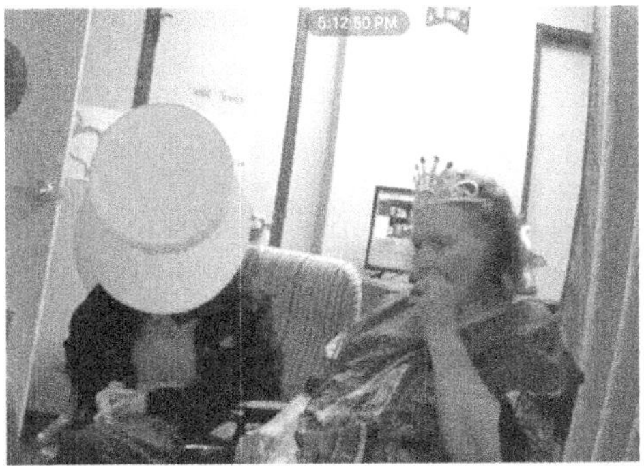

The DON reported she's lost 5 pounds, so hopefully, this will help make sure she's eating.

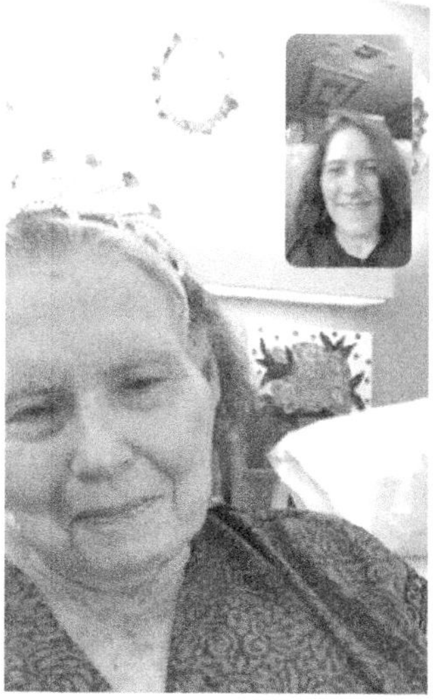

Mom Chronicles April 18, 2020

Tammy just FaceTimed with me so that I could try to encourage Mom to eat. She wanted nothing to do with the pudding but did like the ice cream.

Tammy said they put Mom on the list of residents who need a little more interaction from staff. Staff will stop by more often to say hi or to try and get her to eat.

I put Simi in the camera, and Mom lit up. She was trying to get Simi's attention with little noises. Simi got more interaction than me!!

She was able to say "I love you" twice to me. I'll take it.

Sheila was able to FaceTime next. As always, thank you, Tammy!

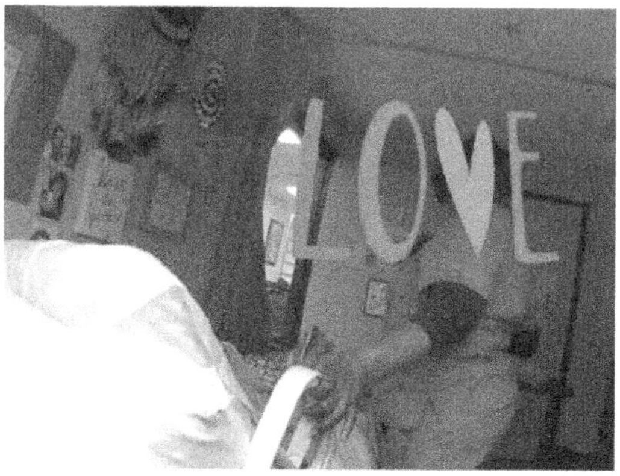

Mom Chronicles April 22, 2020

I can't be there to tell her I love her, but when I hear an aide call her beautiful and say, "I love you," it makes my heart full. Thank you to the nurses and aides who are stepping in for families and letting our loved ones know they are loved and not forgotten.

Mom Chronicles April 23, 2020

She was holding a picture of you today, Joshua. She must have taken it off her wall, or it may have been on her table, and someone gave it to her. I'm not sure, but she was happy looking at your face.

She may not know your name or that you are her grandson, but she knows she loves you. That's all that matters.

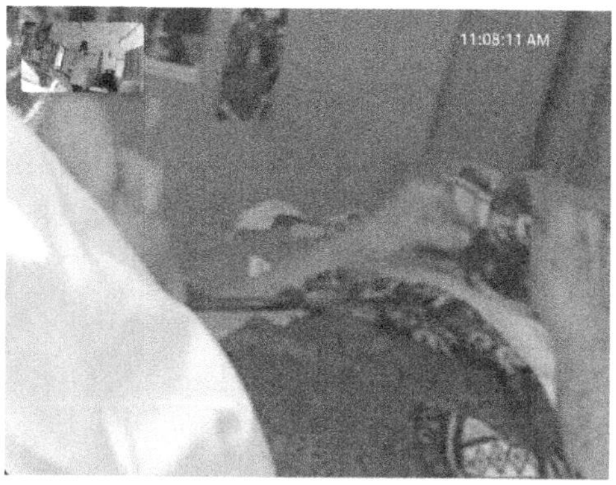

Mom Chronicles April 28, 2020

The speech-language therapist sat with Mom for about an hour at lunchtime today, trying to get her to eat. Finally, she was able to get her to eat some. Mom would refuse some, so she would wait a few minutes or have her take a drink and then try again. Slowly but surely, she was able to get her to take some bites.

Mom also forgot to swallow her food some. So the therapist had to keep reminding her to swallow. Mom did better when she had the bread or brownie or cup of water/juice in her hand. It helped to trigger her brain that she needed to chew/swallow. It didn't always work, but it helped some. Unfortunately, there is no way we can expect an aide to sit with her for a solid hour to help her eat. They have other patients to help. Most of the time, they just try a few times to get her to eat and then give up and get the nutrition shake. I can't blame them. It's hard to watch, but I can't blame them.

I'm not sure if the therapist will make any changes to her diet because of this. I'll just have to keep monitoring through the camera to see. I am grateful that she took the time today to work with Mom to see how she's doing.

This last stage of Alzheimer's is a hard one to watch. (Well - none of them are easy to watch.) I don't like it; I don't like it; I don't like it.

Mom Chronicles April 29, 2020
My friend Jenni, the former director of the memory care center where Mom lived (and more importantly, my friend), just sent this to me. She permitted me to share.

"A thought for you to ponder... What you and your mom are going through is just a season in this life... she's had past seasons, and you will still have future seasons. As you wait for her to move to her next, don't lose focus of YOUR next season on this earth.

People tend to hold their breath and focus on their loved one's ending. When it happens, and the loved one is gone, they get slammed with feelings of 'what do we do now?

While you can, right now, make sure you have a focus that will carry you through that first three months after she passes... a hobby, a work project, a cause, your book.... something that you are so passionate about that it will keep you from feeling both her loss and a 'what now' kind of loss for yourself.... tell Bruce what that is and make him agree now, to push you towards that when she passes."

I have several friends going through this "season," too. Just substitute Bruce's name in the sentence with someone in your life who can agree to push you.

Mom Chronicles May 4, 2020
Miss T was able to video chat with me today. I could get Mom to smile and blow me a kiss but could not get any words out of her. I really couldn't tell if she knew me. She kept looking at Miss T mostly. I wonder what is going through her mind when she sees all the masks on the nurses and staff members.

Through the camera, I saw that she only ate a few bites at breakfast and refused all food and drink at lunch.

I've been struggling this past week, so I'm going to stop with this and just post that I was happy to see her face today. Oh... and I had Miss T take the phone over to Ms. S's room so that I could say hi to her. She is the lady who sat at the next table in the dining hall, and I would always chat with her while helping Mom with dinner. So it was nice to put a smile on her face today too.

Mom Chronicles May 6, 2020
Mom is refusing to eat and drink today, even the shake. So I asked the aide to keep coming back and trying. Update... Another aide came in, and it looks like she could get her to take a few drinks. Hallelujah.

Mom Chronicles May 6, 2020
Long post...

My dear friend Myra Scrabeck shared this with me. She recently went through this journey with her mom and is okay with me sharing. She is an educator like me and wants to help people as much as possible.

"Lori, I just read your post on your mom not eating. I just wanted to let you know what happened when my mom stopped eating. It was similar to what was happening with your mom over the last couple of weeks. Mom ate less and less until finally, she just pretty much stopped. We would try to coax her to eat in any way we could think of, bringing her shakes, watermelon, cake, etc., etc., etc. Every once in a while, she would take a sip of something or a bite of something, but that was usually all. They told us at that time that this is a natural progression of the disease. The body starts shutting down, and they told us not to coax her so much. She stopped being able to digest food easily and started getting very constipated in that kind of thing. I think it would be good if you talked to the head nurse or her doctor and explained what's happening and see what they advise you all in this. This is a very, very hard part of the disease when it starts happening. You want to feed her and get her to drink, but it just might not be possible whether you were able to be with her or not. A doctor would know if she was at that point or not."

I then asked her how long it took for her mom to pass once she quit completely eating and drinking. She said it was less than a week. I know that every person is different, and God has a plan for each soul.

I contacted the nurse to discuss this. Luckily, the doctor was there today, so he took a quick look at her. He is removing the Aricept (the memory medicine) and Cymbalta medications and putting her on a different antidepressant with an appetite stimulant.

She said this could also be situational depression since she can't leave her room and see her family.

If this doesn't work, the doctor said he would consider hospice. But even then, the hospice worker can't go into the building. It can only be through Telehealth, so that is a huge limitation.

All I can say is that today has been rough. I pray the new meds work but, in my heart, I know they won't. Hopefully, I'm wrong.

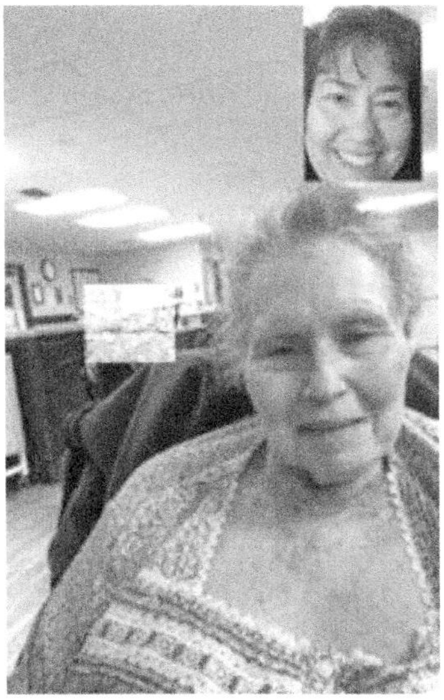

Mom Chronicles May 7, 2020
Blessings, blessings, blessings.

I noticed in the camera that they had taken Mom out of her room about an hour ago. I just got a video call from Tammy. They had wheeled her down to the TV room to change her environment for breakfast. All other patients are in their rooms to reduce any exposure risks.

The aide is with her and has been able to get her to eat two pieces of toast with jelly, and she is drinking her nutrition shake. She is usually more alert in the mornings, so she was able to smile and tell me she loves me.

While she was doing this good, I asked her to try video calling my sister quickly so that she could see her. I'm hoping she was able to get through to her. Sheila and I were struggling last night. We are losing Mom, and we can't be there with her. Update - Sheila was able to video with her!! I don't know if this is a fluke and that she will stop eating again. I'm just grateful they tried something new with her, and it worked this morning. Tammy asked if it was okay to take her out of her room at mealtimes to see if this helps encourage Mom to eat. I said yes, yes, yes!

Mom Chronicles May 7, 2020
The camera is offline now. The lady sweeping the floor accidentally hit the cord and unplugged it. In the past, when this has happened, I've never been able to get it to reset automatically. I asked them to plug it back in for me to try to reset from a distance. I'm not sure if they were able to plug it back in. I contacted two different people.

If it doesn't reset automatically, I will be heartbroken because I won't see my mom through the camera. I may beg them to let me in just for a moment with all my PPE (gloves, masks) and go straight to the room without Mom in it and not touch anything but the camera and hotspot. I don't think they will let me, but it can't hurt to ask. I'll see if Tammy can try rebooting the hotspot to see if that will reset it.

Mom Chronicles May 9, 2020
The head CNA is supposed to meet me at the nursing home this morning to try and get the camera back online. I will stand outside the window and try to walk her through all the different button-pushing steps to get it working today. Fingers crossed! I've hated not checking in on Mom these last two days. Besides the occasional FaceTime calls, this is the only way that Sheila and I can see her.

Mom Chronicles May 9, 2020
My heart is full! The camera is back on, and they brought Mom to the door to let me see her that way. At first, she motioned for me to come in. Tammy and I had to fib and say I was not feeling well and did not want to give her my germs. (She probably didn't understand what we were saying at all.)

She was able to say I love you, and blow me kisses. It was a short visit, but it made all the difference in the world.

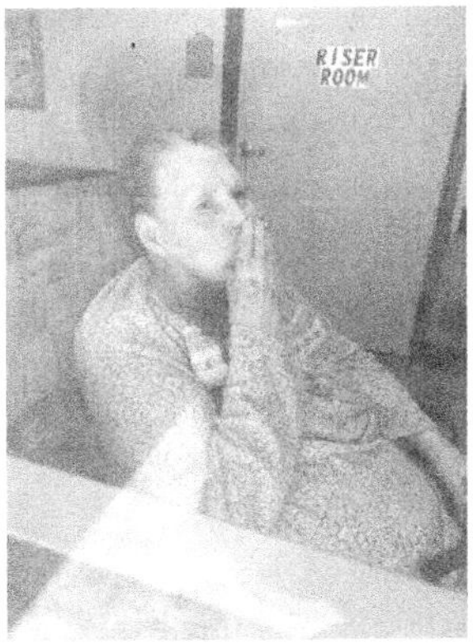

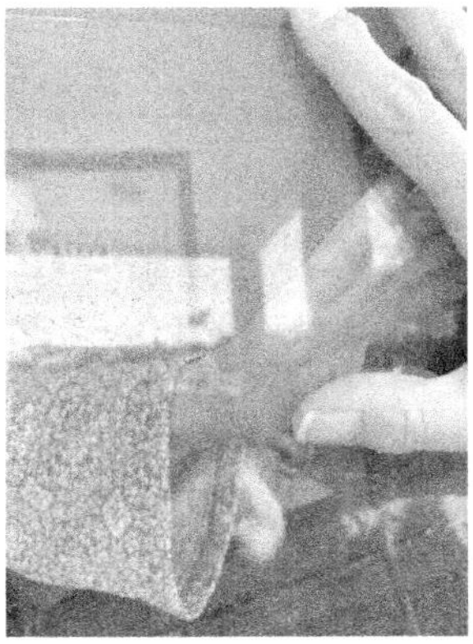
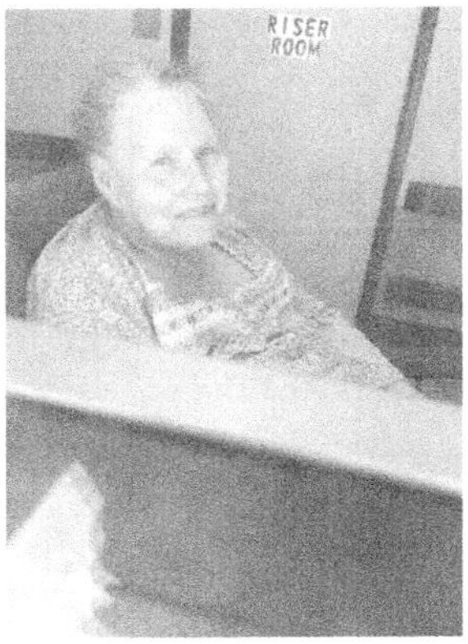

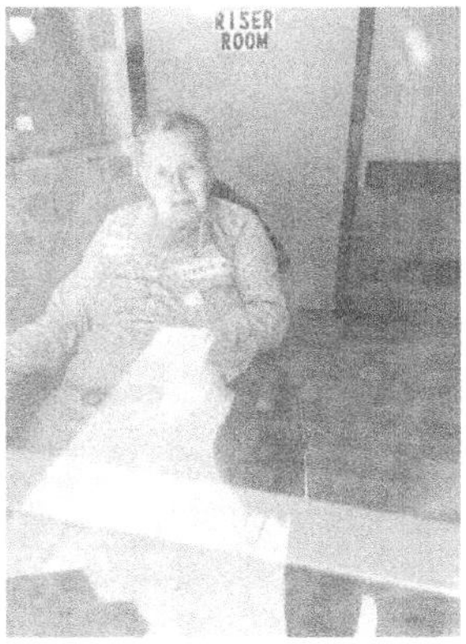

Mom Chronicles May 12, 2020
Mom is persnickety tonight. She didn't eat lunch and only drank her shake. She didn't eat dinner, so the aide brought her a nutrition shake a few minutes ago. She refused it, so he left the drink on her table. After he left, she picked it up, put it to her side, and then promptly dropped it on the floor. When he comes back to check on her, he will have a big mess to clean up! I should be sad that she didn't eat or drink her health shake, but all I could do was laugh. I can just imagine her face when she dropped that drink on the floor. "You can't make me" comes to mind! Oh, and if you were wondering, that is the same face my sister would make when she didn't want to do something. My grandma always said my mom and my sis were just alike!!!

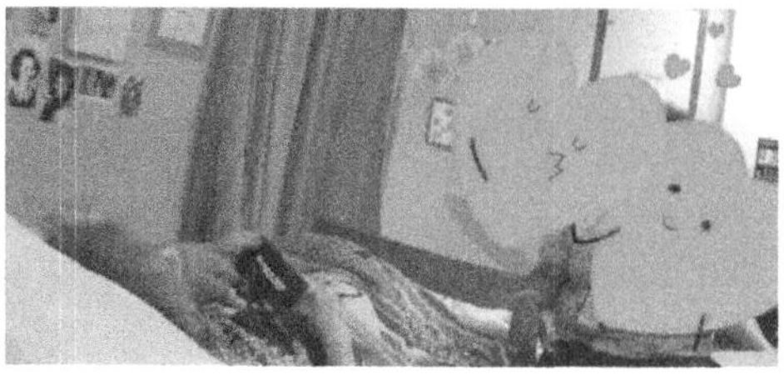

Mom Chronicles May 18, 2020
I checked back through the recording today, and I saw one of the ladies who stayed a little later than usual in there with Mom trying to get her to eat some dinner (she ate a few bites!) and played Elvis music for Mom on her phone. I just love her for genuinely caring for the residents as much as she does.

I also saw the speech therapist work with her in trying to eat a little bit this morning. I've seen her with Mom quite a bit over the last few weeks trying to encourage Mom to eat. Some aides try just a couple of bites and then give up and move on. And then I see folks like these two ladies who keep trying. I'm sure Mom loved the Elvis music.

Mom Chronicles May 20, 2020
The Activities Director stopped by Mom's room to show her a card mailed by Sheila and to play 3 Elvis songs for Mom. Mom was trying to sing, and a few times, she "danced" in her wheelchair. I love people who truly care. She definitely does. She even told Mom, "I love you" several times.

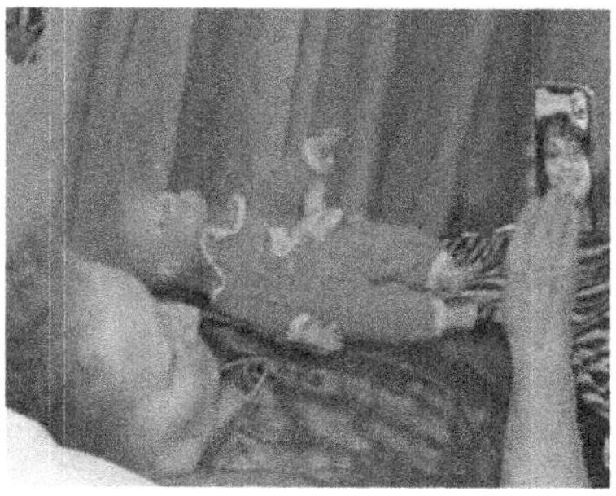

Mom Chronicles May 22, 2020
I looked in on Mom and saw that my sister was able to video chat with Mom for a few minutes. So I grabbed this shot of Mom touching Sheila's face. I will be so happy when we can really touch each other's faces again.

Mom Chronicles May 28, 2020
The Activities Director, Tanzania Wallace, aka Miss T, visited Mom today to play several Elvis songs. She was able to get her to smile some and "dance" a little. What I thought was extremely thoughtful is that she turned Mom around so that we could see her face through the camera. It was great seeing hints of a smile and her dancing slightly. It did strike me, though, that her hair seems so much grayer now from the front. I miss her but am soooo grateful for moments like this.

Mom Chronicles June 1, 2020
I just received a call that Mom tested negative for Covid but that two residents and one staff member have tested positive. None showed symptoms. The staff member has not been there since last week. The residents have been moved to a different hall. They will test all residents again. Please pray for our nursing home that this has not/will not spread. I'm thankful they are keeping family informed.

Mom Chronicles June 3, 2020

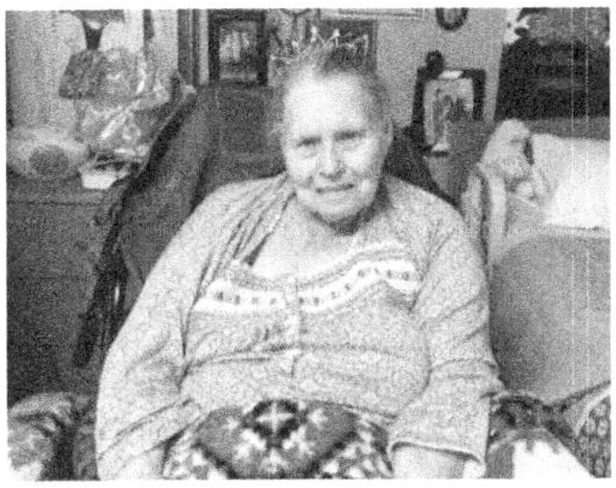

I had a short video call with Mom, and it was wonderful. She was more alert today and able to say "I love you very much" in her garbled way. She also tried to sing our "bushel and a peck" song. I talked briefly with the aide, and she said Mom has been eating and drinking a little better with the appetite stimulant. So maybe, just maybe, she will hang around long enough for Sheila and me to be able to see her again on this earth. I just pray she wasn't exposed to COVID like the others were at the nursing home. I see a glimmer of hope, and I'm holding on to it.

Mom Chronicles June 22, 2020

I'm not happy. I'm trying to find out if something is wrong with Mom. She was brought back from her shower around 11:30, and then she was never served lunch. The aide completely forgot about her. Hopeful the DON will answer me soon.

Edit: the DON had to leave the facility early today but assured me Mom would get her dinner tonight and then would talk to the CNA in the morning.

As an added measure, I contacted the former director of the nursing home, who is now a regional director for this nursing home system. She said she would follow up on this. I don't like going over one's head but not feeding my mom is unacceptable. Even if she's not eating well, I want them to try and give her a few bites or give her the nutrition shake.

Mom Chronicles June 25, 2020

I noticed they put Mom on oxygen this morning. The nurse just called and said her O2 levels were borderline low. They wanted to try the oxygen today to see if it helps. They said they would also run some labs just to check everything out since they noticed a slight decline with her, and she's staying sleepy. They will let me know the results.

Mom Chronicles June 26, 2020

Last night, I asked the nurse via text message how Mom was. She told me Mom was still on oxygen but that her stats were okay. She told me if anything changed overnight, she would call me. When I checked the camera this morning, I saw that the nurse peeped in several times overnight on her, once with a flashlight from the door. I may be wrong, but I think she was checking to see if Mom was still breathing.

Mom's oxygen level came up enough this morning that they were able to take her off oxygen, but her blood pressure was really low. It was 90 something over 50 something. So they took her off her blood pressure meds (Mom has always had high blood pressure), and it has started coming back up.

The CNA tried doing a video call with me, but I was hosting an important meeting via Zoom at work, so I couldn't talk to Mom at the moment. It broke my heart because it's been a few weeks since we've received a video call. She looked horrible for the few moments I saw her. Her face looked haggard, and her jaw was hanging open. I don't think she recognized me. I asked the nurse to try videoing with Sheila instead since I couldn't talk right then. Sheila said that she did get to have the video call.

At lunch, I noticed the aide having a hard time waking Mom up. They are running several tests to see if they can determine what's going on. Hopefully, they will get results soon. I watched the recording when they drew the blood this morning. Normally Mom screams or jerks away when they put the band around her arm and stick her with the needle. She never flinched. She didn't even acknowledge that she was getting her blood drawn. They will be monitoring her stats carefully.

Sheila is coming up this weekend to visit me for the first time since the COVID lockdown. If we see that Mom is better and strong enough to sit up in her wheelchair, we will try and get them to wheel her down the hall to let us see her through the door. Wish us luck and that Mom starts to feel better this weekend.

Mom Chronicles June 27, 2020
We were watching through the camera and saw that they got her out of bed today for lunch. So we hightailed it over to the nursing home to try to see her through the door after they fed her and before they put her back in the bed. It was a shift change, so it took about 30 minutes, but we finally got one of her aides to help us. I gave him my phone number, and we all talked through the speakers on our phones. Mom didn't say anything, but we got some big smiles out of her a few times. This is the first time Sheila has been up here since the lockdown and the first time she saw her through the door. I had seen her once before on Mother's Day weekend.

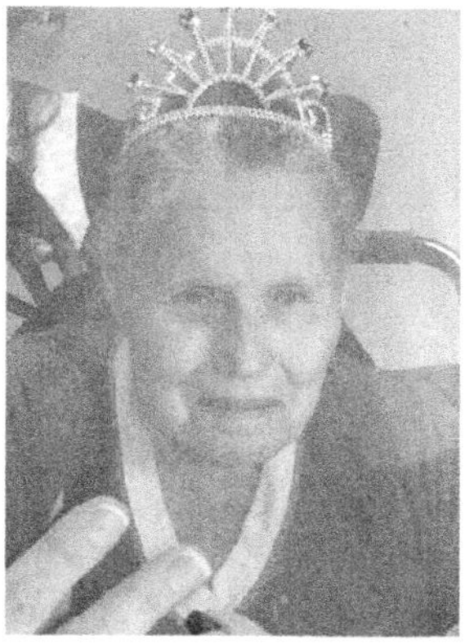
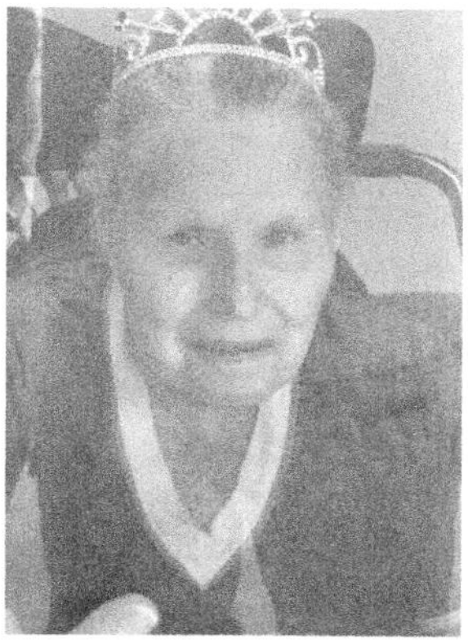
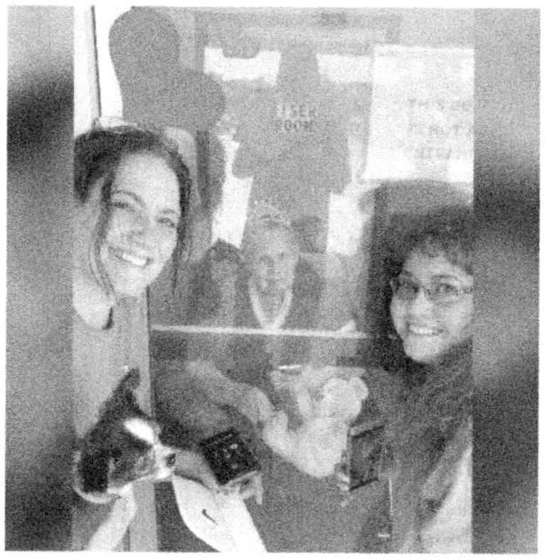

Mom Chronicles June 29, 2020
I heard from the DON this afternoon. Several of Mom's labs came back elevated, including her white blood cell count. They also think she is dehydrated.

They have started an IV to give her fluids and an antibiotic for seven days. They said they would place it "mid-line" to be harder for her to pull out. I had to look that up. It's much longer than a regular IV and can stay in for 7-14 days.

Our camera got knocked offline again today, so hopefully, we'll get it back online tomorrow so that I can keep checking in on her.

I'm praying this treatment snaps her out of not feeling well. Yesterday, I noticed she didn't eat or drink at any of her meals.

Lastly, I learned that there would be a new DON. She started today. I'm praying I will have a good relationship with her too.

Mom Chronicles June 30, 2020
I got a call from the nursing home. They have had a 911 crew pick her up. They are concerned about a possible clot. Because she's nonverbal, one family member can be with her. I'm here at the ER waiting to be

let in to see her. They are checking her in now. I will keep you all posted because I know many of you love my mom as well.

Mom Chronicles June 30, 2020
I'm with her now and have so many mixed feelings. I'm glad to see her, touch her face and hold her hand. But she's nonresponsive. They are running a lot of tests on her. I have been able to get her eyes open a few times but not much. She grinned at least a couple of times.

I can tell she's lost weight since I saw her 3 1/2 months ago. I'm not going to post a photo of her. She looks pretty frail.

Mom Chronicles June 30, 2020
She does not have any blood clots. She does have a slight case of pneumonia, though. So, the doctor is giving her a round of fluids and an antibiotic. Once that's done (in about an hour), she will be discharged back to the nursing home. So, I'm going to love on her for another hour or so while I can.

Mom Chronicles June 30, 2020
Mom was released from the hospital back to the nursing home after a round of fluids and antibiotics.

I was able to spend those precious few hours with her holding her hand, hugging her, kissing her forehead, and singing to her. She would open her eyes every so often, and when she would, I would Skype with Sheila.

Mom doesn't look well at all. I truly believe that was the last time I will see her alive until I see her in heaven.

With COVID, no one is allowed in nursing homes. Not even hospice - at least that's the case at this facility.

Mom is in 14 days of isolation now, so I won't see her through the camera. She was moved to a room away from all the others. So I'm just going to have to trust that they will take good care of her. I'll make sure they have at least taken her doll or bear down there to her. But if she remains in the same shape as she is today, she won't even realize she has the doll or bear.

Pray for her. If it's getting close to her time to transition, please pray that she goes peacefully. But, of course, the good Lord can also surprise me and heal her long enough for us all to get past COVID and see her again. Miracles do happen.

Mom Chronicles July 1, 2020
I found out that when Mom gets down to the last few days of her life, the nursing home will let us in to see her. This is a change in their policy, hallelujah.

They let us see her via FaceTime a few minutes ago. Unfortunately, she's still out of it.

They are working on getting the camera set up in her room. They also brought her bear down there to her room and the CD player with Elvis so that they can play the CD for her often.

We also learned the main aides who are used to taking care of her will still be taking care of her. I love that continuity. Lastly, we were told they would let Sheila and I come in when they see the signs of when/if she's declining. So I'm thankful we may get the chance to see her again. We are still hoping the antibiotics and fluids snap her out of this, though.

Mom Chronicles July 2, 2020
Praise report! The nurse called me a little while ago and said Mom is much better today. She ate 50% of her breakfast, is more alert, and is smiling at them. Hallelujah!

Mom Chronicles July 3, 2020
We were able to FaceTime with her!!! And she lit up when she saw Josh and Bruce. She actually waved then. We were able to get her to blow a kiss. She's looking soooo much better!

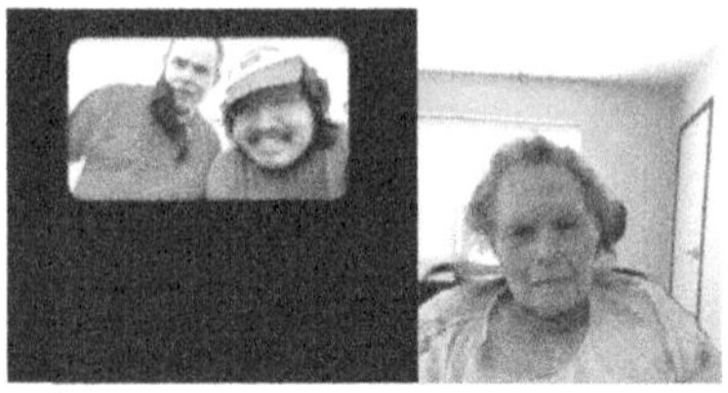

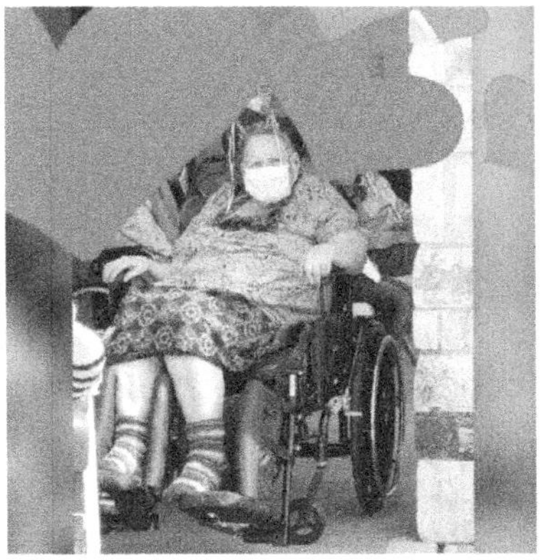

Mom Chronicles July 4, 2020
We are about to do a 4th of July parade at 10:00 at Mom's nursing home! They said they would bring her out to watch the parade. We were afraid they wouldn't since she is in isolation for a couple of weeks. I'll take a photo of her when we drive by her.

Update: we made three trips around. She wasn't out on the first trip.

Many families participated, and the fire department started it off with their fire engine truck with lights and sirens. It was great to see her!!

Thank you, Tammy, for helping to get her outside to let us see her!

Mom Chronicles July 7, 2020
I got a call from the nurse about 30 minutes ago. Mom is weak and lethargic again. The doctor has put her on another round of 7 days of IV fluids to see if that perks her back up again. I don't want to lose her, but I don't want her suffering either. Have I mentioned lately that Alzheimer's bites??

Mom Chronicles July 8, 2020
First - good news. She was more alert this morning.

Second - We are now at the stage of pureed foods and thick nectar liquids for Mom because of her difficulty with swallowing and just remembering "how to eat." The speech therapist called me this morning to report a few things:
1. they noticed Mom does not recognize that she has food left in her mouth (At snack time, they found eggs left tucked into her cheeks from a morning's breakfast.)
2. normal liquids like juice were just dribbling out of the front of her mouth because she can't control it

She fed Mom the pureed breakfast and thick nectar liquid this morning, and she ate 100% of the meal. She only turned her head away once to refuse, so she stepped out for a few minutes and came back to try again. After that, mom didn't refuse anymore. The therapist feels that Mom won't refuse as much anymore since it will be easier to tolerate the food. She also said she educated the staff on how to help Mom with this stage. Each stage is a new experience.

Mom Chronicles July 8, 2020
My heart always stops a moment when I see the nursing home call. This time it was to report someone else has tested positive there at the center. They didn't say if it was a patient or a staff member. They asked permission to test Mom again, so of course, I permitted that.

Mom Chronicles July 8, 2020
Welllll... I received another call from the nursing home. A test just came back showing Mom has a blood clot in her left leg. Apparently, it doesn't call for hospitalization. Instead, she will be given "Eliquis" to dissolve it.

Mom Chronicles July 10, 2020
A friend shared a website with me with jewelry that has the "Bushel and a Peck" lyrics. Mom and Ted used to sing this song to each other all the time. Because Mom was familiar with this song, Sheila and I started singing it with her as well.

I bought three necklaces - one for each of us, although Mom will probably not wear her necklace. I also bought a bracelet that has the lyrics and Sheila's and my name on it. I plan on using mine as the centerpiece of whatever art project I do with her costume jewelry in the future.

[I am wearing the necklace in my author's photo for the book in memory of my mother, and we put one of the necklaces and the bracelet on Mom when we laid her to rest.]

Mom Chronicles July 13, 2020
I received a call from one of the nurses at the nursing home. Mom's skin has taken a sudden turn for the worse and is breaking down in several places. He said this is indicative of something happening internally, which is common towards the end of life.

The doctor recommended palliative care (not quite Hospice yet). He could send her to the hospital today, but they would just discharge her either this afternoon or in the next day or two. Mom would be out of her comfort zone, and the nurses wouldn't know Mom's routine in care. It would give us another opportunity to see her right now, but after talking to Sheila and Bruce, we decided not to send her to the hospital. It would only be for very selfish reasons to do that. She would be put in another 14-day isolation. Palliative care means they will continue to change her, attempt to feed her, and give her meds, but it also allows for medication to keep her comfortable.

We will be making a 3-way call with the new DON tomorrow to find out exactly at what point they will allow family in to see her. The nurse I spoke to, who has been an amazing advocate for Mom since we first moved her there, said he would have eyes on her every day monitoring the wounds, and when he sees that point of the "deep dive," he would let us know. He promised to keep me updated on Mom's condition.

So... we are taking another step forward on her life's path. We mainly want her to be comfortable. It would have been extremely selfish to send her to the hospital and delay that for a few days just for us to see her physically. We just pray that we will get the opportunity to see her at some point before her last breath.

Mom Chronicles July 14, 2020
Sheila and I just got off a group call with the new DON. She was very nice and listened to our concerns.

She will talk to her regional director to see what options they can do about letting us in to see Mom because she is in her "end of life" stage. We will also investigate hospice facility options because, from what we understand, they allow families in without restrictions. She even said that Mom fits all the criteria for hospice and end of life, so we think we have a leg to stand on. The governor's orders even state that families can see loved ones at the end of life. It doesn't specifically say a few hours left. It says end of life, which could be days, weeks, or even a few months. So, wish us luck. And trust me - we want to keep everyone safe in a facility. We can follow all the guidelines that staff follow to keep COVID away from us.

Update: Nope - they still aren't going to allow us in. She isn't "imminent." I have asked what their definition of "imminent" is. I've also sent a message to the nursing home's parent company for their definition of "imminent" and "end of life." The governor's orders say, "compassionate care which includes "end of life." The CDC even says visitors can be allowed for compassionate care. We are just a little frustrated.

Mom Chronicles July 15, 2020

After several text messages, calls, and Sheila contacting the nursing home's ombudsman, we are finally going to get to see Mom. We don't know all the parameters yet, but they are moving Mom to a different hall and are working out the guidelines. We weren't being ugly - because we know they are in between a rock and a hard place - but Mom fits the guidelines from both the governor of our state and the CDC. Compassionate care visits - which include "end of life" - are allowed. It's not just limited to "imminent" status.

We understand that we need to wear full PPE, and we are more than willing to accommodate that. I want to keep the staff and other residents safe as well.

Update: Praise Jesus - we are going to be able to see her before she leaves us!! Sheila is headed up here after work today.

Now we are waiting to hear what their guidelines will be. If it's still not enough, I have a couple of in-patient hospice facilities to call.

Thank you for the prayers on this. Resolutions that can satisfy all parties can be worked out.

♥

If you noticed in this last post, I mentioned an "ombudsman." A Long-Term Care Ombudsman is someone who protects the rights of assisted living and nursing home residents. They will listen to residents and their families when there are concerns, and they will share the rights that the residents and family members have. But, most importantly, which helped our case, they will solve problems and make sure that state regulations and laws are being followed concerning the resident. Without our ombudsman, we don't believe we would have been allowed in by the nursing home. You can find more information about ombudsmen on your state's government site.

Mom Chronicles July 16, 2020

We have a little more information.

1) we can have a 1-hour visit with Mom in full PPE, and we cannot touch her at all. No hand-holding. No kissing her forehead. Nothing. That's better than nothing.
2) we are trying to get her referred to a local hospice facility that allows 24/7 visitation. The only catch will be that they must determine she qualifies for general inpatient care. Medicare will pay 100% for the care. Otherwise, we would have to pay $375 a day. We just can't do that. I'm praying they will determine she qualifies for GIP.

Mom Chronicles July 16, 2020

We have been blessed with a visit and an understanding director, nursing staff, etc. Once Mom's COVID test comes back (hopefully first thing tomorrow), she will be moved to a hospice facility where we can spend

24/7 with her until... She is no longer eating or drinking. She opened her eyes for us earlier. We played Elvis music, and we swear we thought we saw her "dance" for a brief moment.

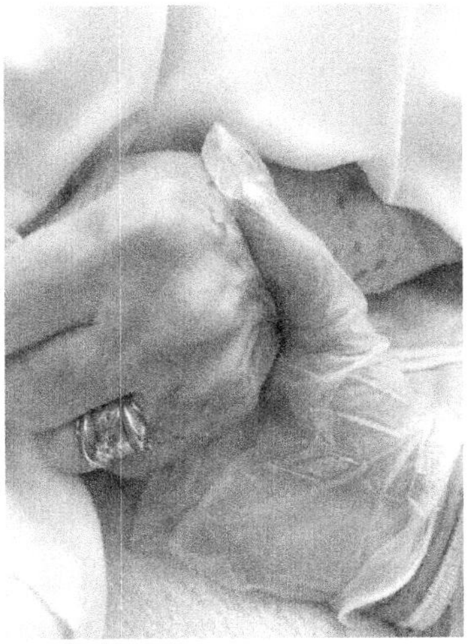

We are required to wear gloves, a gown, and a mask. At first, we were told we could not touch her or hold her hand. However, they did change their mind on that as long as we kept our gloves on. When we get to the hospice center, we will be able to take our gloves off.

I have the utmost respect for everyone working in this environment. This gown is soooo hot, and yet they do their job with love and care. They have a fine-tuned system for checking in for all staff. I was really impressed. Everyone has truly been amazing.

Mom Chronicles July 16, 2020
I'm always trying to find humor in any situation. So here is our "funny" for the day.

She takes turns holding our hands. With Sheila's hand, she tries to give her kisses. Then, with MY hand, she tries to bite it!! What's up with that??? Aren't you NOT supposed to bite the hand that feeds you?? Oh, Momma... we are gonna have to talk about this someday!!

Mom Chronicles July 16, 2020
This woman still has some spunk left in her!! For the last hour, she has been making faces at us and sticking her tongue out at us periodically. And then sometimes she grins right after. She never ceases to amaze me.

Mom Chronicles July 17, 2020
We are with her and still waiting for COVID results before we can get her transported to the hospice facility.

She is no longer able to eat or drink. We are just swabbing her mouth with the swab wet with cold water. She keeps trying to bite down on it.

They have also started her on morphine to keep her comfortable.

She has kissed our hands quite a bit. She has tried biting a few times but mostly gives kisses.

Mom Chronicles July 18, 2020, 6:37 am
Let's talk about caregiver guilt for a moment while I can.

One of the common things I learned over the years in support groups is that it's very natural to want your loved one to go ahead and die. It's very selfish, but it is also very natural.

I'm being very honest, raw, and blunt here for a minute. We started this journey 5 1/2 years ago when she moved in with us. When that happened, our life was put on hold. We stopped hanging out with dear friends and going on group vacations. We worked extra jobs and started a business just to make ends meet for her care. We made the difficult decision to sell our beautiful home and leave our wonderful neighbors so that she could get excellent care at a memory care center during the middle part of her Alzheimer's journey. We made lots of sacrifices. But.... as we stand here with this door about to close, I am sticking my foot in the door, trying to stop it. Yes, she needs this earthly body to go because she's suffering and not truly living. But I don't want her to go. I feel so guilty (and I know I shouldn't) for ever wanting her to die. For all the sacrifices, there have been huge blessings. New friends I would have never known, adventures in our RV, my sister and I growing so much closer than ever before, and most importantly, I have had the precious time I needed to heal a relationship with my mom. Sheila and I were reminiscing yesterday evening by her bedside about our childhood. 1) to give us something positive to do and 2) so that she would hear our voices and our laughter. We've been told that hearing is one of the last senses to go. I found that we were talking about all the positives and that I was able to gloss over the negatives that had me disliking her for many years. I always loved her, but she made some decisions that made me dislike her many times. That's gone now. All I want is my mommy back. I don't want that door to close.

We got a call around midnight last night, and when I saw the caller ID, it was the nursing home. All I could say was no, no, no. Luckily, it was the new nurse on duty for the day, just saying how much she was declining. I asked if we needed to get back up there right away, but he said no. He just wanted me to be aware.

So, I was able to breathe a sigh of relief. And one last blessing... As I am typing this, the nursing home just called and said her COVID results are negative, so I'm going to hop off and get hold of my hospice contact to try and get her moved ASAP. She also said Mom's status is the same.

Love and blessings, my friends.

Mom Chronicles July 18, 2020, 1:53 pm - The End

Today my mom went to sleep here on earth and woke up seeing Jesus face to face. We were able to be with her during her last breath here on earth. As our good friend Jenni told me, as she was taking her last breath here, she took her first breath in heaven. She is no longer suffering from Alzheimer's, which is an absolutely horrible disease. This disease took my mom away from me, starting about six years ago when we first started noticing the signs of her memory loss. We knew it was coming because my grandma had Alzheimer's as well.

When Bruce and I first decided to bring her home from California, we weren't looking forward to the level of care this would take. All I can say is that as tough as it was and all the sacrifices we made (including my sister, who drove 3 hours up here every other weekend), it was a complete blessing. It allowed me to remember the Mom I had when I was young and rebuild a relationship that I would have missed out on if she had passed in California. Instead, I had 5 1/2 years of smiling, laughing, crying, beating my head against a wall, endless doctor appointments, weekly nail appointments, keeping my husband from losing his sanity, growing closer to my sister, and loving my mom. I also learned to become a stronger person by advocating for people with dementia who don't have a voice anymore.

I actually started writing this before today so that I could write it from a place not as emotional. I knew we were counting down to the end because I had seen her eating less and less and sleeping more and more.

For the last few weeks, I have been mourning a loss that hadn't happened yet. It's hard to explain, but I knew I was losing her and couldn't do a darn thing about it. I couldn't be there to try and coax her to eat, play Elvis music, fix her nails, give her blingy rings, talk to her, or hold her hand. I knew she was slipping away, and I would constantly look at the camera to see if she was still with us each day, all throughout the day and night. The last month or so has been horrible with not being able to see her through the camera. It got accidentally unplugged, and I never could get anyone to help me get it restarted.

My family and I want to thank you for your kind words, thoughts, prayers, and support over the years while we chronicled this journey. This "journal" became so much more than just a way for us to share our thoughts and feelings. It allowed us to share things we had learned about how to help someone with Alzheimer's and how to help caregivers. We tried to use humor along with the very raw feelings we were experiencing.

Most importantly, thank you for loving our mom along with us through the years.

Mom - I love you. You are no longer in pain or confused. You are safe now. Thank you for doing the best you could. Plant a beautiful garden with your green thumb. Tell Dad, Grandpa and Grannie Clark, Grandpa, and Grandma Parsley, Bubba, and Margaret, and Ted hello for me and that I love them all very much. And if the evil stepdad (you know which one) is there by chance - kick him in the shins extremely hard - I mean really, really hard - if Jesus will let you. 😉

I'll see you when my season here is over.

Marylin Yvone Clark Parsley
August 20, 1941 - July 18, 2020

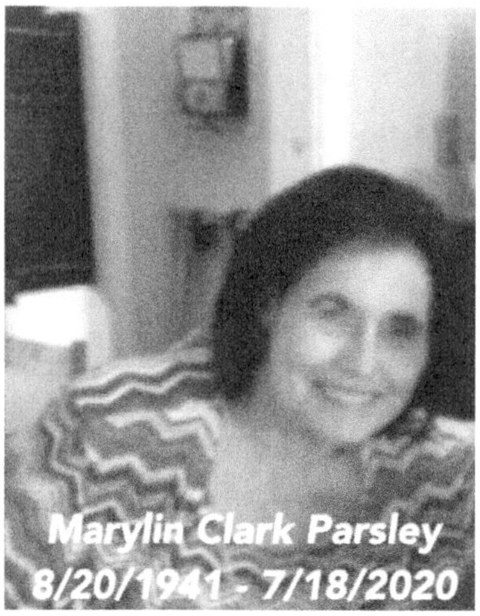
Marylin Clark Parsley
8/20/1941 - 7/18/2020

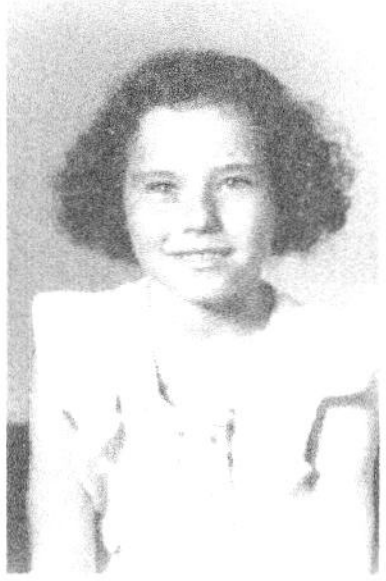
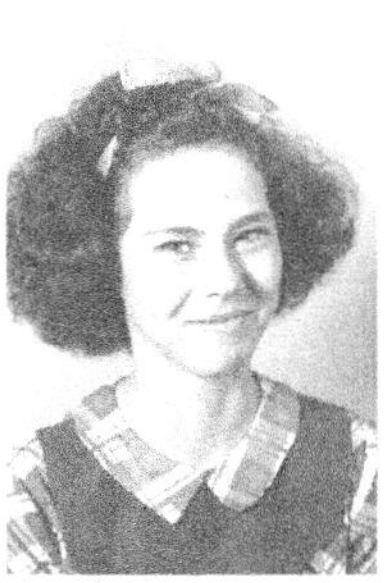
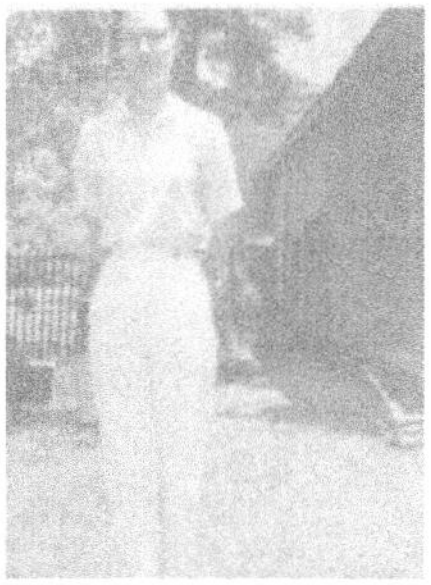
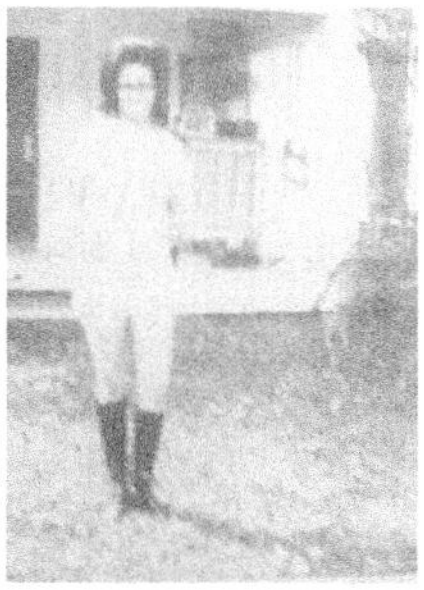
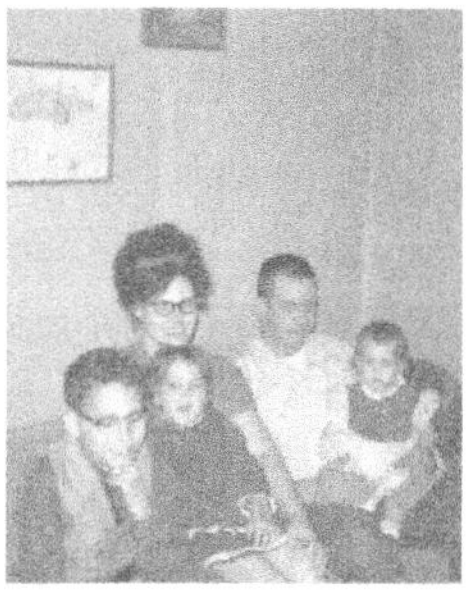

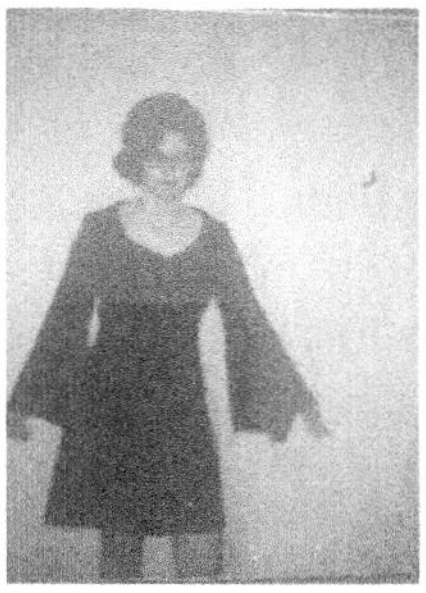
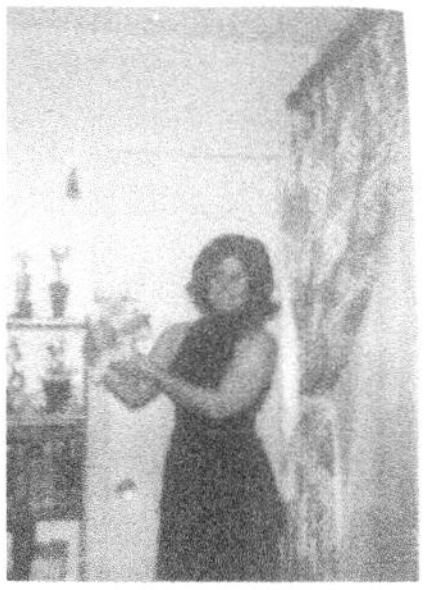
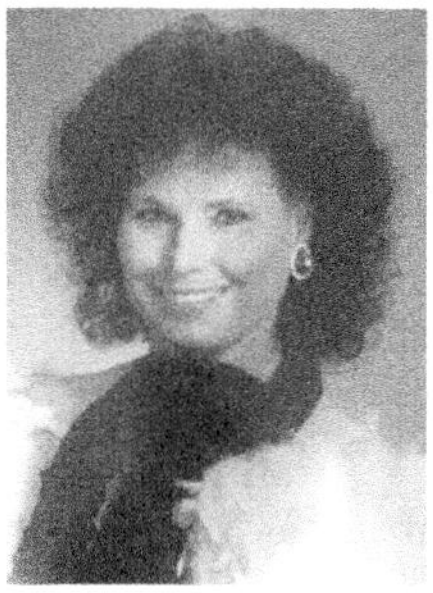
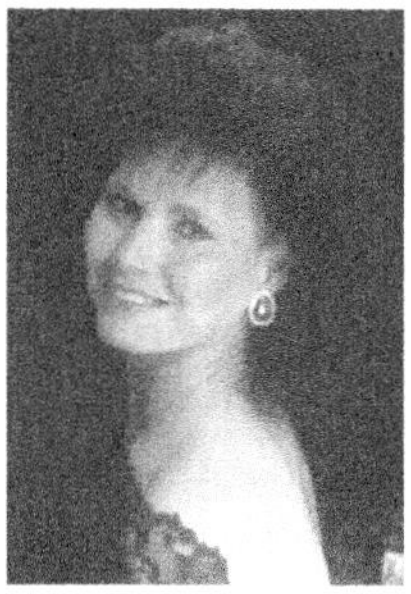
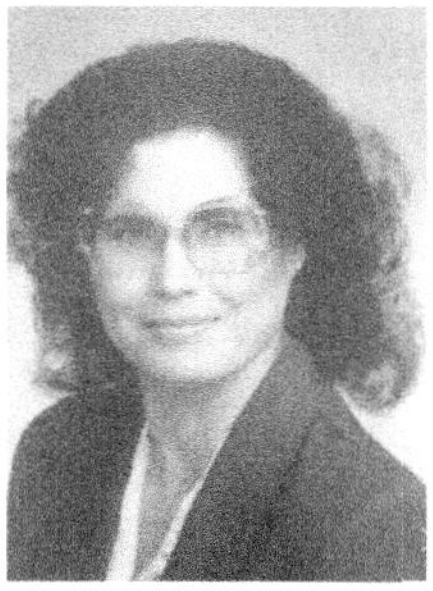

CHAPTER 6: AFTERWORD

My precious mother is perfectly healed from Alzheimer's in heaven as my family, and I firmly believe as Christians. This disease ravaged her brain and body for a little over six years. It was hard to watch her diminish over the years to the shell she was on her final days. Now it was time to lay her to rest. As you can guess by now, we made sure she was honored in death as she was in life. She deserved bling, bling, and more bling - and we made sure she got it!

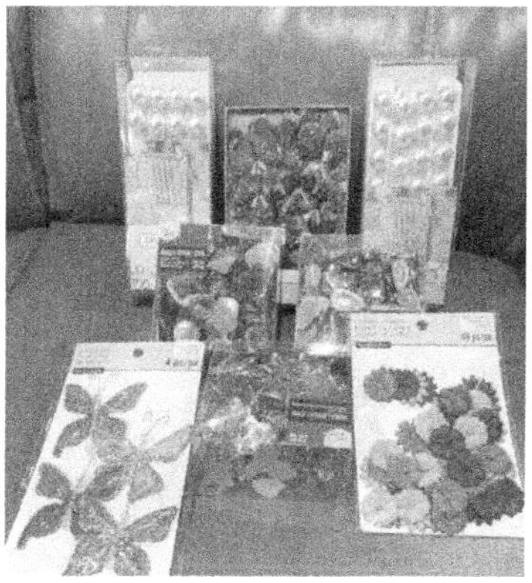

Mom Chronicles July 19, 2020
Alrighty, my friends. We worked with the Dallas Casket company and are getting a PINK casket for half the price. Now guess what we are going to do with all this??!!

Mom Chronicles July 21, 2020
So far, the obituary for Mom is only posted on the Sam Houston Memorial Funeral Home website. The Charles W Smith & Sons Funeral Home should have it posted soon. SHMFH will handle the graveside service down in Coldspring, Tx, where my dad and Bruce's parents are resting. The Charles W Smith & Sons Funeral Home will handle the local arrangements here in the Dallas area.
www.shmfh.com/m/obituaries/Marylin-Clark-Parsley/Memories

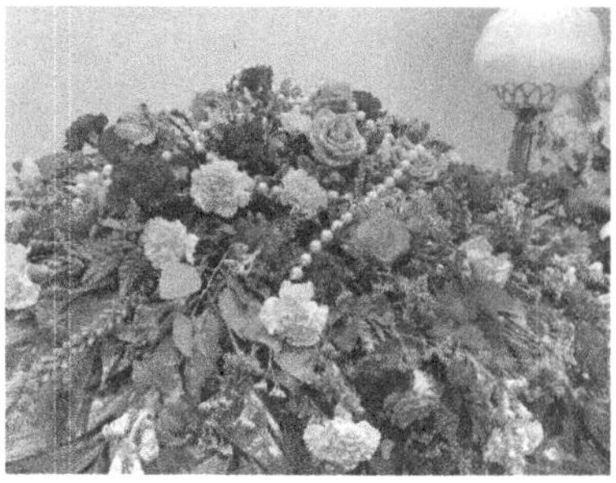

Mom Chronicles July 22, 2020

The Wylie Flower Shop did a fantastic job with the flowers we ordered for Mom. We took "pearls" to them to include in the arrangements. The other flowers and plants that have arrived from our friends are beautiful as well. Thank you!

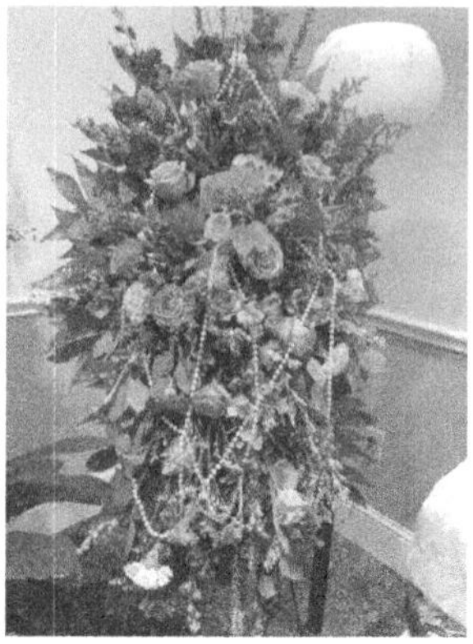

Mom Chronicles July 22, 2020

I do not like to take pictures of a deceased body, but I will share the "blinging" going on of the casket. I have her cropped or blurred out in the photos. It's going to be beautiful!! We are saving a section for Josh when he gets off work today. Jenni Knutson, Shauna Sweetser, and Lynda Hart got in on the action when they stopped by for the visitation by helping add some bling as well!! We think Mom is happy with this!!

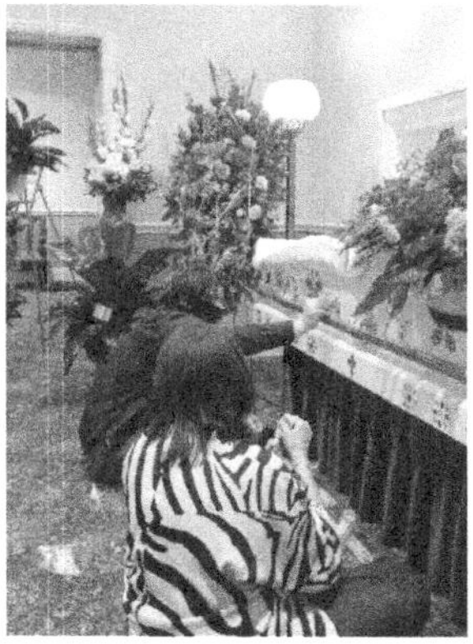
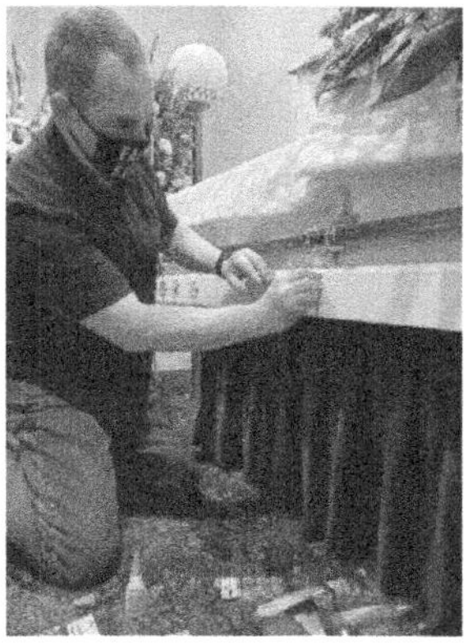
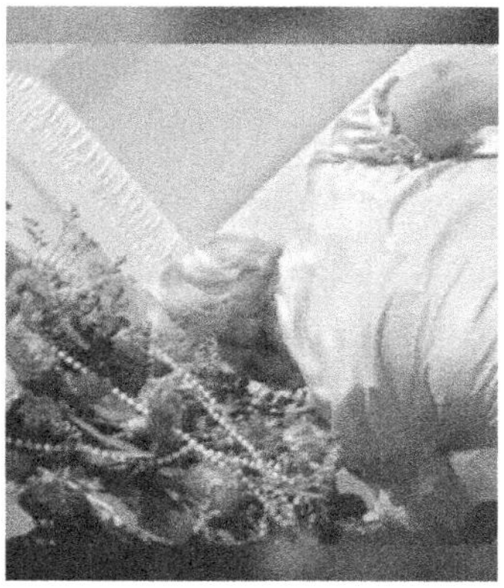
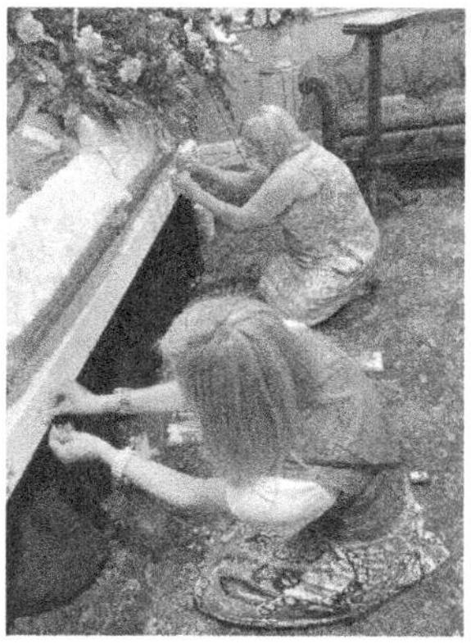

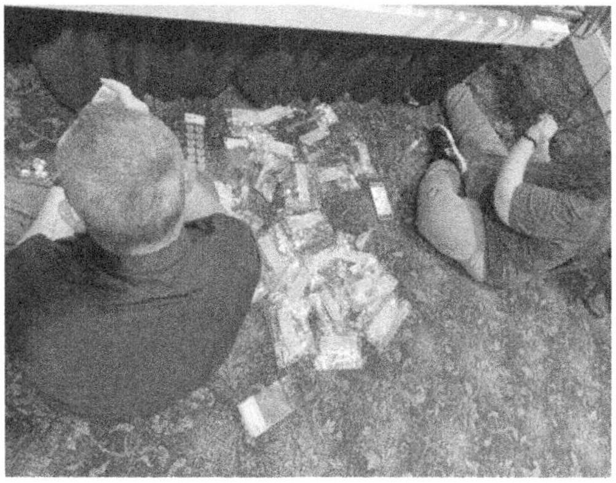
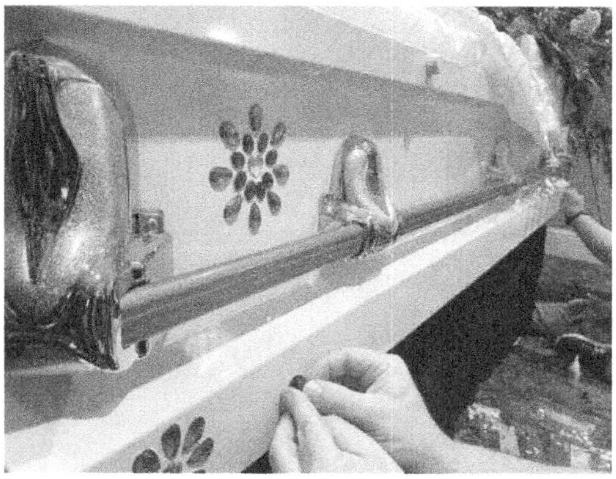

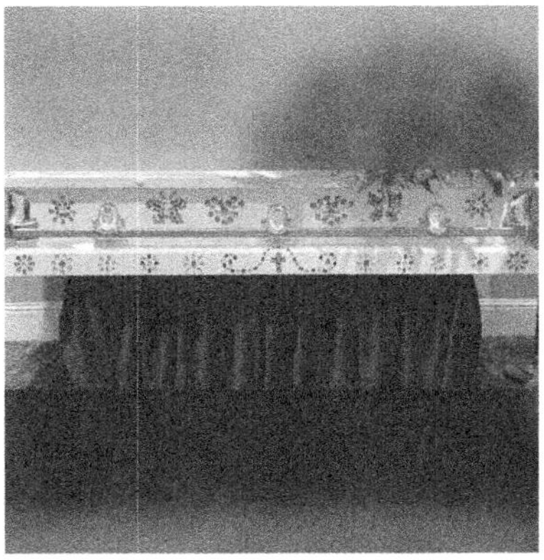
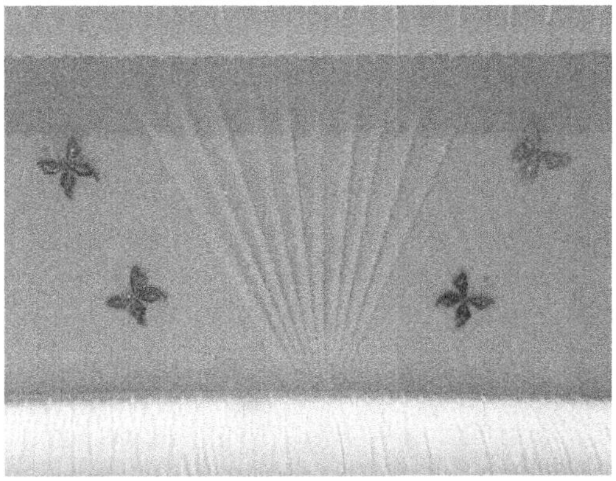

Mom Chronicles July 23, 2020
Because of the pandemic, we kept Mom's service small and limited to just the family. I know many of our church family and friends wanted to be there, so we live-streamed it. We were told the service was beautiful. We played a couple of Elvis' spiritual songs and Il Divo's "Amazing Grace" for music. Because Elvis helped me reach Mom so much through music the last few years of her life, he needed to be part of the service!

Bruce spoke during the service to share his memories of Mom. Sheila was not emotionally able to share her thoughts. I knew the service was going to be hard for her. She is really struggling with losing her.

I read the following passage until the very last paragraph, and then I broke. Bruce and Josh hopped up and finished it for me. I couldn't have gone through this whole journey without them. They have been my rocks.

My Words at Mom's Funeral

You guys know our family. We love to use humor whenever we can, so let's start this remembrance of Mom off the right way!!

Marylin Yvone Clark Davis Parsley Massengill Buvinghausen Barnes McCombs Davis Clark Parsley was a force to be reckoned with. She gave Elizabeth Taylor a run for her money on the number of marriages. Officially there were seven marriages. Unofficially there were 8. She and Ted, her last "husband", and we all will admit was the absolute love of her life, albeit late in life, were not officially married in the eyes of the law in California. The cool thing was that his last name of Clark was her maiden name as well, so it worked out perfectly.

Mom just didn't have a lot of luck in the love department until meeting Ted. She did love my dad, but he was an alcoholic. She tried for ten years to make it work, and when she saw that he wasn't able to beat that demon, she went from being a stay-at-home mom with only a GED to earning her real estate license and broker's license to provide a living for my sister and me. She does have a son from her first marriage, but as life sometimes deals rotten hands, there were complications in that relationship, so we will pray that someday in heaven, we will all be able to heal that relationship.

Hubby number 3 was a total jerk. I'm refraining from saying bad words here in church out of respect for our Lord and Pastor Ken. He was verbally abusive, controlling, and sometimes physically abusive to her. We were finally able to escape him, and I mean literally escape him. You see, she knew she had to time it just right. One day when the evil stepdad had an early morning appointment, she came and checked Sheila and me out of school, and we hurried back to the house to pack as many of our belongings in our two cars as we could. I had just earned my learner's permit, but I didn't know how to drive the stick-shift car yet, so I got to drive her car with the automatic transmission. We hid out in a hotel that first night and the next day secretly moved to a small lake home in the Coldspring Terrace for three months that husband #4 helped us find. The only positive thing that came out of that relationship is that I met Bruce in school there in the town where we were hiding out. The only reason I mention this story is to prove how strong of a woman she was and that she would protect her family in all ways. Did she make some bad decisions along the way? Yep. But really, who doesn't?? And she was a fierce protector of her dad. If he was in the hospital in pain, her Irish temper would come out, and she would be one of those persistent family members who kept bugging the nurses until they gave him pain meds.

Now let's talk about some fun stuff. Growing up, we would drive to Ennis from Houston many times to visit my grandparents. This was when CB radios were popular. She LOVED to cut up and carry on with the truckers and other drivers. Just guess what her CB handle was… Her handle was "Mischief Maker." Soooo appropriate! She was very, very social, as you can only imagine.

Her hobbies included playing the piano when she was younger, fishing, reading, dancing, traveling, gardening, and oil painting. I have a cherished painting that she painted of me holding Josh when he was a baby. She could grow any kind of flower with her green thumb. Our backyard in our childhood home in Houston looked like a jungle. She had a goldfish pond and banana trees, shrubs, and all kinds of flowers growing there. Sheila has a memory of our dad trying to plant rose bush cuttings exactly according to the Gardening 101 instructions, digging the hole in the precise dimensions, adding the fertilizer in the exact quantities, and so on. Mom would just plop the rose bush stem in the ground. Dad's rose bushes would die. Mom's roses would thrive. Daddy would get soooo mad!

Mom loved her kids. She did as much as she could to help Sheila and me grow into strong, independent women. She put us in beauty contests so that we could learn to be comfortable in front of crowds and become confident in our own skin. She let us play in girls' softball leagues and participate in drill teams. She kept us active. She was our room mother in elementary school in most of our classes and was loved by all our friends. I still have a dear friend from junior high named MaryHelen who loved her like a mom as well. If you are watching this, Maryhelen – she loved you dearly!

And boy, oh boy, did she love her grandson Josh. She thought he hung the moon. When he was about four years old, she bought him a HUGE stuffed bear. It was probably about 4 feet tall and 3 feet wide. She had a Porsche at that time with a sunroof. She drove that giant bear all the way up from the south of Houston to Huntsville with the bear's head sticking out of the sunroof. I can only imagine the looks she got on the drive. And knowing her, she was eating it up and waving to everyone. He adored her as well and would visit her and Ted most summers out in California.

When she met Ted online – yes online – she just knew he was the one. She made the hard decision to leave Texas and her family to move out to California to be with him around 2001. That was probably the happiest she has ever been in her entire life. I never heard one cross word about Ted. All the other hubbies – you betcha. There were tons of cross words. But never Ted. And let's face it, Mom had a little bit of a temper, so you know those cross words weren't always their fault. If you have ever seen Sheila pout, it's because she got it from Mom. She wanted things her way or not at all.

She was totally relaxed and at ease out there in California. They loved taking photographs and printing tons and tons of pictures they took. It kind of got to be a joke amongst all of us. We would get photo albums each Christmas full of these printed photos. She did win an award once for a photo she took of an old country water tower. She was so proud of that award. I want to make a special mention of Robin Nikula and her precious family. Robin is Ted's daughter and she, along with her children and grandchildren, was special to Mom as well. She thought of them as her own even though they didn't get to see them very much since they lived so far away.

In 2002, my grandmother needed full-time care from her Alzheimer's. I was taking care of her since both my mom and uncle were living out of state. I was about to lose my job with all the doctor appointments, so I moved her to live with Mom. Mom faithfully cared for her for four years before she passed. I don't know if Mom realized there was a high chance she would suffer from Alzheimer's or not. She never mentioned it to me. In 2014, we started seeing the signs in her. There was the constant repeating of stories on the phone, and then she got lost going to the nail salon one day. That was the turning point. We decided to move her and Ted back to Texas. Ted went to live with Robin, and Mom moved in with Bruce and me. Over the last several years, you all have learned about our mom through the Mom Chronicles. Thank you for going along with us in this journey through Alzheimer's.

I hope you learned she was a very loving woman who loved us and her bling. She also loved to have her nails as beautiful as possible. She could no longer talk clearly– she had lost the ability to speak real words to us for the most part for about a year or two ago, but she would communicate the best way she could. She would blow kisses and smile. She was spunky, even right up to the day before she passed. She would stick out her tongue and try to grin. Bruce and Josh were able to experience this spunkiness one last time through FaceTime.

On her last day, we finally got approval to move her to a hospice facility. We knew the time was close, so Sheila rode with her in the ambulance while I followed. As soon as we arrived at the hospice facility, the medics removed her from the ambulance, and she drew her last breath out in the sunshine. Sheila was right by her, and I had just walked up to the stretcher. Robin helped me realize that Mom didn't pass away in a nursing home or a hospice facility. Instead, she passed from this earth with the sunshine on her face.

My friend Jenni told me that when she drew her last breath here on earth, she took her first breath in heaven.

I did have to laugh when I asked Pastor Ken which hubby she would be with in heaven. She had a lot to choose from, you know. I'll keep his answer private because I'm still not quite sure if he was joking with me or not since he kind of gave me a sideways glance when he said it.

So, I'm going to close this with part of my last Mom Chronicle's entry:

Mom – I love you. You are no longer in pain or confused. You are safe now. Thank you for doing the best you could. Plant a beautiful garden with your green thumb. Tell Dad, Grandpa and Grannie Clark, Grandpa, and Grandma Parsley, Bubba, and Margaret, and Ted hello for me and that I love them all very much. And if the evil stepdad (which would be hubby # 3) is there by chance – kick him in the shins extremely hard – I mean really, really hard – if Jesus will let you. I'll see you when my season here is over.

Josh will come up now and read a poem he wrote the night that his grandmother passed. He has such a beautiful gift with words, and I wanted people to hear his expression of grief if you didn't see it on Facebook. Then he will share the scripture readings for the service.

Hollow Anger

Hollow anger is all I feel.
An empty rage, that cannot be channeled.
There is nothing to channel.
Empty, hollow, sacred nothing.

My soul screams to the sky,
There is no sound that escapes my lips.
Empty, hollow anger.
Nothing.

I was not the best. Nor was I the worst.
I simply was, and that's all there is.
I love you Grandma. I will miss you.
You were loved. You are loved.

I feel so cold, so empty, so broken.
There is nothing wrong with that.
It simply is what it is.
Fear not my child is what I hear.

Lord grant me your strength.
I need it now, I needed it then.
Grant me your life, your love.
Hold me with Your hallowed arms.

The tears come.
I fight them away.
What should I do?
Strength, from within or without?

Save me, Lord God,
From that which I do not know.
Help me, O' King.
Guide my family.

Protect them.

Joshua Aden 7/18/2020

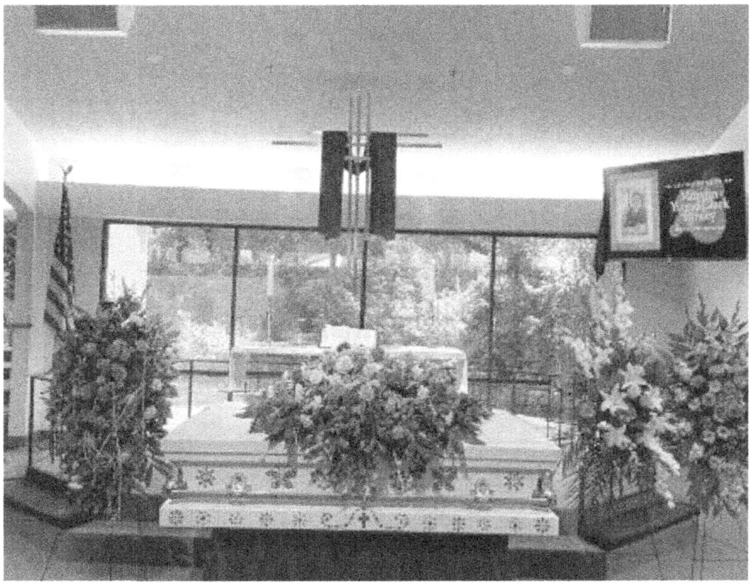

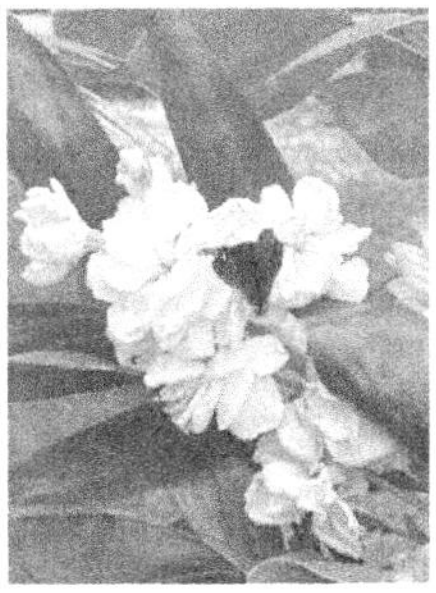

Mom Chronicles July 24, 2020

The plot we bought a few years ago is right next to our dad. We had asked for one near him when I bought it sight unseen. We didn't realize there was one still available right next to him. Margaret and Bubba (Bruce's parents) are close too. Our parents are all next to each other here in Coldspring. I am soooo happy! And to top it off, a butterfly and a hummingbird flew in during the graveside service. We believe Mom was telling us that she's okay. Thank you, Larry Graves, for being our voice today at the graveside and Pastor Ken Krippner for sending words that we included in the service.

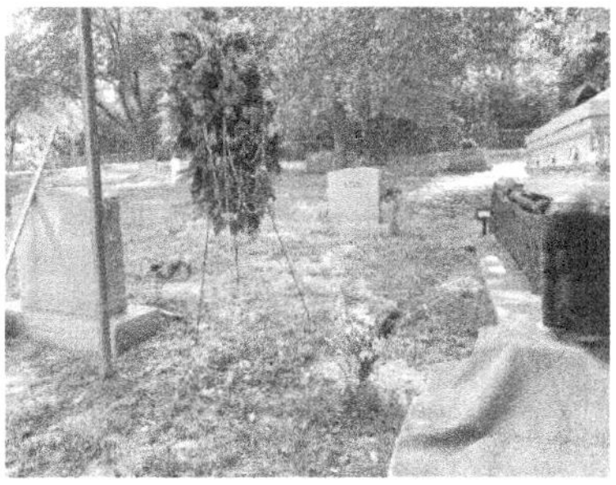

November 21, 2020

Part 1 of the bling project is in the books. We were running out of daylight, so we decided to stop. Sheila will design a frame around the hummingbird and then come back and finish it out. We put the Christmas flowers out for all the family lying in rest here. We will drop some off at my grandparents in Ennis tomorrow.

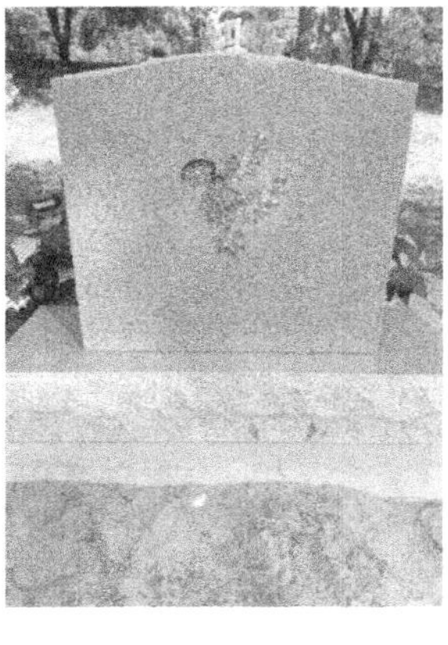

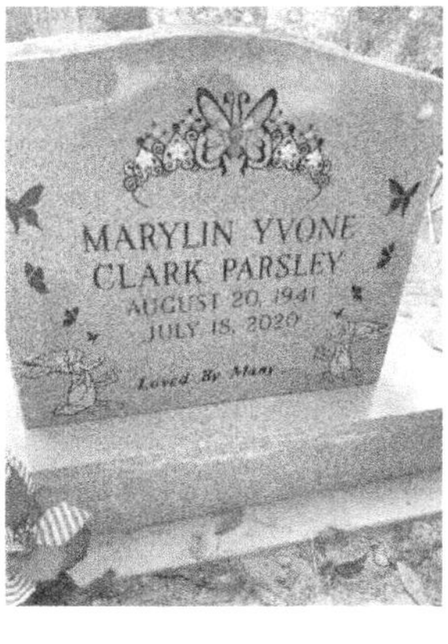

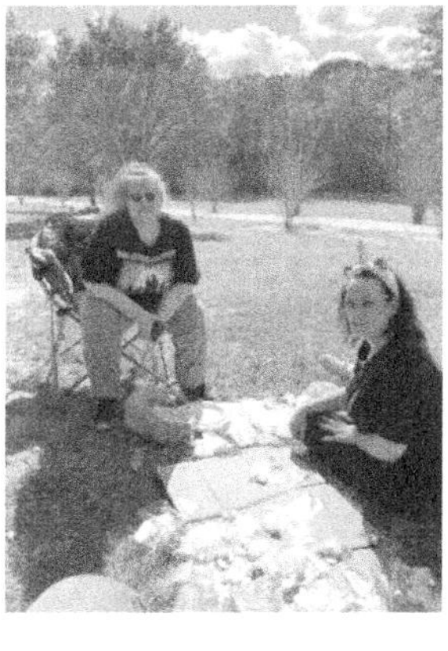

November 22, 2020
After placing flowers on my grandparents' graves in Ennis, I realized that Mom and Grannie Clark (Mom's mom) both passed away on July 18, just 14 years apart from Alzheimer's. Coincidence? I don't believe in coincidences.

December 25, 2020
I did "a thing" for my sister and me. I took Mom's ring guard from her wedding band from Ted that she wore until her last breath and had it separated into two matching rings for Sheila and me. Then I took another ring she had and had it split into two matching necklaces with her birthstone added. I wanted to do something special with some of her jewelry. I think this worked.

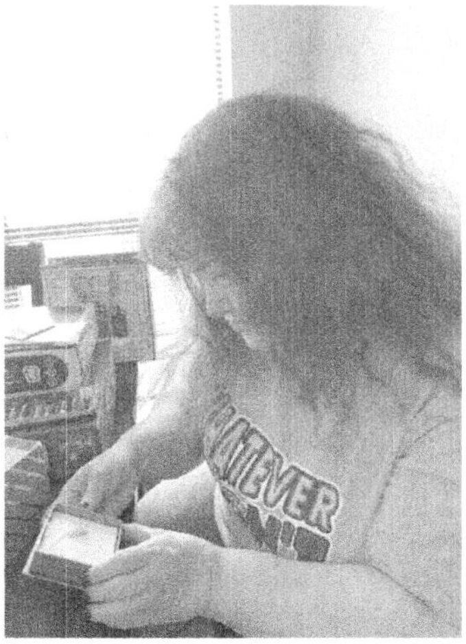

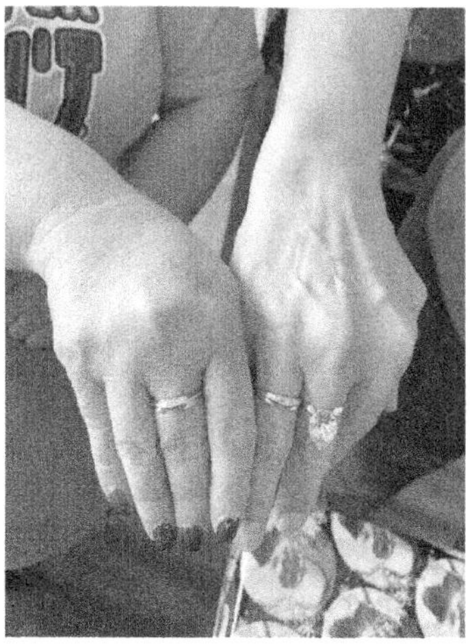

January 9, 2021
My sister outdid me this year. Her Christmas present for me was a little late and came in today. She made Bruce promise to record me when I opened it. I'm now a blubbering mess. This necklace is my mom's handwriting from a greeting card that says:

I love you.
Mom

Thank you, Sheila. I will treasure this always!

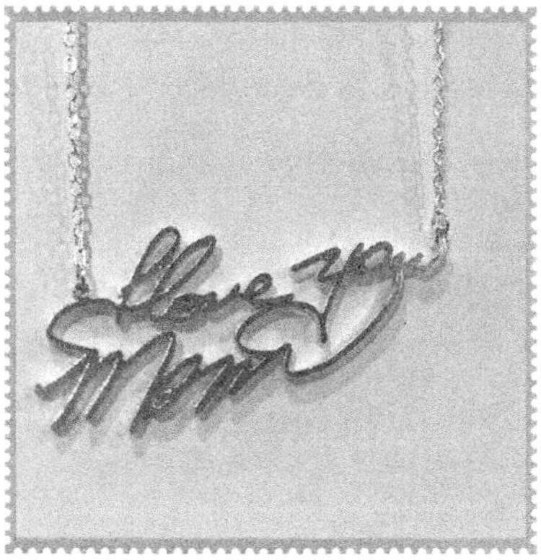

♥

I hope you have enjoyed the Mom Chronicles. I pray that it helped you understand how to care for or connect to someone who has Alzheimer's. I also hope that it helped you see a glimpse of how it is possible to let go of some hard feelings for someone in your life and cherish the time you do have left on earth with them. Being Mom's caregiver was hard, but I would not have wished for anything else for those 5 ½ years. I was given a chance that many others do not get - I had time to reconnect with my mother and love and care for her unconditionally for the last season of her life.

This book did not list every single idea that could help with the various stages of Alzheimer's. As technology, research, and creativity expand each year, more ideas are always coming out. Please bookmark the resources shared and find support groups both in-person and online to grow your knowledge base. What worked for Mom may not work for others in many instances, so keep digging until you do find the one thing that may work for your loved one.

Always keep my mom's words in your heart when you ask your loved one if she remembers something or someone, but she struggles for that vague memory that is slipping away from her mind:

"I remember me."

CHAPTER 7: ♥ RESOURCES

These are the resources that were helpful to me as I was going through this journey with Mom and researching information for this book.

Websites:

www.agingcare.com

www.alz.org

www.alzheimers.gov

www.alzheimers.net

www.alzheimersweekly.com

www.bladderandbowelfoundation.org/bladder/bladder-conditions-and-symptoms/alzheimers-and-incontinence

www.cdc.gov/aging

www.onpluto.org

www.secondwind.org

www.teepasnow.com

www.webmd.com/alzheimers/guide/alzheimers-disease-stages

Books:

The 36-Hour Day by Nancy L. Mace and Peter V. Rabins

Creating Moments of Joy Along the Alzheimer's Journey by Jolene Brackey

Here are questions to ask a nursing home before moving a loved one there.
(Source: Medicare.gov.)
Basic information:

- Is the nursing home Medicare certified (Certified means the home passed an inspection conducted by a state government agency)?
- Is the nursing home Medicaid certified?
- Are the nursing home and current administrator licensed in my state?
- Does the nursing home have a bed available? (Note-Medicare beds and Medicaid beds are NOT the same. Nursing homes only allocate a certain number of beds for Medicaid patients.)
- Does the nursing home offer specialized services, like a special care unit for dementia patients or ventilator care?
- Is the nursing home located close enough for friends and family to visit?
- Are there resident policies I must follow? Will I get a written copy of these policies?
- Are there extra charges for other services like beauty shop services?
- Will the nursing home tell me in writing about their services, charges, and fees before I move into the home?

Safety and Care

- Have you checked the nursing home's star ratings on Medicare.gov?
- Is the nursing home taking action to improve quality or staffing as needed?
- Can residents still see their personal doctors? If needed, does the facility help arrange transportation for this purpose?
- Does the nursing home have an arrangement with a nearby hospital?
- Are care plan meetings held with residents and family members at times that are convenient and flexible whenever possible?
- Does the nursing home's inspection report show quality of care problems or other citations?
- Has the nursing home corrected all citations on its last state inspection report?

Preventing Abuse

- Does the relationship between staff and residents appear to be warm, polite, and respectful?
- Does the nursing home check to ensure they don't hire staff members with a finding or history of abuse, neglect, or mistreatment of residents in the state aid registry?
- Does the nursing home have policies and procedures on prohibiting and reporting abuse and neglect?
- Is the nursing home taking action to keep residents safe from abuse, neglect, mistreatment, or exploitation?
- Is there information about how to report concerns about the care and safety of residents? (There should be notices in the facility on how to contact the home's ombudsman.)
- Is there information about how the facility responds to concerns that are reported?
- Has the nursing home been cited for issues related to abuse in the last year or two? If so, you will see an icon that looks like a red circle with a white hand located next to their name on the Medicare.gov site.

Nursing Home Appearance

- Are residents clean, well-groomed, and appropriately dressed for the season or time of day?
- Is the nursing home free from overwhelming unpleasant odors? (The one we chose made sure to remove soiled bedding and throw out dirty or wet diapers immediately. They were never left in the patient's room.)
- Does the nursing home appear clean and well kept?
- Is the temperature in the nursing home comfortable for residents?
- Does the nursing home have good lighting?
- Are the noise levels in the dining room and other common areas comfortable?
- Is the furniture sturdy yet comfortable and attractive?

- Are exits clearly marked?
- Are there quiet areas where residents can visit with friends and family?
- Does the nursing home have smoke detectors and sprinklers?
- Are all common areas, resident rooms, and doorways designed for wheelchairs?
- Are handrails and grab bars appropriately placed in the hallways and bathrooms?

Menus and Food

- Do residents have a choice of food items at each meal? Do they serve foods your loved one likes?
- Can the nursing home provide for special dietary needs (like low-salt or no-sugar-added diets)?
- Are nutritious snacks available?
- Does the staff help residents eat and drink at mealtimes, if needed?

Staff

- Do staff knock on the door before entering a resident's room?
- Do staff refer to residents by name?
- Does the nursing home offer a training and continuing education program for all staff?
- Is there licensed nursing staff 24 hours a day, including a Registered Nurse (RN) present at least 8 hours per day, 7 days a week?
- Do Certified Nurse Aides (CNAs) help plan the care of residents?
- How many nurses, including CNAs, will be available to help my loved one during the day, at night, and on weekends?
- Is there a person on staff assigned to meet my loved one's social service needs?
- Will staff call the doctor for my loved one if she has a medical need?
- Has there been a turnover in administrative staff in the past year?
- Does the staff speak my loved one's primary language? If not, is there an interpreter?

Resident's Rooms

- Can residents have personal belongings and furniture in their rooms?
- Does each resident have storage space in their room?
- Does each resident have a window in their bedroom?
- Do residents have access to the internet, a computer, a personal phone, and a television? (Don't forget to ask about cable and who pays for it.)
- Do residents have a choice of roommates?
- Are there policies and procedures to protect residents' possessions, including lockable cabinets and closets?

Activities

- Can residents choose to take part in a variety of activities? (Be sure to ask if residents will be wheeled down to the activity if they can't wheel themselves.)
- Do residents help plan or choose the activities that are available?
- Does the nursing home have outdoor areas for resident use?
- Is staff available to help residents go outside?
- Does the nursing home have an active volunteer program?
- Does the resident get to choose what time to get up, go to sleep, or bathe?
- Can the resident have visitors at any time - even early or late hours?
- Can the resident leave the facility for a few hours with a family member? Are their procedures for leaving the facility?
- Does the nursing home offer religious or cultural support?

Caring for Residents with Dementia

- Does the nursing home have specific policies and procedures for residents with dementia?
- If so, does the policy include the use of non-medication-based approaches to care as a first attempt to respond to behavioral symptoms?
- What percentage of residents who have a dementia diagnosis are currently prescribed an antipsychotic medication?
- What's the nursing home's current rate of antipsychotic medication use?
- Does the nursing home participate in any efforts related to reducing antipsychotic medication use in nursing homes (like the National Partnership to Improve Dementia Care)?

WORKS CITED

10 commandments of Alzheimer's Caregiving. (n.d.). Retrieved from Alzheimer's Reading Room: http://www.alzheimersreadingroom.com/2016/07/alzheimer-care-10-commandments-of-alzheimers-caregiving.html#more

10 Early Signs and Symptoms of Alzheimer's. (n.d.). Retrieved from Alzheimer's Association: https://www.alz.org/alzheimers-dementia/10_signs

A Simple Way to Document the Medical Care. (n.d.). Retrieved from Advance Directive for Dementia: https://dementia-directive.org/

Agnvall, E. (2011, March 1). *Mother's Alzheimer's Increases Your Risk*. Retrieved from AARP: https://www.aarp.org/health/brain-health/info-02-2011/health-discovery-mothers-alzheimers-increases-your-risk.html

Albert, F. R. (2014, August). *Hearing Loss and Dementia – Who's Listening?* Retrieved from US National Library of Medicine National Institute of Health: https://www.ncbi.nlm.nih.gov/pmc/articles/PMC4075051/

Alzheimer's Caregiving: Bathing, Dressing, and Grooming: Alzheimer's Caregiving Tips. (n.d.). Retrieved from National Institute on Aging: https://www.nia.nih.gov/health/bathing-dressing-and-grooming-alzheimers-caregiving-tips

Botek, A.-M. (2020, May 26). *Alzheimer's and Sleep Disorders: Expert Answers to 6 Common Questions*. Retrieved from Aging Care: https://www.agingcare.com/articles/alzheimers-and-sleep-expert-answers-to-6-common-questions-156720.htm

Coping with Agitation and Aggression in Alzheimer's Disease. (n.d.). Retrieved from National Institute on Aging: https://www.nia.nih.gov/health/coping-agitation-and-aggression-alzheimers-disease

Dementia: Eating and drinking at the end of life. (n.d.). Retrieved from Social Care Institute of Excellence: https://www.scie.org.uk/dementia/advanced-dementia-and-end-of-life-care/end-of-life-care/eating-drinking.asp

Duggan, S. (2019, May 8). Stolen Memories. *C&S Media Publications - Wylie News*, p. C1. Retrieved from https://bit.ly/3fW4HK2

Heiser, K. G. (n.d.). *Personal Care Agreements: A Must for Caregiver Compensation and Medicaid Planning.* Retrieved from AgingCare: https://www.agingcare.com/articles/personal-care-agreements-compensate-family-caregivers-181562.htm

Hospice Eligibility. (n.d.). Retrieved from Pathway Hospice: https://pathwayhospice.net/wp-content/uploads/2020/04/HospiceEligibility.pdf

Hospice Eligibility Criteria Dementia. (n.d.). Retrieved from Crossroads Hospice: https://www.crossroadshospice.com/hospice-care/hospice-eligibility-criteria/dementia/

Is Alzheimer's Genetic. (n.d.). Retrieved from Alzheimer's Association: https://www.alz.org/alzheimers-dementia/what-is-alzheimers/causes-and-risk-factors/genetics

Late-Stage Caregiving: Infections and Pneumonia. (n.d.). Retrieved from Alzheimer's Association: https://www.alz.org/help-support/caregiving/stages-behaviors/late-stage

Marcel, J. (n.d.). *What Do I Do If My Elderly Parent Refuses to Go to the Doctor.* Retrieved from AgingCare: https://www.agingcare.com/articles/aging-parent-refuses-go-to-doctor-133384.htm

Meredith Fields Lawler, L. (2016, June 28). *The Five Love Languages of Caregiving.* Retrieved from Crossroads Hospice Charitable Foundation: https://crhcf.org/Blog/the-five-love-languages-of-caregiving/

Middle Stage Caregiving. (n.d.). Retrieved from Alzheimer's Association: https://www.alz.org/help-support/caregiving/stages-behaviors/middle-stage

Sauer, A. (2019, September 5). *Why Is Alzheimer's More Likely in Women?* Retrieved from Alzheimers.net: https://www.alzheimers.net/8-12-15-why-is-alzheimers-more-likely-in-women

Second Wind Dreams. (n.d.). Retrieved from https://www.secondwind.org/.

Sleep Issues and Sundowning. (n.d.). Retrieved from Alzheimer's Association: https://www.alz.org/help-support/caregiving/stages-behaviors/sleep-issues-sundowning

Trowbridge, J. (2020, February 12). *50 Tips on Transitioning a Loved One to Memory, Dementia, or Alzheimer's Care.* Retrieved from Senior Link: https://www.seniorlink.com/blog/50-tips-on-transitioning-a-loved-one-to-memory-dementia-or-alzheimers-careyour-blog-post-title-here

VISN 21 MIRECC. (n.d.). Retrieved from US Department of Veterans Affairs: https://www.mirecc.va.gov/visn21/pdf/CV_208_reisberg_b_franssen_eh_clinical-stages-

AD_atlas_1999.pdf

What is Alzheimer's Disease. (n.d.). Retrieved from Alzheimer's Association: https://www.alz.org/alzheimers-dementia/what-is-alzheimers

ABOUT THE AUTHOR

Lori Aden is an educator by trade with over 28 years of experience in K12 and higher education, with a master's degree in Educational Technology and a doctorate in Teacher Leadership. In addition to running a successful home-based business, she works full-time as a program coordinator for one of Texas's largest education service centers and part-time as an adjunct instructor for a community college. However, her proudest roles are wife, sister, mom, bonus mom, and bonus nana. Most importantly, she is the proud daughter of Marylin, who is the inspiration behind this book.

www.irememberme.life

ACKNOWLEDGEMENTS

Book Cover: ....Designed by Connie Swiderski

Book Cover Silhoutte Image: ....Designed by Kreativkolors / Freepik

Chronicle Contributions:...Written by Sheila Parsley

Author Photo: ....Taken by Bruce Aden

Videos: ....Edited by Joshua Aden

Made in the USA
Middletown, DE
04 November 2026

36560127R00150